EMERGENCY NURSING

A Practice Guide

EMERGENCY NURSING

A Practice Guide

JEAN H. ROGERS, RN, MSN, CEN

Associate Executive Director of Nursing
City Hospital Center at Elmhurst
Queens, New York

HAROLD H. OSBORN, MD, FACEP

Director, Department of Emergency Medicine
Our Lady of Mercy Hospital
Bronx, New York
Professor of Clinical, Community and Preventive Medicine
New York Medical College
Valhalla, New York

LIDIA POUSADA, MD

Department of Medicine
Montefiore Medical Center
Bronx, New York
Assistant Professor of Medicine
Albert Einstein College of Medicine
Bronx, New York

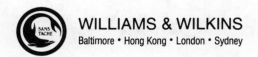

WILLIAMS & WILKINS
Baltimore • Hong Kong • London • Sydney

Editor: Susan M. Glover
Associate Editor: Marjorie Kidd Keating
Copy Editor: Bill Cady
Design: Dan Pfisterer
Illustration Planning: Ray Lowman
Production: Raymond E. Reter

Copyright © 1989
Williams & Wilkins
428 East Preston Street
Baltimore, Maryland 21202, USA

Accurate indications, adverse reactions, and dosage schedules for drugs are provided in this
book, but it is possible that they may change. The reader is urged to review the package
information data of the manufacturers of the medications mentioned.

Printed in the United States of America

Library of Congress Cataloging-in-Publication Data

Emergency nursing.

   Includes bibliographies and index.
   1. Emergency nursing. I. Rogers Jean H. II. Osborn, Harold H. III. Pousada,
Lidia. [DNLM: 1. Critical Care—nurses' instruction. 2. Emergencies—nursing.
3. Emergency Service, Hospital—nurses' instruction. WY 154 E5234]
RT120.E4E4745   1989   610.73'61   88–37850
ISBN 0–683–07322–2

89   90   91   92   93
1 2 3 4 5 6 7 8 9 10

*This book is dedicated to the staff and
patients of the city hospital, an institution
that has provided a site for learning for
generations of health practitioners and
has offered equal health care to all
regardless of their ability to pay.*

PREFACE

The goal of this manual is to provide nurses with a practical guide for assessment of and intervention for commonly encountered clinical problems. This manual is not a theoretical text on emergency care; rather, it is a direct-care reference based on years of experience in busy city hospital emergency departments.

It is our hope that this manual will be of value to both experienced emergency nurses and those just entering the field.

Written from the perspective of the nursing process, this manual provides information on patient assessment, diagnostic procedures, nursing and medical intervention, emergency department discharge planning and patient teaching. We use a holistic approach to patients, with the appreciation that patients are part of a dynamic family and cultural and social network.

We wish to express our gratitude to Grace H. Johnston, who typed, proofread, and provided needed support and encouragement; and to Kenlyn Morris, RN, who provided insightful comments and suggestions; and to Celia, for her patience and understanding (H. H. O.).

Jean H. Rogers, RN
Harold H. Osborn, MD
Lidia Pousada, MD

CONTENTS

Chapter 1

CARDIOVASCULAR EMERGENCIES

Chapter 2

RESPIRATORY EMERGENCIES

Chapter 3

NEUROLOGIC EMERGENCIES

Chapter 13

OPHTHALMOLOGIC EMERGENCIES

Chapter 14

PSYCHIATRIC EMERGENCIES

Chapter 15

SOCIAL AND LEGAL CONCERNS

Chapter 16

EMERGENCY PROCEDURES

APPENDICES

INTRODUCTION TO EMERGENCY NURSING

TRIAGE

ED* triage is a variation on military or disaster triage. It is a process of sorting or classifying patients according to the need for emergency treatment and potential for further injury. The word *triage* is French for to sort into three groups.

The number of ED visits has dramatically increased since the 1950s, and the trend is expected to continue. The ever-increasing number and severity of conditions of patients seen make triage one of the most important activities in the ED. An ED without triage has little control over the effects of patient volume and acuity.

To assess or to establish a triage system, the following factors should be taken into consideration:

1. Number of ED visits per day
2. Times of peak activity
3. Number of qualified triage staff and availability of consultation staff
4. Presence of a walk-in clinic or other treatment areas outside the ED
5. Logistic and administrative concerns

Goals of triage may include:

1. See the patient shortly after arrival, prior to registration.
2. Obtain a brief account of the present complaint and objective data, i.e., vital signs.
3. Perform a brief physical assessment.
4. Prioritize patient care, with critical patients being seen first.
5. Determine the area or level of primary provider, i.e., clinic, gynecologic area, minor OR, physician assistant.
6. Initiate therapeutic and/or diagnostic interventions, i.e., selected laboratory tests, acetaminophen for an elevated temperature, urinalysis for a patient with dysuria, etc.

---

*See "Appendix A" for definition of common abbreviations used in the text.

7. Greet and promote positive public relations—set the tone of the ED visit.
8. Provide documentation of time, condition, and initial treatment.

Certain patients must be brought directly into the ED (without triage) where a nursing assessment may be done. These patients include all those arriving with life-threatening conditions, external blood loss, chest pain, asthma, or seizures.

Triage Systems

ED triage, which has been in use for 20–25 years, exists in a variety of forms. Triage by a receptionist or ED clerk is still in use in many hospitals. On the basis of the patient's statement the clerk will notify the ED staff if he or she deems the patient to be an emergency. Obviously, this system does not meet the major goals of a triage system. It leaves a difficult or less-than-obvious judgment to the member of the ED staff least able to make such a decision. If this form of triage is in use, the time between registration and being seen by an ED physician or nurse must be closely monitored.

Triage by a MD has the advantage that patients with minor injuries may be treated and/or referred directly from triage. It is questionable whether MD triage is, under most circumstances, necessary, cost-effective, or practical staffing. In many facilities the triage function is performed by registered nurses. In most instances, nurse triage is the most comprehensive in design and most expansive in scope.

Triage should be assigned to a nursing staff member with at least 2 years of clinical experience. The triage nurse should receive formal triage orientation and ongoing education in triage decision making. A good triage officer also needs good communication skills and common sense, although these are difficult to measure and more difficult to instill. The use of a triage protocol book will facilitate correct decision making by all those involved with triage.

Concerning the location and structure of the triage area, much will depend on the function and goals of triage within the hospital. The following will need to be considered:

1. Triage should be easily accessible to the ED entrance and treatment area.
2. Telephone and intercom are needed for consultation, referrals, and emergencies.
3. Triage area should provide a view of those persons waiting for triage and, optimally, the waiting room.
4. Pediatric and adult triage areas should be separate, if possible.

5. Privacy should be commensurate with the functions performed in triage, i.e., interview, taking of vital signs, listening for lung sounds.
6. A stretcher and wheel chair should be available in or immediately adjacent to the triage area.
7. Equipment for immediate emergency treatment, i.e., airway, bag/mask device, 4 × 4-inch gauze, etc., should be available.
8. A sink for hand washing should be available.

Triage Process

1. Obtain a brief account of chief complaint and related history. Evaluate the complaint or problem and ask questions to obtain information needed to make the triage decision. Give consideration to the cause of the problem; e.g., a facial laceration from a fall could possibly be the result of syncope. Avoid asking leading questions, such as "Did the pain also travel down your arm and back?" If the patient presents stating a diagnosis, e.g., "I've got a stomach ulcer," ask what symptoms he or she is experiencing.
2. In addition to obtaining the patient's subjective account of the problem, observe for gait, speech, indications of anxiety, dyspnea, discomfort, etc.
3. Determine as quickly as possible whether the situation is emergent, and if so, bring the patient into the treatment area and turn him or her over to an ED clinician. (See Appendix B, "Classification of Patients by Acuity Level.")
4. According to the goal of triage within a particular hospital, the triage assessment may include:
   a. Assessment of vital signs including orthostatic signs, as indicated
   b. Data collection and observation
   c. Use of touch and palpation, i.e., skin temperature, crepitus, induration
   d. Auscultation, i.e., lung sounds, wheezing
   e. An advanced triage system in which selected diagnostic tests are performed or initiated by the triage nurse, e.g., blood glucose by Dextrostix, drawing CBC and electrolytes, an x-ray request for the patient with a minor limb injury. Advanced triage is commonly based on written triage protocols or guidelines. Benefits of advanced triage include: decreased patient waiting time; the feeling by patients that they have received attention shortly after arrival; and decreased patient treatment time, since the triage nurse has a more direct role in initiating therapeutic intervention. On the negative side, the performance of tests by the triage nurse may cause delays in patient triage. Advanced triage is only beneficial when it does not interfere with the major role of the triage nurse, which

is the timely assessment and categorization of patients needing immediate treatment. If staffing permits, assignment of a licensed practical nurse or a technician trained in phlebotomy to assist the triage nurse will prevent the delays inherent in advanced triage.

f. Periodic reassessment of selected patients should be considered part of the triage process particularly if waiting time is prolonged.

5. One of the primary goals of triage is to prioritize the need for emergency care. This is often accomplished by a 3- or 4-category rating of patients. The following is an example of a 3-category system:

Emergent - Patients who require immediate treatment and/or evaluation, e.g.,

Cardiopulmonary arrest	Drug overdose
Acute chest pain	Hemorrhage
Profuse vaginal bleeding	Serious arrhythmia
Attempted suicide	Seizure in progress
Respiratory distress	Shock

Urgent - Patients with serious illness or injury who require intervention and/or evaluation in 20 minutes to 2 hours, e.g.,

Fractures without neurovascular compromise
Acute abdominal pain
CVA/TIA
Significant alteration in vital signs
Vomiting

Nonurgent- Patients with minor injuries and nonacute conditions who may be triaged to a walk-in clinic, e.g.,

Strain or sprain	Urinary frequency
Minor burn	Soar throat
Cough/nasal congestion	Low back pain

Triage Standards

Written protocols or algorithms provide a valuable adjunct for triage decision making and triage orientation. The use of protocols improves the quality and consistency of triage and provides a basis for evaluation and quality assurance review. The following is an example of a triage algorithm (see Appendix C for further examples):

Triage Algorithm for Chest Pain

Severe chest pressure/pain	→	Emergent category
Angina-like pain		Immediate MD exam-
Abnormal vital signs		ination, ECG,
Gunshot or stab wound to chest		start IV and O$_2$
Hx of angina or CHF		

Triage Algorithm for Chest Pain (continued)

Nonradiating chest pain	→	Urgent category
Hx of blunt trauma		ECG, x-ray, ABG
Pleuritic chest pain		
Normal vital signs		
Cough	→	Nonurgent category
No cardiac symptoms or Hx		
Muscular-skeletal discomfort		

Documentation

A formal record of triage assessment and initial treatment should be started in triage (see Fig. I.1). Ideally, the patient should be seen by the triage nurse prior to registration. Therefore, the triage form is commonly a separate form that will be included in the total ED chart once the registration process is completed. For emergent patients the nursing triage/assessment record may be the sole means of documenting care until the ED chart is generated. Having key information preprinted on this form will alert the staff to documentation standards. Figure I.1 is an example of a nursing triage/assessment form that is initiated in triage and used to document patient assessment and intervention throughout the course of ED treatment.

ASSESSMENT OF VITAL SIGNS

The measurement of vital signs (blood pressure, temperature, respirations, pulse rate) is an essential component of patient assessment in the ED. Vital signs should be taken during triage and used along with the patient's history and physical examination to determine the level of acuity. Although the triage nurse's assessment will be based on a single set of values, vital signs are most significant when they are taken serially and when trends can be viewed in light of the clinical situation. Variations or incongruities in a patient's vital signs need to be analyzed. The following should be considered when assessing vital signs:

1. The patient's previous medical record will aid in assessing the current values.
2. The patient and/or family may have information on the patient's usual blood pressure or pulse rate.
3. If no additional information can be found, compare the patient's pres-

```
NURSES NOTES                    │ registration plate
                                │ name, age

Date_____ Time_____ Information received from _____
BP_____Pulse_____Resp_____Temp_____

                    NURSING HISTORY

CHIEF COMPLAINT & HX OF PRESENT ILLNESS_____
_____
_____

PAST MEDICAL HX_____
_____
_____

MEDICATION TAKEN & TIME_____
_____
_____

ALLERGIES--NONE KNOWN-- LIST_____   LMP_____
                             _____

COMA SCALE_____
                                                            PUPILS-
EYES       SPONTANEOUSLY        4      │ pupil key
OPEN       TO SPEECH            3      │ + reaction       RT-size_____
           TO PAIN             2      │ -no react.        reaction___
           NONE                1      │ c eye closed      LT-size_____
                                                          reaction___

BEST       ORIENTATED           5
VERBAL     CONFUSED             4       INDICATE AREAS OF INJURY
RESPONSE   WORDS
             INAPPROPRIATE      3          Anterior    Posterior
           INCOMPREHENSIBLE
             SOUNDS            2
           NONE                1

BEST       OBEYS COMMANDS        6
MOTOR      LOCALIZES PAIN       5
RESPONSE   FLEXION-WITHDRAWAL   4
           FLEXION-ABNORMAL     3
           EXTENSION            2
           NO RESPONSE          1

PUPIL SCALE  in mm.

●8  ●7  ●6  ●5  ●4  ●3  •2  •1          Right   Left   Right


                                       _____  R. N.
```

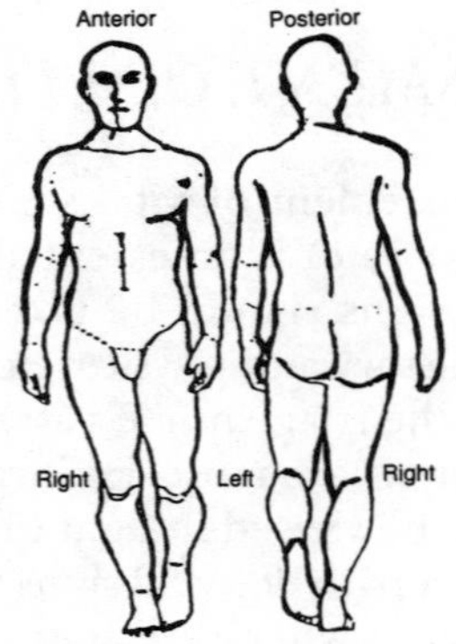

Figure I.1.   Nursing triage/assessment form.

ent vital signs with the normal values for a patient of the same age and in the same general condition.

4. Environmental conditions such as room temperature and recent exercise will affect vital signs.
5. Fear and stress will affect values. Retake vital signs after obtaining the patient's history and providing appropriate reassurance.
6. Use the initial vital signs, history, and physical examination to determine the frequency of subsequent vital sign measurements.
7. Be sure to have appropriate equipment on hand, e.g., a variety of blood pressure cuff sizes and oral and rectal thermometers.
8. Verify and report abnormal signs.

Temperature

The body's normal core temperature is maintained within 1°F of average temperature (98.6°F) by the hypothalamus. When heat reduction is necessary, the hypothalamus signals vasodilatation and stimulates sweat glands. Heat is thereby lost by radiation and evaporation. Heat production and conservation responses include vasoconstriction, increased metabolic rate, shivering, and inhibition of sweat glands. Premature infants and the elderly are more sensitive to hypothermia, as they have less ability to produce heat.

Temperature determination is an essential part of patient assessment. The measurement of temperature may be temporarily deferred in some emergency situations, but it must be noted that any severe fluctuation in body temperature constitutes a life-threatening emergency.

A temperature reading is required on any patient with altered mental status (see Chapter 6, "Heat Stroke" for a further discussion of causes of temperature alteration and interventions). Physical signs and symptoms seen in concurrence with temperature alteration include: skin response (warm, dry, shivering, diaphoretic); alteration in heart rate (bradycardia or tachycardia); and altered mental status (restlessness, lethargy, coma). Interventions such as administration of cold IV solution (e.g., blood), inspiration of cold gas, and certain drugs (alcohol, diuretics, tranquilizers) increase the risk of temperature alteration.

Question the patient about medication that can alter the temperature (aspirin, acetaminophen) or the pulse and blood pressure (beta blockers and antihypertensives).

Temperature can be accurately measured by using an electronic or glass thermometer. A temperature probe and a thermocouple or thermistor should be used for patients for whom the use of glass is unsafe and for those with extreme temperatures (hypothermia and hyperthermia). Refer to the manufacturer's instructions for proper use of electronic thermometers. It is important to note that some patients (diabetics, immunosuppressed, dehydrated, uremics, cirrhotics, etc.) may be seriously infected but have little, if any, temperature elevation.

Appropriate Temperature Measurement

Site and method	Special considerations
Oral - Place a glass thermometer under the patient's tongue in the posterior sublingual pocket. Have the patient keep it in place 3–8 minutes with lips closed.	Method is convenient and accurate but is contraindicated in small children; in patients with altered mental status, facial trauma, or seizure disorder; following smoking or the drinking of hot or cold liquids; during oxygen administration by cannula or mask; and during respiratory distress.
Rectal - For an adult, insert lubricated thermometer 1½ inches into the anus. Do not force thermometer. Keep thermometer in place for 2–4 minutes.	Method provides accurate core temperature and is indicated for mouth breathers and patients suspected of having a serious infection. Stool may impair accuracy. It is contraindicated following rectal surgery or injury and in patients with hemorrhoids.
Axillary - Place the thermometer into center of axilla and hold it in place for 5–10 minutes.	This least accurate method has no place in the ED setting.

Pulse

A radial or peripheral pulse is obtained by lightly compressing the artery against an underlying bone or muscle. The pulse wave is caused by the ejection of blood from the left ventricle during systole. Each pulse wave felt is a reflection of stroke volume.

The heart rate is determined by the intrinsic firing rate of the sinoatrial node with modification by the parasympathetic and sympathetic nervous systems. Determination of pulse rate and quality is an integral part of a cardiovascular assessment. Heart rate is a major determinant of cardiac output, as indicated by the following equation:

$$\text{Heart rate} \times \text{Stroke volume} = \text{Cardiac output}$$

At unusually fast or slow rates cardiac output is primarily determined by heart rate. Under normal circumstances there is a compensatory relationship between heart rate and stroke volume. This compensation is clearly seen in mild hypovolemic shock in which a decreased stroke volume is balanced by an increased heart rate and the cardiac output remains constant. Heart rate is a more effective compensatory mechanism than stroke volume. When assessing a patient with tachycardia of 120/min or above, the nurse should consider the following:

1. Tachycardia may be in response to decreased stroke volume (hypovolemia, cardiac failure, pericardial effusion).
2. Tachycardia may result from a variety of causes, e.g., thyroid disease, fever, hypoxemia, fear, sepsis, exercise, age (infant: 100–160/min; child: 80–120/min; adult: 60–100/min).
3. Tachycardia (>160/min) without an obvious cause may indicate a primary cardiac event (e.g., supraventricular tachycardia). Tachycardia increases the work load of the heart. Cardiac output decreases in extreme tachycardia due to inadequate time for diastolic filling.

In addition to rate, pulses should also be assessed for amplitude or force (weak, thready), rhythm (equality of interval), and contour (unusually sharp or jerky). The pulse rhythm can aid in determining the presence of cardiac arrhythmias and in assessing the effect on cardiac output. Consider a patient with an apical rate of 100/min and an irregular radial pulse of 60/min. There is a pulse deficit of 40 beats/min. With 40 beats/min this patient does not have an adequate stroke volume to result in a radial pulse. A potential nursing diagnosis for this patient would be alteration in cardiac output related to irregular cardiac arrhythmia (e.g., atrial fibrillation).

Respirations

Assessment of the vital sign respirations includes rate, depth, and pattern of respirations. Respirations are best taken after the pulse, with the patient sitting in a comfortable resting position. Count the respirations while still feeling the patient's radial pulse; this will decrease the possibility of the patient consciously trying to control breathing. Assess the respiratory rate in light of signs and symptoms of respiratory compromise: cyanosis, restlessness, orthopnea, dyspnea, abnormal breath sounds. Respiratory rates are normally affected by age (infant: 30–60/min; child: 20–30/min; adult: 12–20/min), exercise, smoking, medications, and emotional factors. Observe the chest movement to assess the depth of respirations (shallow, normal, or deep). By palpation, the equality and degree of chest wall expansion can also be determined. Note paradoxical motion of the chest wall, especially in the trauma patient. The depth of respiration or tidal volume is normally 300–500 ml/breath in an adult at rest. A rapid respiratory rate does not necessarily mean that the patient is moving an increased amount of air. Alterations in breathing patterns are as follows:

Condition	Description
Apnea	Intermittent (10–60 seconds) or persistent (respiratory arrest) cessation of respirations
Biot's	Random irregular depth of respirations
Bradypnea	Slow, regular
Cheyne-Stokes	A gradual increase and decrease in the depth of respiration with a period of apnea between each phase
Dyspnea	Difficult breathing that requires increased effort and use of accessory muscles
Hyperventilation	Increase in rate and depth of respirations in excess of metabolic demand
Hypoventilation	Rate and depth of respirations that are below normal
Kussmaul's	Excessively deep breathing that is seen in diabetic ketoacidosis

Blood Pressure

Systolic blood pressure is a function of the force of ventricular contraction exerted on the aorta during systole. Diastolic pressure is a function of vasoconstriction (vascular resistance). The lowest pressure reached during ventricular diastole is the diastolic pressure. The difference between the systolic and diastolic pressure is the pulse pressure, an important hemodynamic indicator. Pulse pressure is affected by stroke volume and peripheral resistance, as indicated by the following equation:

Blood pressure = Cardiac output × Peripheral vascular resistance

A normal adult blood pressure ranges from 100 to 135 mm Hg systolic and from 60 to 80 mm Hg diastolic. A wide variety of factors can affect blood pressure, including age (4 years: 85/60; 6 years: 95/62; 12 years: 108/67; 16 years: 118/75; and adult: 120/80 mm Hg), body position, and cuff size. Patients particularly at risk for blood pressure alterations are those with cardiac disease, renal disease, diabetes, hypovolemia, or head or spinal cord injury.

An improperly fitting blood pressure cuff will produce inaccurate results. A blood pressure cuff should be 20% wider than the patient's arm diameter with a bladder that completely encircles the arm without overlapping.

A normal blood pressure in the ED should not be considered a clear indication of stability. Healthy, young patients are particularly able to compensate for a fluid volume deficit. Patients at risk for hypovolemia should be evaluated for postural vital sign changes.

Orthostatic Vital Signs

To obtain orthostatic vital signs, take the blood pressure and pulse with the patient supine, and repeat the procedure with the patient in a standing position. Those patients unable to stand should be evaluated while they are sitting on the stretcher with their legs dangling over the side. A decrease of 10 mm Hg or more in systolic pressure or an increase in heart rate of 10 beats/min or more upon sitting is indicative of hypovolemia. Subjective signs of hypovolemia upon position change include dizziness, weakness, blurred vision, and syncope. Heart rate is a more sensitive indicator than blood pressure unless the patient has cardiac disease or is on a medication such as beta blockers. Normal blood volume is approximately 70 ml/Kg or 4900 ml (roughly 5 liters) in a 70-Kg person. With hypovolemic losses of 500 ml or less, no change in orthostatic vital signs is detectable. With losses of 500–1000 ml, orthostatic tachycardia should be seen. With losses of 1000–1500 ml, orthostatic tachycardia and hypotension are seen. With losses of >30% of blood volume (>1500 ml), hypotension and a weak pulse in all positions should be detected.

Vital signs provide an easily obtainable indication of the patient's condition. To be used optimally they must be viewed collectively and serially along with the patient's level of consciousness, results of the physical examination, and the illness history.

FAMILY CRISIS AND GRIEVING

In most cases, a time for the patient's family and friends in the ED is minimal. Staff time is limited, space is at a premium, and patient care must always be the first priority. But from another perspective, the patient and family are a unit, an emotional, social, financial unit. Members of the nursing staff need to consider the patient's family and close friends in planning the patient's care and, to whatever extent possible, have them participate in the caring process.

Family Notification

If family members do not arrive with the patient, attempt to contact them as soon as possible. You may be aided in this process by police, admitting office staff, or social worker. Full details of the patient's condition should not be given over the phone. Verify to whom you are talking and their relationship to the patient. Advise them that the patient is being treated and that the family should come to the ED. Often the relatives' distress and anxiety are obvious over the phone; ask them to repeat the directions to the hospital and encourage them to come with another family member or close friend. It is not advisable to make notification of death over the telephone and should only be done when no other options are available.

Keep the Family Informed

If the patient is in critical condition or resuscitation is in progress, the nurse will make the initial contact with the family. Ask about the patient's medical history, medications, allergies, etc., if not already known. Tell the family, in basic terms, the patient's condition and the treatment in progress. Be honest and direct about the patient's condition. If the patient is in serious or critical condition, say so. Let the family know that a number of ED staff members, physicians, and nurses are caring for their relative. Tell the family where to wait and that you will keep them informed on the patient's progress. It is not the amount of time you spend with the family that is most important; rather, it is the caring and concern you feel for the patient, that you convey while talking with the family, that is most important. Even within the brief time allowed, you can show a caring manner by addressing the patient and family by name, acknowledging the family's feelings and concerns, telling them the name of the physician treating their relative, using touch, and providing clear explanations of the patient's progress. Whenever possible, provide a moment, regardless of how brief, when the family can see, talk with, or touch the patient. The nurse can bring the family to the area outside x-ray or to the elevator the patient will take on the way to emergency surgery, so that the family have what may be a last opportunity to contact their loved one. Ask the family if they would like a member of the clergy to see and talk with the patient. Encourage a lone family member to call someone to come to the hospital and stay with them.

Notification of Death

If the patient dies in the ED, the primary physician and nurse or social worker should take family or friends to a private area to inform them. At this time they should be told about the patient's treatment and what basic measures have been employed, e.g., medications, use of a ventilator, pacemaker. This information from the physician who treated the patient will reinforce to the family that everything possible was done. Before they leave the hospital, give the family the physician's name and a telephone number they can call if they have questions at a later time. Much of the information they receive in the ED will be felt more than remembered. The initial grief response may vary from shock and disbelief to extreme emotion. No one response is normal or the right way to grieve. Be prepared for relatives who, in their distress, may express anger at the hospital and staff for the patient's death. Often, there is little you can say to the family at this time; just be supportive and take time to listen. As family members start the work of grieving, they may want to tell you something about the patient, his or her achievements, and their life together. Do not rush the family out of the hospital; they need this time to come to grips with what has happened. When dealing with a large number of family members, try to concentrate on one or two group members who are acting as group supports and organizers.

Viewing the Body

Family members often need to view the body to believe or accept what they have been told by the ED staff. Before this viewing, prepare the body by removing resuscitation equipment, washing off blood or body fluids, and covering the body with a clean sheet. Provide the family time and privacy to say goodbye, to kiss or touch their loved one. Prepare the family in advance that the deceased, particularly the trauma victim, does not look the way they remember.

Explain any necessary paper work and forms to be signed; inform them of the medical examiner's regulations, if they apply, and of the need to contact a funeral director. A request for autopsy can be made at this time. Included in the discussion should be the purpose of the autopsy, the effect on the deceased's appearance, and the time period involved. Considering the family's response and the patient's physical condition, a request for organ donation, e.g., eye, skin, can be made to the family. Do not offer sedation; it provides no cure or comfort. Encourage a surviving spouse to have a family member or friend stay with him or her for the next few days. Consider a 24-hour follow-up telephone call to a lone spouse or close relative.

Some families need a prolonged time before they are ready to leave the hospital. Try to let them set the pace; they need this time to collect their thoughts and make some short-range plans. They may want to use the phone to call other family members or friends. Enlist the assistance of the ED social worker, clergy, or bereavement counsellor if you are unable to stay with the family during this time.

SUGGESTED READINGS

Triage

Butler WR. ED patient classification matrix: development and testing of one tool. J Emerg Nurs 1986;12:279–290.

Maughan MD, Gross PL, Fox SS. Emergency ward triage. In: Wilkins EW, et al, eds. MGH textbook of emergency medicine. Baltimore: Williams & Wilkins, 1983:879–890.

Molitor L. Triage dilemmas and decisions: a tool for continuing education. J Emerg Nurs 1985;11:40–42.

Rund AR, Rausch TS. Triage. St Louis: CV Mosby, 1981.

Thompson JD, Dains JE. Comprehensive triage, a manual for developing and implementing a nursing care system. Reston, Virginia: Reston Publishing, 1982.

Wilson M. Setting up an effective ED triage system. Nursing 1988;18:55–56.

Patient's Family Crisis and Grieving

Archer DN, Smith AC. Sorrow has many faces. Nursing 1988; 18:43–45.

Baker HM. Behavioral issues, some thoughts on helping grieving families. J Emerg Nurs 1987;13:359–362.

Bluhm J. Helping families in crisis hold on. Nursing 1987; 17:44–46.

Dubin WR, Samoff JR. Sudden unexpected death: intervention with the survivors. Ann Emerg Med 1986;15:54–57.

Sohl R. When your patient is acutely ill: how to comfort and guide the family. Nursing 1987;17:63–64.

Chapter 1

CARDIOVASCULAR EMERGENCIES

CARDIOPULMONARY ARREST

Cardiopulmonary arrest, commonly associated with MI,* is also seen in a wide range of other medical-surgical emergencies, including airway obstruction, drowning, electrolyte imbalance, electrocution, and trauma. Deaths from coronary artery disease that occur within 2 hours of the onset of symptoms are called "sudden death" and are primarily the result of cardiac arrhythmias. Many of those who die from sudden death do not have a MI, and it is presumed that if basic life support or advanced life support (BLS/ACLS) was readily available, a significant number of sudden deaths could be prevented. All ED staff must be trained in CPR, and ACLS should be standard for professional staff members.

Immediate Assessment and Treatment

Rapidly assess the patient to ascertain the absence of pulse, BP, and breathing. Because scant initial history accompanies the majority of patients who have suffered acute arrest, most patients are given the benefit of the doubt, and resuscitation is initiated. Exceptions to this rule (as determined by a physician) include patients with obvious lethal injuries and those with a clearly defined do-not-resuscitate status. Signs of death include rigor mortis, dependent lividity, tissue decomposition, and fixed, dilated pupils.

Physical Findings
Airway - Open the airway by tilting the patient's head (unless contraindicated by cervical trauma) and ventilate with oxygen via a bag/mask de-

---

*See "Appendix A" for definition of common abbreviations used in the text.

vice until endotracheal intubation can be accomplished. Always use an oxygen reservoir with the bag/mask device, to provide close to 100% oxygen. Have suction readily available; gastric distention and vomiting are common occurrences with bag/mask ventilation.

Check pulse and cardiac rhythm - Institute cardiac compression. Monitor the effectiveness of cardiac compression by checking femoral and carotid pulses at regular intervals. Use "quick look" paddles on the defibrillator to check the rhythm. This can save precious time early in the resuscitation effort. The ECG machine can be attached as soon as possible thereafter.

Establish at least one IV line - If possible, obtain blood for SMA when an IV line is started. Any well-running peripheral line will be adequate, but if it is difficult to start, prompt placement of an internal jugular, subclavian, or femoral line is indicated.

Announce a cardiac arrest to obtain assistance, if necessary - Many hospitals assign a particular team to cover arrests. The cardiac arrest team will usually report to the site within minutes, at which time the direction of the resuscitation may be assumed by the team leader. Each member of the arrest team should be assigned a role, such as medication preparer, recorder, etc. Quiet and order are of paramount importance. Other personnel not assigned to the team or needed for the resuscitation effort should return to their usual assignments. If members of the ED staff participate in the resuscitation, at least one staff member must be left to make regular rounds on all other patients until the resuscitation is completed.

Assessment

History

Once the resuscitation is in progress, it is often the role of the nurse to approach the family concerning the events immediately preceding the cardiac arrest and pertinent medical history. The patient's history may contain information that is crucial to the resuscitation effort, such as the patient has previously suffered chronic renal failure or severe anemia or is an insulin-dependent diabetic. Obtaining a brief history also provides an opportunity to communicate with the family concerning the patient's critical status and the resuscitation efforts in progress. Let them know that all possible efforts are being made, e.g., "A team of doctors and nurses is caring for your husband," "A pacemaker is being inserted." Encourage lone family members to call a friend or relative to stay with them during this crisis. If possible, have a nurse or social worker stay with the family and provide them with periodic progress reports.

Diagnostic Tests

ABGs - Check ABGs repeatedly; results provide the basis for assessing ventilation and determining whether bicarbonate administration is necessary.

SMA - Do a Dextrostix for blood glucose immediately. Send a specimen for stat electrolytes, especially K^+ and cardiac enzymes.

CBC - Spin a stat Hct if bleeding or trauma is suspected.

ECG - A continuous ECG is needed until the patient is stabilized.

Intervention

1. Monitor the patient constantly - Regularly assess the patient's response to treatment. After intubation, check for bilateral lung sounds. Provide 100% oxygen and suction as indicated. Blood gas results of hypoxemia (low pO_2) and/or hypercapnia (high pCO_2) warrant reassessment of endotracheal tube placement, oxygen delivery system, and the need for suctioning. Place the patient on a cardiac monitor and make frequent vital sign determinations. Placement of a nasogastric tube may be indicated to reduce gastric distention and decrease the risk of aspiration.

2. Drug therapy - Prepare expected resuscitation drugs including epinephrine, atropine, lidocaine, and sodium bicarbonate. All resuscitation drugs may be given in a good peripheral or central IV line. Intracardiac administration is not recommended. Avoid administering sodium bicarbonate with epinepherine or any catecholamine, as it will inactivate the catecholamine. Epinephrine, atropine, and lidocaine can be administered intratracheally, via the endotracheal tube, if an IV line has not been established. One nurse should be assigned to record frequency and amount of drugs. It is also important for the medication nurse to notify the team when the recommended dosage limit has been reached, e.g., 2 mg atropine. It is advisable to use a flow sheet with columns for time, medication, other treatment, and patient response. This type of a CPR flow record can be reviewed at a later date as part of the quality assurance process. (See Appendix D for use of emergency drugs.)

3. Defibrillation - The recommended energy for initial defibrillation is 200–300 J (watt-sec) with a maximum of 360 J. Higher energy levels are no more effective and may precipitate AV block and myocardial damage. (See ventricular fibrillation algorithms in this chapter.) Subsequent energy levels are increased, and three successive defibrillations are given at the onset. (See "Electrical Defibrillation and Synchronized Cardioversion" in Chapter 16.) It is vital that the team member assigned to defibrillate is experienced in the procedure and

applies all necessary safety precautions. Reassess the patient's cardiac rhythm and pulse after each defibrillation.

4. Acid-base balance - Cardiopulmonary arrest will result in both metabolic and respiratory acidosis. Respiratory acidosis (pH < 7.35, pCO_2 > 45) will develop rapidly after an arrest and will respond just as rapidly after treatment. Ventilation by bag/mask device, intubation, and clearing the lungs of secretions should dissipate excess pCO_2. Metabolic acidosis develops more slowly. During severe respiratory insufficiency and failure, as the body cells continue to function without adequate oxygen, the process of anaerobic metabolism results in the production of lactic acid. Treatment of lactic acidosis should be guided by results of blood gas analysis. Immediate use of sodium bicarbonate during a resuscitation is no longer recommended by the American Heart Association. Correction of acidosis with sodium bicarbonate may be a more pressing need in patients with a history of an acidosis-related disease such as renal failure, diabetic ketoacidosis, and alcoholism and for those who continue to show a profound acidosis (pH < 7.2) despite adequate ventilation.

5. Electromechanical dissociation - EMD is determined when the heart's electrical conduction does not result in a sufficient mechanical response to generate a palpable pulse. This will usually be seen as a sinus or junctional rhythm with no pulse. Since this condition results in inadequate perfusion, CPR must be continued. Treatment consists of epinepherine, bicarbonate, calcium, and isoproterenol. Other conditions to be excluded before a diagnosis of EMD can be made include shock (septic, cardiogenic), hypovolemia, cardiac tamponade, cardiac rupture, tension pneumothorax, right ventricular infarction, and pulmonary embolus.

6. Stabilization after successful resuscitation - Review ongoing therapy and monitoring with the goal of supporting the patient's cardiopulmonary status and preventing complications. Particular attention should be paid to correction of hypotension with fluids or dopamine, if necessary. The patient must have adequate fluid volume for dopamine to be effective. An arterial and/or pulmonary artery catheter may be inserted. An antiarrhythmic infusion (lidocaine) and a follow-up bolus, if necessary (check total dosage), should be started to prevent recurrence of ventricular tachycardia or fibrillation.

ED Discharge Planning

A physician and nurse or social worker should meet with the family after the resuscitation to discuss the patient's treatment, present status, and prognosis. This meeting should take place in an area that affords privacy and an opportunity for the family to ask questions. A staff member should be assigned to stay with those who have lost a close friend or family member. The presence of a bereavement protocol will facilitate the management of grieving friends and family and will increase staff sensitivity. If the patient's transfer to the ICU is delayed, prepare the family to see the patient briefly in the ED.

In the ICU, priorities include:

1. Assessment and provision for oxygenation.
   a. Provide oxygen delivery by mask, T bar, or ventilator, as indicated.
   b. Observe for signs of hypoxia, e.g., in the nailbeds and lips.
   c. Suction and maintain a patent airway.
   d. Place the patient in a mid-Fowler's position.
   e. Monitor blood gases.
   f. Decrease oxygen requirements by maintaining rest (medicate with diazepam or morphine, if indicated), reduce anxiety, and treat temperature elevation.
2. Assess and support cardiac output and tissue perfusion.
   a. Provide continuous invasive or noninvasive pressure monitoring, and regulate fluids and/or vasopressor drugs to maintain blood pressure at 100 mm Hg.
   b. Observe level of consciousness and urinary output (at least 30 ml/hr) as indicators of perfusion.

Study the following algorithms for cardiac dysrhythmias (Figs. 1.1–1.7[†]).

[†]Figures 1.1–1.7 are reproduced with permission from the American Heart Association and Albarran-Sotelo R, et al. Textbook of advanced cardiac life support. Dallas, Texas: American Heart Association, 1987.

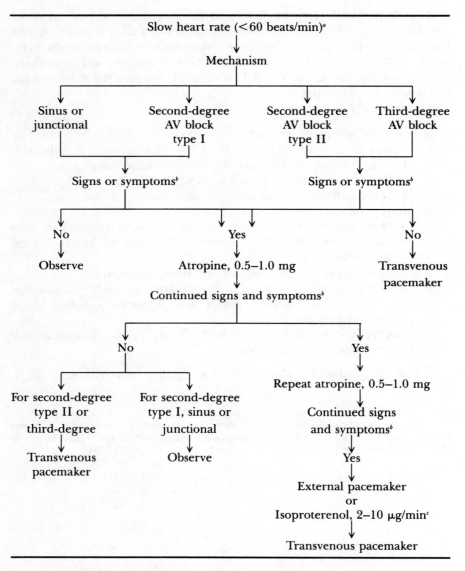

Figure 1.1. Algorithm for bradycardia. This sequence was developed to assist in teaching how to treat a broad range of patients with bradycardia. Some patients may require care not specified herein. This algorithm should not be construed to prohibit such flexibility. *AV*, atrioventricular.

[a]A solitary chest thump or cough may stimulate cardiac electrical activity and result in improved cardiac output and may be used at this point.

[b]Hypotension (BP < 90 mm Hg), premature ventricular contractions, altered mental status or symptoms (e.g., chest pain of dyspnea), ischemia, or infarction.

[c]Temporizing therapy.

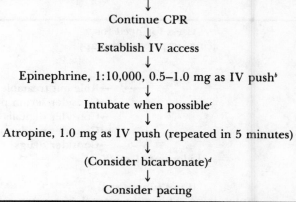

If rhythm is unclear and, possibly, VF, defibrillate as for VF. If asystole is present,[a]

↓

Continue CPR

↓

Establish IV access

↓

Epinephrine, 1:10,000, 0.5–1.0 mg as IV push[b]

↓

Intubate when possible[c]

↓

Atropine, 1.0 mg as IV push (repeated in 5 minutes)

↓

(Consider bicarbonate)[d]

↓

Consider pacing

Figure 1.2. Algorithm for asystole (cardiac standstill). This sequence was developed to assist in teaching how to treat a broad range of patients with asystole. Some patients may require care not specified herein. This algorithm should not be construed to prohibit such flexibility. Flow of algorithm presumes asystole is continuing. *VF*, ventricular fibrillation.

[a] Asystole should be confirmed in two leads.

[b] Epinephrine should be repeated every 5 minutes.

[c] Intubation is preferable; if it can be accomplished simultaneously with other techniques, then the earlier the better. However, CPR and use of epinephrine are more important initially if the patient can be ventilated without intubation. (Endotracheal epinephrine may be used.)

[d] Value of sodium bicarbonate is questionable during cardiac arrest, and it is not recommended for the routine cardiac arrest sequence. Consideration of its use in a dose of 1 mEq/Kg is appropriate at this point. Half of original dose, if used, may be repeated every 10 minutes.

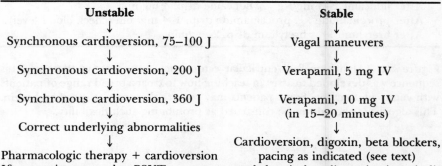

Unstable	Stable
↓	↓
Synchronous cardioversion, 75–100 J	Vagal maneuvers
↓	↓
Synchronous cardioversion, 200 J	Verapamil, 5 mg IV
↓	↓
Synchronous cardioversion, 360 J	Verapamil, 10 mg IV (in 15–20 minutes)
↓	↓
Correct underlying abnormalities	Cardioversion, digoxin, beta blockers,
↓	pacing as indicated (see text)
Pharmacologic therapy + cardioversion	

If conversion occurs but PSVT recurs, repeated electrical cardioversion is *not* indicated. Sedation should be used as time permits.

Figure 1.3. Algorithm for paroxysmal supraventricular tachycardia (*PSVT*). This sequence was developed to assist in teaching how to treat a broad range of patients with sustained PSVT. Some patients may require care not specified herein. This algorithm should not be construed as prohibiting such flexibility. Flow of algorithm presumes PSVT is continuing.

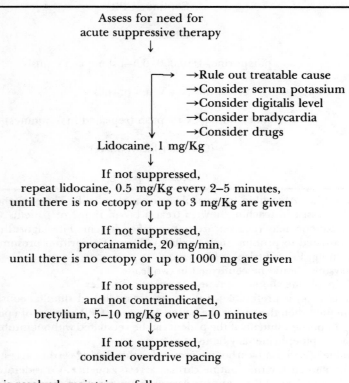

Assess for need for
acute suppressive therapy
↓

→Rule out treatable cause
→Consider serum potassium
→Consider digitalis level
→Consider bradycardia
→Consider drugs

Lidocaine, 1 mg/Kg
↓

If not suppressed,
repeat lidocaine, 0.5 mg/Kg every 2–5 minutes,
until there is no ectopy or up to 3 mg/Kg are given
↓

If not suppressed,
procainamide, 20 mg/min,
until there is no ectopy or up to 1000 mg are given
↓

If not suppressed,
and not contraindicated,
bretylium, 5–10 mg/Kg over 8–10 minutes
↓

If not suppressed,
consider overdrive pacing

Once ectopy is resolved, maintain as follows:
    After lidocaine, 1 mg/Kg . . . lidocaine drip, 2 mg/min
    After lidocaine, 1–2 mg/Kg . . . lidocaine drip, 3 mg/min
    After lidocaine,2–3 mg/Kg . . . lidocaine drip, 4 mg/min
    After procainamide . . . procainamide drip, 1–4 mg/min (check blood level)
    After bretylium . . . . bretylium drip, 2 mg/min

Figure 1.4.   Algorithm for ventricular ectopy: acute suppressive therapy. This sequence was developed to assist in teaching how to treat a broad range of patients with ventricular ectopy. Some patients may require therapy not specified herein. This algorithm should not be construed as prohibiting such flexibility.

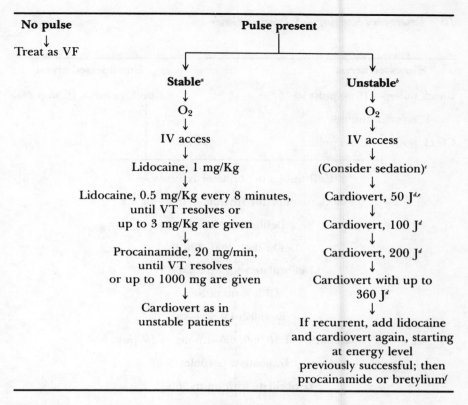

Figure 1.5. Algorithm for sustained ventricular tachycardia (*VT*). This sequence was developed to assist in teaching how to treat a broad range of patients with sustained VT. Some patients may require care not specified herein. This algorithm should not be construed as prohibiting such flexibility. Flow of algorithm presumes that VT is continuing. *VF*, ventricular fibrillation.

[a] If patient becomes unstable (see Footnote b for definition) at any time, move to "Unstable" arm of algorithm.

[b] Unstable indicates symptoms (e.g., chest pain or dyspnea), hypotension (systolic BP < 90 mm Hg), CHF, ischemia, or infarction.

[c] Sedation should be considered for all patients, including those defined in Footnote b as unstable, except those who are hemodynamically unstable (e.g., hypotensive, in pulmonary edema, or unconscious).

[d] If hypotension, pulmonary edema, or unconsciousness is present, unsynchronized cardioversion should be done to avoid delay associated with synchronization.

[e] In the presence of hypotension, pulmonary edema, or unconsciousness, a precordial thump may be employed prior to cardioversion.

[f] Once VT has resolved, begin IV infusion of an antiarrhythmic agent that has aided resolution or VT. If hypotension, pulmonary edema, or unconsciousness is present, use lidocaine if cardioversion alone is unsuccessful, followed by bretylium. In all other patients, recommended order of therapy is lidocaine, procainamide, and then bretylium.

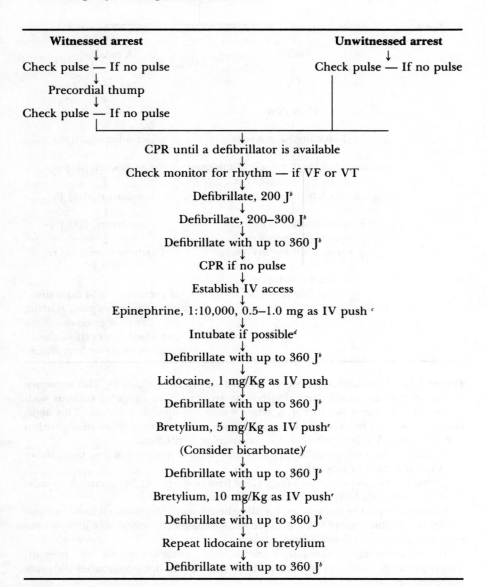

Figure 1.6. Algorithm for ventricular fibrillation (*VF*) (and pulseless ventricular tachycardia (*VT*)).[a] This sequence was developed to assist in teaching how to treat a broad range of patients with VF or pulseless VT. Some patients may require care not specified herein. This algorithm should not be construed as prohibiting such flexibility. Flow of algorithm presumes that VF is continuing.

^aPulseless VT should be treated identically to VF.

^bCheck pulse and rhythm after each shock. If VF recurs after transiently converting (rather than persists without ever converting), use whatever energy level has previously been successful for defibrillation.

^cEpinephrine should be repeated every 5 minutes.

^dIntubation is preferable. If it can be accompanied simultaneously with other techniques, then the earlier the better. However, defibrillation and epinephrine are more important initially if the patient can be ventilated without intubation.

^eSome may prefer repeated doses of lidocaine, which may be given in boluses of 0.5 mg/Kg every 8 minutes to a total dose of 3 mg/Kg.

^fValue of sodium bicarbonate is questionable during cardiac arrest, and it is not recommended for routine cardiac arrest sequence. Consideration of its use in a dose of 1 mEq/Kg is appropriate at this point. Half of original dose may be repeated every 10 minutes if it is used.

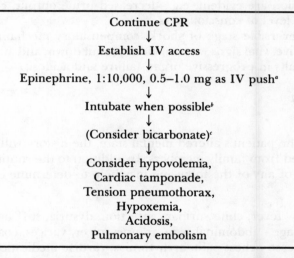

Continue CPR
↓
Establish IV access
↓
Epinephrine, 1:10,000, 0.5–1.0 mg as IV push^a
↓
Intubate when possible^b
↓
(Consider bicarbonate)^c
↓
Consider hypovolemia,
Cardiac tamponade,
Tension pneumothorax,
Hypoxemia,
Acidosis,
Pulmonary embolism

Figure 1.7. Algorithm for electromechanical dissociation (*EMD*). This sequence was developed to assist in teaching how to treat a broad range of patients with EMD. Some patients may require care not specified herein. This algorithm should not be construed to prohibit such flexibility. Flow of algorithm presumes that EMD is continuing.

^aEpinephrine should be repeated every 5 minutes.

^bIntubation is preferable. If it can be accomplished simultaneously with other techniques, then the earlier the better. However, epinephrine is more important initially if the patient can be ventilated without intubation.

^cValue of sodium bicarbonate is questionable during cardiac arrest, and it is not recommended for routine cardiac arrest sequence. Consideration of its use in a dose of 1 mEq/Kg is appropriate at this point. Half of original dose may be repeated every 10 minutes if it is used.

SHOCK

Shock is a clinical syndrome that results when there is inadequate circulatory perfusion to provide for the metabolic needs of the cells. The types of shock include septic, cardiogenic, hypovolemic, drug-induced, neurogenic, and anaphylactic.

Shock may be divided into three stages: early, intermediate, and irreversible. In the early stage of shock, compensatory mechanisms are in operation. This condition is potentially reversible. The pulse is increased, and BP may be somewhat higher or lower than the patient's normal pressure. There is orthostatic hypotension, and the skin is cool and pale.

In the intermediate stage of shock, tachycardia and hypotension are pronounced, and respirations are shallow and rapid. Signs of decreased tissue perfusion are evident, e.g., decreased urine output, cold clammy skin, altered level of consciousness.

In the irreversible stage of shock, compensatory mechanisms are no longer effective, vital signs worsen, kidneys shut down, and anaerobic metabolism results in progressive organ failure and acidosis.

Assessment

History
Because of the patient's altered mental state, the history will often need to be obtained from family members. In addition to the routine information, history of any of the following may help to determine etiology and treatment:

1. Infection - fever, chills, urinary infection, dysuria, stiff neck
2. Hemorrhage - abdominal pain, trauma, ulcer, varices, coagulopathy
3. Heart disease - chest pain, arrhythmias, cardiac medication
4. Diabetes - diet or medication regulation
5. Exposure - extreme heat or cold
6. Drug overdose - suicide attempts
7. Pregnancy - abdominal pain, vaginal bleeding
8. Trauma - head or neck injury, numbness, paralysis
9. Allergies - recent administration of drugs, food allergies

Physical Findings
Vital signs - Frequent monitoring with particular attention paid to the following vital signs is necessary.

Blood pressure - Usually <90 mm Hg. BP alone, however, is a poor indicator of shock. Initially, BP should be taken every 5 minutes. An automatic BP machine with alarm may be used, but be aware that results tend to be less reliable when pressure is very low. A Doppler monitor can be used if the BP can not be auscultated.

Pulse - In an attempt to maintain cardiac output the heart rate increases to compensate for low stroke volume. Tachycardia, 120–150/min, with a weak, thready pulse is common in all types of shock except neurogenic shock and shock due to bradydysrhythmias.

Respirations - Tachypnea of >40/min and shallow is commonly seen.

Temperature - An elevated or below normal temperature may be seen in septic shock. Regardless of the cause, an elevated temperature increases metabolic demands and oxygen consumption.

Lungs - Listen for rales or signs of consolidation.

Cardiovascular system - Check for rate, rhythm, murmur, and extra sounds.

Skin - Observe for rashes, edema, petechiae, signs of trauma. Skin is cool and clammy to touch.

Head - Level of consciousness and neurologic status is an important indicator of cerebral perfusion. Observe for signs of trauma. Check pupils for size and reaction. Pupils may dilate in the late stages of shock, but constricted pupils (miosis) are indicative of narcotic overdose. If the level of consciousness is variable, the patient may be restless or somnolent.

Neck - Observe for neck vein distention. Neck veins (external and internal jugular) should not be observable when the patient is at a 45° or greater angle. Distended neck veins are seen in cardiogenic shock, tamponade, tension pneumothorax, and CHF. Flat veins, when the patient is in a horizontal position, are seen in hypovolemia. CVP determinations will correspond to neck veins; i.e., the determinations will be elevated (>15 cm H_2O) in cardiogenic shock and below normal (<5 cm H_2O) in hypovolemic shock.

Abdomen - Feel the abdomen for guarding, rebound, tenderness, and masses (a pulsatile mass is indicative of an aneuyrysm).

Extremities - Feel for coolness and claminess. Make sure pulses are equal. Estimate capillary refill time.

Rectal examination - Test for occult blood.

Diagnostic Tests

Laboratory tests - Spin a stat Hct and send for CBC, differential, platelets, and PT. If the Hct is <30, send for a type and cross-match; if not, send for a type and hold. Do a stat Dextrostix for serum glucose. Check the electrolytes and PT.

Drug levels - Send a specimen for appropriate toxicology screening if overdose or poisoning is suspected.

ABGs - Monitor for acid-base imbalance, primarily for acidosis and hypoxia. Results of an analysis of mixed venous blood gas may be helpful in making an early diagnosis.

Urinalysis - Check for ketones and glucose. Insert a Foley catheter to obtain urine for C&S and to enable monitoring of hourly urine output.

ECG - Obtain an ECG as soon as possible to check for signs of myocardial ischemia (ST wave changes) and arrhythmias.

X-ray - A chest film should be obtained. Usually, a portable flat plate of the abdomen or a decubitus view may be ordered if abdominal pain or trauma is present. A cross-table lateral view is indicated if an abdominal aortic aneurysm is suspected.

Culdocentesis - Should be performed on a female patient of childbearing age who has a positive pregnancy test or a history of a missed period, to rule out ruptured ectopic pregnancy, if she presents with unexplained shock and abdominal pain. (See "Ectopic Pregnancy" in Chapter 10.)

Intervention

The following elements are used in common in the treatment of septic, cardiogenic, hypovolemic, and drug-induced shock:

	Septic	Cardiac	Hypovolemic	Drug-induced
Check airway and respirations and give O_2	Yes	Yes	Yes	Yes
Start large-bore 14–16-gauge IV line	Yes	Yes	Yes	Yes
Spin Hct and check stool guiac	Yes	Yes	Yes	Yes
Rapid fluid administration of lactated Ringer's solution	Yes	No	Yes and blood, if needed	Yes
MAST suit	Yes	No	Yes	Yes
ECG monitor	Yes	Yes	Yes	Yes

Generally Used Protocol

1. Airway/breathing - All patients in shock require supplemental oxygen. If a patient shows signs of respiratory failure with an increased pCO_2

and a decreased pO_2 and tidal volume, intubation is indicated. Hypoperfusion of the lungs may lead to ARDS. To maintain acceptable ABG values, a higher-than-usual ventilator setting may be required, i.e., a tidal volume of 10 ml/Kg or higher, an oxygen setting (F_IO_2) of 60–100%, and a PEEP of 5–30 cm H_2O. Placement of an nasogastric tube will decrease gastric distention and reduce the possibility of aspiration.

2. Fluid administration - Large-volume fluid administration (1–2 liters in 30 minutes) is indicated in all but cardiogenic shock. Initially, crystalloid solutions such as lactated Ringer's or NS should be administered for rapid volume replacement. Colloid solutions may be administered if further volume expansion is needed. Colloid solutions including Plasmanate, dextran, and hetastarch (Hespan) expand volume by increasing colloidal osmotic pressure, thereby pulling interstitial fluid into the intravascular space. Hypotension in cardiogenic shock is often treated with low-dose dopamine (2–10 μg/Kg/min). Fluid challenge and Swan-Ganz PAP monitoring are commonly used to clarify the patient's volume status. Strict monitoring of hourly intake and output is critical, with urine output being one of the most reliable indicators of perfusion and response to treatment. Position the patient flat in bed. Elevation of the patient's legs will increase venous return, but use of the Trendelenburg position is not advised.

3. Blood transfusion - Hypovolemic shock from blood loss, a common occurrence in trauma, is treated with immediate transfusion of type-specific blood. For rapid administration, place the blood in a pressure bag and connect this to a warmer. Mix packed cells with 100–200 ml of saline to decrease viscosity and increase the infusion rate. Run blood in a separate large-bore line so that one line is available for simultaneous administration of fluid and drugs. Two units of fresh frozen plasma and 1 ampule of calcium chloride are given for every 6 units of blood.

4. Cardiac arrhythmias - All patients in shock, regardless of cause, have decreased perfusion and are prone to cardiac arrhythmias. Arrhythmias may be an indication of hypoxia.

5. MAST suit - Acts to increase peripheral vascular resistance and elevate the patient's BP. The MAST suit is contraindicated in cardiogenic shock. Note: Many authorities now question the efficacy of the MAST suit. Its role, if any, in the treatment of shock states requires future clarification.

Specific Protocol for Drug-induced Shock
1. Administer naloxone (Narcan), 5 ampules, in an IV push. If patient shows a clinical response, 5 more ampules are given IM, and an naloxone IV drip of 10 ampules/liter is started and titrated to wakefulness.

2. Insert a large-bore 36-gauge orogastric tube and lavage the stomach; smaller tubes will not lavage pill fragments. When lavage is clear, activated charcoal (60 gm) and FLEET Phospho-soda are given. (For further details, see "Drug Overdose: A General Approach" in Chapter 7.) Caution: If the patient is hypothermic, treat as indicated under "Hypothermia" in Chapter 6.

ED Discharge Planning

The mortality from shock remains high. In order to provide maximum monitoring and specialized therapy, placement in the ICU is indicated. A Swan-Ganz catheter may be inserted in the ED or on admission to the ICU. The resulting PAP readings will serve as a guide to fluid balance regulation and cardiac function. The PCWP reading, normally 6–12 mm Hg, reflects the left ventricular end-diastolic pressure. The PCWP is closely monitored during rapid fluid administration and is essential in determining fluid requirements in cardiogenic shock. Cardiac assist devices may be used in the treatment of cardiogenic shock. An intraaortic balloon pump may be inserted to improve coronary artery blood flow and augment cardiac function by decreasing afterload.

SYNCOPE

Syncope is a sudden, spontaneous, transient loss of consciousness. Etiologies include inadequate oxygenation, hypoglycemia, seizures, drug or alcohol intoxication, pulmonary embolus, infection, cerebrovascular disease, hypotension, and psychogenic unresponsiveness.

A vasovagal event (classical fainting) is the most common cause of syncope. During the acute phase of a fainting spell, virtually all patients exhibit pallor, a slow pulse, and hypotension. After a short recovery period, all signs return to normal. Patients who do not recover quickly after lying supine with their feet elevated should be examined thoroughly.

Assessment

History
Because the numerous etiologies for syncope are so varied and range from benign to catastrophic illness, any history is valuable. Of special importance are accurate descriptions of the presence or absence of a prodrome and the patient's activity at the time of the attack. The presence of associated symptoms, such as seizure activity, loss of continence, chest pain, dyspnea, diaphoresis, headache, palpitations, or emotional out-

bursts, should be noted. A general history should include similar past events, medications, and drug or alcohol consumption.

Physical Findings

Vital signs - Include a rectal temperature and assessment of orthostatic changes (heart rate and BP of the patient both lying and standing). Correlate the pulse with the patient's general condition; note that patients on beta blockers may not be able to mount a tachycardia despite volume depletion. Note pulse irregularities and pulse deficit.

Head and neurologic signs - Check the pupils, and observe for signs of trauma, respiratory pattern, motor activity, and level of consciousness.

Lungs - Listen for equal breath sounds, wheezes, or rales.

Cardiovascular system - Listen for regularity of rhythm, murmurs, and gallops.

Diagnostic Tests

CBC - Obtain a spun Hct and send for WBC and differential.

SMA - Check Dextrostix for serum glucose and electrolytes; send for toxicology as indicated.

ABGs and x-ray - Request x-ray and check ABGs if indicated.

ECG - An ECG is always indicated.

Rectal examination - Test the stool for occult blood loss.

Intervention

1. Take vital signs and ensure adequate airway and breathing. Provide oxygen and suction as needed.
2. Start an IV of lactated Ringer's or plasma expander to support BP. If vital signs are stable or cardiac origin is suspected, run an IV of D5W at keep-open rate.
3. Place the patient on a cardiac monitor and obtain an ECG.
4. If the patient remains unconscious or a Dextrostix indicates hypoglycemia, give 1 ampule of D50W IV. Thiamine, 100 mg IM, should precede D50W if the patient has a history of or shows signs of alcohol abuse or malnutrition.
5. Give 5 ampules of naloxone in an IV push.
6. Orient the patient to his or her surroundings. Obtain further history as the patient's level of consciousness improves.

ED Discharge Planning

Life-threatening emergencies, such as acute MI, profound bradyarrhythmias, massive GI bleeding, pulmonary emboli, diabetic coma, uremia, overdose with cardiopulmonary depression, sepsis, meningitis, or intracranial lesions, obviously require admission. The cause of many syncopal episodes (transient losses of consciousness), however, remains obscure after ED treatment. The following factors favor a further evaluation on an inpatient basis:

1. Older age (over 40 years)
2. Associated illness, especially cardiac disease
3. Significant findings on physical examination
4. Metabolic, hematologic, or cardiac abnormalities
5. Lives alone and has no one available to check on patient at periodic intervals

Most fainting episodes do not require admission. A brief observation period is appropriate before discharge from the ED. The patient should be accompanied by family or friend when leaving the ED.

ED Discharge Instructions
Appropriate instructions should be given to the patient and/or family on discharge, including:

1. Information on the possible cause or precipitating event and possible means of avoiding a recurrence
2. Home care for a syncopal episode, which consists of keeping the patient in a reclining position and not forcing food or drink
3. Returning to the ED if there is a recurrence
4. Need for further medical evaluation, clinic appointment, or laboratory tests

CHEST PAIN

The main goal of the evaluation of chest pain in the ED is to distinguish between the many minor causes of chest pain and the few potentially life-threatening causes. The triage nurse in many instances will not be able to determine whether the cause of chest pain is minor or serious but will be on solid ground in his or her thinking if all patients with chest pain who look ill and those for whom there is not a definite minor cause of the pain are triaged as emergent.

Assessment

History
It is essential to obtain a clear description of the patient's pain. The mnemonic PQRST may be helpful:

P-What *provokes* the pain? What makes it better or worse?

Q-What is the *quality* of the pain? Have the patient describe the pain, i.e., burning, stabbing, etc.

R-Does the pain *radiate*? Where is the pain located?

S-How *severe* is the pain? Have the patient rate pain on a scale of 1–10.

T-How long (*time*) has the pain lasted? What was taken (*treatment*) to relieve the pain?

A past medical history should be obtained, including previous cardiac and lung disease, hypertension, diabetes, and current medications.

Physical Findings

Vital signs - Check BP and pulse. Note hypotension or hypertension, irregular pulse, elevated temperature, and breathing rate and rhythm.

Neck - Check the trachea in midline.

Lungs - Observe for signs of trauma. Auscultate for breath sounds, rales, wheezing, and pleural rub. Note bruises or tenderness.

Heart - Note distant heart sounds, murmurs, gallops, and friction rub.

Abdomen - Does the patient complain of nausea and/or vomiting. Palpate for a mass or tenderness.

Extremities - Look for clubbing, cyanosis, or edema. Check for pulses in the extremities.

Diagnostic Tests

CBC - Check CBC and WBC with differential.

SMA - Send for electrolytes and, if indicated, cardiac enzymes. Creatine phosphokinase isoenzyme (CPK-MB) begins to rise in 2–6 hours.

ABGs - Analysis of ABGs may be clinically indicated.

ECG - All patients with chest pain that is not clearly of a noncardiac etiology should have a cardiogram. Look for signs of ischemia and inflammation, i.e., ST and T wave changes. See "Myocardial Ischemia and Infarction" in this chapter and "Pericarditis" in Chapter 9 for further details.

X-ray - A chest x-ray or rib films may be indicated, depending on the clinical picture.

Differential Diagnosis of Chest Pain

Serious Causes of Chest Pain

The following are considered serious causes of chest pain. The triage and ED nurse needs to be knowledgeable about the symptoms and implications of these conditions, not to make a diagnosis but to seek immediate medical intervention for those that are emergent.

Unstable angina - The first episode of angina or a previously stable angina that is increasing in frequency or duration, that now occurs with rest as well as exercise, or that is now unrelieved by nitroglycerin. The pain usually lasts less than 30 minutes. Be sure to check the age and condition of the patient's nitroglycerin tablets.

MI - Indicated by a crushing retrosternal pain lasting longer than 30 minutes, unrelieved by rest or nitroglycerin. This is discussed later in this chapter.

Acute pericarditis - Indicated by pleuritic retrosternal pain of gradual onset, which is often relieved by leaning forward. Fever, distant heart sounds, or pericardial friction rub may be noted. See Chapter 9 for further information on pericarditis.

Dissecting aortic aneurysm. Classically, indicated by an excruciating tearing retrosternal back pain that is sudden in onset and may radiate to the head, back, or abdomen. A detailed discussion of aortic aneurysm may be found later in this chapter.

Pneumonia - Indicated by pleuritic pain with a productive cough. Fever, dyspnea, and rales may be noted. Chest x-ray shows infiltrate. See Chapter 2 for further discussion of pneumonia.

Pulmonary embolus - Indicated by pleuritic or crushing chest pain of sudden onset, which is associated with dyspnea, dry cough, and hemoptysis. The pain increases on inspiration. See Chapter 2 for more detail on pulmonary embolus.

Pneumothorax - Indicated by pleuritic or crushing pain with dyspnea of sudden onset. Decreased breath sounds or tracheal shift may be noted. A detailed discussion of pneumothorax is provided in Chapter 2.

Less Life-threatening Causes of Chest Pain

There are numerous causes of chest pain that are not life-threatening and may be triaged as urgent or delayed on the basis of the chief complaint, history, and assessment findings. The following comprise the most common causes:

Stable angina - Retrosternal chest pressure lasting a few minutes, relieved by rest and nitroglycerin within 5 minutes. The patient often gives a history of previous episodes. The ECG may show ST depression or T wave inversion during pain.

Noncardiac causes - Musculoskeletal strain, calcific tendonitis, costochondritis, rib fractures, GI problems, tracheobronchitis, and pleurisy.

ED Discharge Planning

All patients with serious or uncertain causes of chest pain should be monitored in the ED with frequent vital sign determinations. Start oxygen and an IV line and reassess the patient's condition at frequent intervals. You can expect that patients who are diagnosed as having a serious cause of chest pain will be admitted, with some requiring ICU care. One exception in this category should be noted: Pneumonia in a healthy adult will be treated on an outpatient basis. Patients with minor causes of chest pain will be sent home with appropriate therapy and followed on an outpatient basis.

ED Discharge Instructions

Appropriate instructions should be given to the patient on discharge, including:

1. Any necessary curtailment in activity
2. Diet modifications, e.g., a bland diet for patients with gastritis
3. Specific teaching about prescribed medications
4. Need for further treatment or evaluation

MYOCARDIAL ISCHEMIA AND INFARCTION

Myocardial ischemia results from an imbalance between the supply and demand of oxygen to the heart muscle. This usually occurs as a result of an absolute decrease in blood flow to an area of muscle, but it may also be related to increased myocardial oxygen demand seen in times and conditions of stress. In the majority of cases, atherosclerosis is responsible for the decrease in supply. Supply may also be diminished when there is inadequate oxygen-carrying capacity (e.g., carbon monoxide poisoning or profound anemia). Myocardial ischemia regardless of the exact mechanism may result in transient pain known as angina pectoris or in MI from tissue necrosis.

Assessment

History

The triage and the later determination that a patient is suspected of having an acute MI is made primarily on the history. Since the presentation of severe or unstable angina is so similar to that of MI, both entities are included in the assessment and ED intervention. Three factors need to be looked for in the history:

1. Pain - It is important to inquire about the presence and characteristics of the chest pain. Follow the PQRST key (p. 19) and ask the patient to describe the pain relative to the following features: provocation, quality, radiation, severity (on a scale of 1–10), time (duration), and treatment response (relieving factors). The pain of a MI is typically substernal, severe, "heavy," or "tight" and may radiate to the left arm (inside part) or to the jaw, back, or shoulder. In most instances, the

pain lasts longer than 30 minutes and is not relieved by rest or nitrates. However, up to 25% of patients with acute MI have little or no pain. These "silent" MIs are most common in diabetics and the elderly.

2. Associated symptoms - These include shortness of breath, palpitations, weakness, and apprehension with sweating, nausea, and vomiting.
3. Cardiac risk factors - History includes previous MI or angina, hypertension, family history of coronary artery disease, diabetes, hyperlipidemia, history of smoking, and use of cocaine or "crack."

It should be mentioned that coronary artery spasm resulting in variant or Prinzmetal's angina presents a slightly different pattern. These patients typically have chest pain at rest, frequently in the early morning, and at the same time each day. The pain may radiate, and associated symptoms may include dyspnea, syncope, palpitations, and arrhythmias. It responds well to nitroglycerin and calcium entry blockers such as nifedipine and verapamil.

Physical Findings

General - Physical assessment findings depend on the extent of myocardial damage. In patients with small subendocardial infarctions the physical examination may be normal, whereas in patients with a large transmural (full wall thickness) infarct, the examination may reveal pulmonary edema or cardiogenic shock. The patient is often agitated, pale, restless, and diaphoretic. Nausea and vomiting are particularly common in inferior wall MI.

Vital signs - Respiratory rate is often rapid and shallow. Heart rate may be tachycardiac with an irregular rhythm related to ectopic beats. Patients with suspected inferior wall MI (ST elevations in leads II, III, and aVF) should be watched for bradycardia and AV block. BP is variable. It may be elevated related to a sympathetic response, but ventricular dysfunction, arrhythmias, concomitant hypovolemia, nitrates, or analgesics (morphine) may cause hypotension. Elevated temperature is common after 24 hours.

Lungs - Listen for rales that warn of left ventricular failure.

Heart - Observe for distended neck veins that may indicate right heart failure or right ventricular infarct. Auscultate for rate and rhythm; listen for additional sounds S_3 and S_4 (gallop rhythm) and for murmurs that may indicate serious complications such as ventricular septal defect or papillary muscle dysfunction or rupture.

Diagnostic Tests

ECG - Should be done immediately upon suspicion of acute MI (see Fig. 1.8). The characteristic sequence of changes seen with transmural infarct (any of which may be seen at the time of presentation) are as follows:

1. Early development of peaked T waves in the leads corresponding to the site of injury.
2. ST segment elevation with or without deep flipped T waves in leads facing the injury. Reciprocal leads (leads opposite the site of injury) show ST depression. Significant Q waves (at least 0.04 seconds in duration and one-fourth of the QRS voltage) usually signify a MI at least a few days old. Note: With ECG changes consistent with an inferior wall MI, always use right ventricular leads (V_3R, V_4R).

Other patterns include:

1. Nonspecific ST and T wave abnormalities (especially with subendocardial MI).
2. Inversion of the R/S ratio (increase in size of R wave and decrease in size of S wave) in leads V_1 and V_2 (may be the only ECG abnormality with posterior wall MI).
3. Normal ECG - This does not rule out an MI. Patients with a history and physical examination suggestive of MI should be admitted regardless of a normal ECG.

Laboratory studies - CBC with differential, ESR, SMA, PT, PTT.
Cardiac enzymes with isoenzymes - CPK-MB, LDH_1 and LDH_2. Elevations of CPK-MB and LDH_1 (LDH_1 and LDH_2 flip) occur within 12 and 24 hours, respectively, and are relatively specific for necrosis of cardiac cells.
ABGs - Should be drawn in patients with preexisting lung disease, CHF, or acid-base disturbances.

Intervention

1. IV line - Establish an IV line and run D5W at a keep-open rate. To avoid possible fluid overload, use microdrip, IV pump, or heparin lock.

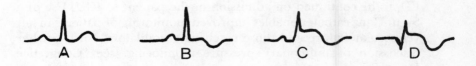

Figure 1.8. ECG changes in MI. *A*, Normal pattern. *B*, Ischemia pattern—T wave inversion. *C*, Ischemia and injury pattern—T wave inversion and ST segment elevation. *D*, Myocardial necrosis indicated by Q wave.

2. Oxygen - Due to alteration in tissue perfusion, oxygen is given via nasal cannula at 3–4 liters/min regardless of whether the patient is experiencing any respiratory difficulty. If the patient has a history of COPD, a lower flow rate to 1–2 liters/min is used, and ABG values are monitored.
3. Vital signs and cardiac monitoring - Initially, vital signs should be taken every 5–15 minutes. Place the patient on a cardiac monitor. Arrhythmias are most likely to arise during the first hours after a MI. Check and set alarm limits and observe for significant arrhythmias and rate changes.
4. Alteration in comfort - Attempt to eliminate pain and anxiety. Relief of pain can comfort and reassure the patient, as well as decrease the myocardial oxygen demand caused by tachycardia. Position the patient in mid-Fowler's if the patient is not hypotensive.
   a. Nitrates - The pain of a MI may be relieved by nitrates. If the patient does not respond to sublingual tablets, 1 inch of Nitropaste may be used. Monitor BP after nitroglycerin administration. Hypotension can develop with any route.
   b. Morphine - This is the drug of choice for severe pain unless the patient is hypotensive or bradycardiac. Give IV in 2–4-mg increments until pain diminishes. Monitor BP closely.
   c. Meperidine (Demerol) - This is as good an analgesic as morphine, causes less vomiting, and is preferable for patients with bradycardia. Give IV in 25-mg increments until pain remits, followed by 25-mg every 3–4 hours.
   d. IV nitroglycerin - May be used to treat continuing pain despite aggressive therapy. Start with 5–10 μg/min via an infusion pump with special tubing. Nitroglycerin (Tridil) is absorbed into regular IV tubing, diluting the solution. Dosage may be increased by 5–10 μg every 5–10 minutes as needed. Remember that patients with normal or low left ventricular filling pressures may become hypotensive and tachycardiac, and increased IV fluid may be needed to support their pressure. Careful and continuous monitoring of the patient is necessary.
   e. Monitoring PAP via a Swan-Ganz catheter may be initiated in the ED, to be continued on admission of the patient to ICU. Use of a Swan-Ganz catheter enables improved monitoring of patients in left ventricular failure and those receiving vasodilators. For a further discussion of pulmonary pressure monitoring, see "Congestive Heart Failure" in this chapter.
   f. Intraaortic balloon pump catheter - This type of catheter is usually not placed while the patient is in the ED, but it may be inserted for cardiogenic shock and intractable chest pain upon admission to the CCU.

g. Coronary artery reperfusion - Streptokinase, tissue plasminogen activator (t-PA), or other thrombolytic agent may be started in the ED. Given by IV drip (or intracoronary artery in the cardiac catheterization laboratory), thrombolytic therapy is considered in patients with ST elevations and recent onset of chest pain (<4–6 hours). The patient requires close monitoring of drug infusion, vital signs, IV site, possible allergic reaction, peripheral pulses, and ventricular arrhythmias, with bleeding being the commonest complication.

5. Antiarrhythmics - Routine pharmacologic antiarrhythmic prophylaxis for ventricular arrhythmias in cases of suspected or known MI is controversial but reasonable in our opinion. Recommended treatment is lidocaine at 1 mg/Kg (50–100 mg) as an IV bolus, followed by a continuous infusion at 2–4 mg/min. Rebolus again after 5–10 minutes; those with resistant ectopy may require up to 3 mg/Kg as the total loading dose. Patients over 65 years of age have a low incidence of primary ventricular fibrillation and do not require prophylaxis. Use a reduced dosage in elderly patients and in those with CHF, liver disease, and hypotension.

6. Pacemaker insertion - For symptomatic bradycardia and heart block (Mobitz type II and third-degree). Have equipment on standby.

7. Provide rest and reassurance for patient and family - The ED is neither the time nor the place for a detailed discussion of MI, but conditions permitting, brief explanations of aspects of care (e.g., IV line, pain medication, cardiac monitor, admission to CCU) with built-in support and reinforcement are important. If BP is stable, let the patient know that pain relief is a positive sign, and help him or her to interpret what is happening to them. Remember that anxiety presents a physical as well as a psychologic stress and causes tachycardia and BP elevations.

8. Limit injury - When reviewing interventions for a patient with a MI, keep in mind that one of the main goals is to limit infarction size. Nursing care activities aimed at limiting infarction size by increasing myocardial oxygen supply while decreasing demand include:
   a. Comfort measures and relief of pain; encourage patients to notify the nurse when pain starts and not to wait until it is severe.
   b. Monitor patient for tachycardia and provide intervention when rate increases due to pain, psychologic stress, or fever.
   c. Provide a calm, quiet environment.
   d. Limit the patient's physical activity.

9. Right ventricular infarction - Occurs more commonly than previously thought and often in conjunction with inferior wall MI, since both receive their blood supply from the right coronary artery. The patient may present with signs of right ventricular failure, including neck vein distention (with clear lungs) and systemic hypotension from decreased

preload. If right ventricular MI is suspected, the ECG should include V_3R and V_4R (right chest) leads. Intervention is primarily aimed at increasing left ventricular output by administration of plasma expanders and IV fluid. Diuretics are to be avoided, because they will decrease circulating fluid volume and venous return (preload).

Complications

The early complications of MI must be watched for diligently. ED nurses need to be knowledgeable about and be prepared to intervene when potential complications such as the following occur:

1. Arrhythmias, including ventricular tachycardia and fibrillation, as well as rapid atrial arrhythmias
2. Conduction abnormalities, including AV block and bilateral bundle branch block with large left ventricular and right ventricular infarcts
3. Left ventricular failure, sometimes progressing to pulmonary edema and cardiogenic shock
4. Right ventricular failure
5. Persistent pain
6. Hypotension secondary to pharmacologic agents

ED Discharge Planning

All patients suspected of having a MI must be admitted to a monitored bed, preferably in the CCU or ICU. Patients with new or unstable angina should also be admitted.

CONGESTIVE HEART FAILURE

Congestive heart failure is a syndrome in which the heart is unable to pump an adequate amount of blood to meet the metabolic needs of the tissues. CHF may be either acute or chronic, with acute CHF and pulmonary edema the conditions that require prompt ED treatment. Commonly, acute CHF is caused by failure of the left ventricle which, when severe or chronic, may lead to right heart failure. Causes include:

Left heart failure	*Right heart failure*
Hypertensive heart disease	Left heart failure
Coronary artery disease	Chronic pulmonary disease
Rheumatic heart disease	Cardiomyopathy
Congenital heart disease	Constrictive pericarditis
Cardiomyopathic heart disease	Pulmonary embolus
Miscellaneous	Right ventricular infarct

Assessment

History

The patient may present with a chief complaint of shortness of breath on exertion, fatigue, or pedal edema. Inquire specifically as to the previous existence of nocturia, orthopnea (number of pillows), paroxysmal nocturnal dyspnea, or angina. Note previous history of cardiac disease or the presence of the important cardiac risk factors: diabetes, hypertension, previous infarct, family history of heart disease in a patient under age 60, hyperlipidemia, or smoking. Note current medications including names and dosage.

A worsening of preexisting CHF or new-onset CHF may be related to:

1. increased salt intake
2. decrease or failure to take medications

Physical Findings

Vital signs - Take a full set of vital signs. BP may be low or elevated, with hypertension being common in CHF with pulmonary edema. Tachypnea and tachycardia are in compensation for poor gas exchange and diminished cardiac output (cardiac output = stroke volume × heart rate). A pulsus alternans (beat-to-beat variation in systolic pressure) suggests left ventricular failure.

Neck-jugular vein distention - Examine neck veins with the patient in the sitting position. Full or pulsating veins in this position are indicative of elevated CVP and possible right heart failure.

Lungs - Auscultate for fine and course crackling (rales and wheezes), so-called "cardiac asthma."

Heart - A third heart sound (S_3) heard early in diastole is common in CHF. The sound is low pitched and often difficult to hear. A combination of tachycardia and S_3 and possibly S_4 results in a gallop rhythm, so named because it resembles the sound of galloping hoofbeats.

Abdomen - Note distention, possibly ascites. Presence of a "fluid wave" will indicate the distention is due to fluid. To test, have an assistant or the patient press his or her hand vertically on the abdomen midline, to prevent vibration from passing along the abdomen wall. With a palm on one flank, tap the other flank; if the distention is fluid, the tapping will be clearly transmitted to the other palm. Note hepatomegaly.

Extremities - Examine for peripheral edema particularly in dependent parts of the body, i.e., arms, legs, feet, sacral area. Check peripheral pulses and for cyanosis.

Diagnostic Tests

Laboratory studies - CBC, SMA, PT, and PTT.

ABGs - Should be done immediately in acutely dyspneic patients to establish pO_2 and acid-base status.

ECG - Obtain an ECG. Changes may indicate MI, pulmonary embolus, pericarditis, pericardial effusion, or arrhythmia.

X-ray - Patients with acute respiratory distress or unstable vital signs should have a stat portable chest x-ray taken. Interstitial edema and alveolar edema can be seen on x-ray, and it will aid the physician in differentiating CHF from other causes of dyspnea.

Intervention

General Considerations

Preload - The force exerted on the ventricle, primarily by the venous return, which causes it to fill, is called preload. Preload or LVEDP can be measured by using a Swan-Ganz pulmonary artery catheter. According to Starling's law, an adequate preload is necessary to maintain stroke volume. A low preload from low circulating fluid volume may result in a decreased stroke volume. Tachycardia is a compensatory mechanism to maintain cardiac output. It should be noted that although CHF is usually seen in conjunction with a high volume state and elevated preload, dehydration with a low preload can also result in decreased stroke volume and CHF. The goal is to have an adequate but not excessive preload.

Afterload - The force required for emptying of the left ventricle during systole is termed afterload. The amount of tension has a direct correlation to cardiac work and oxygen consumption. Afterload in CHF is usually elevated due to increased sympathetic tone, circulating catecholamines, renin release, arteriolar wall thickening, and increased blood volume. The goal of therapy is to reduce afterload.

Reduction of preload and afterload - When the patient is acutely ill, a Swan-Ganz catheter will be inserted so that the response to treatment can be constantly monitored. The measurement of PAP and, more specifically, PCWP provides a direct reflection of the pressure and therefore the function of the left ventricle. In less acutely ill patients and those treated as outpatients the principles of treatment are the same, but therapy is less aggressive, with response evaluated on the basis of more general parameters.

1. Measures to reduce preload include:
   a. Restricting fluid intake
   b. Running an IV with a microdrip or using volumetric pump
   c. Keeping careful intake and output records
   d. Reducing sodium intake in IV and diet
   e. Reducing circulating fluid volume via diuretics

2. Vasodilator therapy - Nitrates affect venous capacitance vessels and preload; hydralazine and diazoxide affect afterload. In addition, nitrates have some arteriolar dilating properties and will thus reduce afterload. Vasodilators should only be used when the patient has an adequate BP. With hypotension, vasodilation could cause a further drop in pressure and precipitate myocardial ischemia, as indicated in the following:

	Preload (venous capacitance)	Afterload (arteriolar tone)
Nitrates	\/\/\/	\/
Hydralazine, dioxide		\/\/
Nitroprusside	\/\/\/	\/\/\/
Diuretics	\/\/	<---->
Morphine	\/\/	\/

3. Digitalis - Acts to strengthen cardiac contraction (positive inotropic action) and slow heart rate (negative chronotropic action) with a net effect of increasing stroke volume and reducing LVEDV. Digitalis may be given PO (digoxin) or IV (ouabain, Cedilanid-D, or digoxin) if rapid action is needed.
4. Diuretics - In conjunction with restricting fluid and salt intake, PO or IV diuretics will decrease preload. Monitor potassium levels particularly if patient is also receiving a digitalis preparation.

Pulmonary edema - When pressure from a failing left ventricle backs up and causes an increase in PAP and leakage of fluid out into the alveoli, the condition is termed pulmonary edema. The patient in pulmonary edema is in severe distress, is extremely anxious and restless, and has a heart rate above 150/min and pink-frothy sputum. Pulmonary edema is a medical emergency; prompt treatment, which consists of the following, usually results in rapid improvement:

1. Oxygenation - Give 100% oxygen via a face mask. If ABG results do not improve or the patient shows signs of respiratory failure and exhaustion, intubation is indicated.
2. Position the patient in a high Fowler's position with arms elevated on pillows or over a bed table. This position will ease breathing and permit greater lung expansion.
3. Morphine - This will cause venous dilation and venous pooling (reduced preload) and decreased sympathetic tone (reduced afterload).
4. Furosemide (Lasix) - A dosage of 20–40 mg as an IV push may be

ordered to reduce preload. Connect a urimeter for hourly output measurement.

5. Rotating tourniquets - May be applied manually or with an automatic tourniquet machine; they act to decrease venous return (preload). Place cuffs on three extremities and rotate them every 15 minutes. Cuff pressure should be regulated so venous return isimpaired, but arterial perfusion is not. Check for arterial pulses. Use with caution on extremities with peripheral IV or circulatory impairment. When disconnecting tourniquets, remove one at a time every 15 minutes. Rapid removal will flood the circulation and exacerbate the failure.

6. Aminophylline - May be given to treat bronchospasm but is infrequently used in pulmonary edema due to serious side effects.

7. Vasodilators - Nitroglycerin IV and nitroprusside (Nipride) both act to decrease preload and afterload. Drug needs to be administered via IV pump with dosage titrated according to hemodynamic parameters (PCWP).

ED Discharge Planning

Patients with pulmonary edema and/or myocardial ischemia or infarction should be admitted to a CCU. Patients with less severe CHF and no myocardial ischemia can be discharged.

ED Discharge Instructions

1. Reduce dietary sodium intake by eliminating use of table salt in cooking or at the table. Patient needs to know what foods are high in sodium and should be encouraged to read labels on packages. Consider referring the patient or responsible family member to the dietician for follow-up instructions.

2. Medication - Review the basic action and precautions for each drug, i.e., "water pill" to be taken early in the day and need to have adequate intake of dietary potassium if a potassium supplement is not ordered. Patients taking digitalis need to be closely monitored. The patient and/or family should know to take the patient's pulse daily and withhold the medication until they contact the physician for a pulse >100/min or <60/min unless otherwise specified. Instruct the patient to seek medical attention promptly for signs of digitalis toxicity (anorexia, nausea, vomiting, visual disturbances).

3. Activity level - Although activity tolerance is very individual, patients with CHF should be counselled to gradually resume activities following ED treatment. In general, strenuous activities should be avoided, and activities of daily living should be paced to provide periods of rest (watching TV, reading, etc.).

4. Follow-up medical care - Stress that the patient has a chronic condition

that can be controlled by medication and diet but cannot be cured. The patient should have outpatient follow up and needs to know to contact a physician or return to the ED for shortness of breath, chest pain/pressure, unusual fatigue, leg edema, and need for increased pillows to sleep.

HYPERTENSION

Hypertension is a major health care problem. The American Heart Association estimates that 37,990,000 American adults have high BP. Incidence of hypertension increases with age, and it affects blacks almost twice as often as it affects whites.

Essential (primary) hypertension - Sustained BP elevation with no known cause. The commonest form of hypertension (90%), it usually develops slowly over years with relatively few symptoms.

Malignant - An accelerated form of hypertension in which there are hemorrhages and exudates in the fundi, evidence of organ involvement, and a diastolic pressure over 140 mm Hg.

Secondary - Elevation of BP is related to a specific disease process, with renal disease being the commonest cause.

Hypertensive encephalopathy - Usually accompanies a sudden increase in BP and is manifested by headache, nausea, vomiting, apprehension, confusion, or seizures. Focal neurologic signs may accompany hypertensive encephalopathy, but they tend to wax and wane. It is usually associated with papilledema.

Hypertensive emergencies include:

1. Malignant hypertension
2. Hypertensive encephalopathy
3. Hypertension complicated by CHF or aortic dissection
4. Hypertension in the face of an acute MI
5. Toxemia of pregnancy
6. Catecholamine excess due to pheochromocytoma, monoamine oxidase inhibitors, or abrupt discontinuation of clonidine therapy

Assessment

History
The patient may present with vague symptoms that, when correlated with an elevated BP, indicate sustained hypertension. Obtain history of the present illness, including nature of onset and length and severity of symptoms. Typical symptoms include headache, nausea, vomiting, palpitations,

and postural syncope. Ask the patient about previous medical treatment for hypertension, medication, and diet. Note that patients often decrease their medication or stop it completely when they have been asymptomatic for a period of time, so ask the patient what medication he or she took yesterday.

Physical Findings
Vital signs - Take the BP in both arms with the patient in a supine and a standing position. Since anxiety related to an ED visit may cause BP to rise, recheck the BP once or twice more prior to discharge.
Eyes - Check pupils. Examination of fundus may show hypertensive retinopathy (hemorrhages, exudates, and papilledema).
Neurologic signs - Check for carotid bruits and neurologic deficits.
Heart - Listen for S_3 and S_4 and gallop rhythm.
Lungs - Auscultate for crackling (rales) and wheezes that may warn of heart failure.
Extremities - Check for equality of pulses in all four extremities if aortic dissection is a possibility.

Diagnostic Tests
ECG - Check for signs of ischemia (ST and T wave changes) or evidence of left ventricular hypertrophy.
Laboratory studies - CBC, BUN, creatinine, and electrolytes.
Urinalysis - Send and Chemstrip for hematuria and proteinuria.
X-ray - A PA chest x-ray will aid in determining cardiac and aortic size, as well as in examining the lung fields.

Intervention

1. Pharmacologic treatment of essential hypertension includes:
   a. Diuretics - Chlorothiazide, 500–1000 mg/day; hydrochlorothiazide, 50–100 mg/day; and furosemide, 40–80 mg/day.
   b. Sympathetic nervous system inhibitors - Reserpine 0.1– 0.25 mg/day; methyldopa (Aldomet), 500–2000 mg/day; clonidine (Catapres), 0.2– 0.8 mg/day; parzosin (Minipress), 20–40 mg/day; propranolol (Inderal), 40–320 mg/day; and metoprolol (Lopressor), 100–450 mg/day.
   c. Direct vasodilators - Hydralazine (Apresoline), 100–200 mg/day; and minoxidil (Loniten), 10–40 mg/day.
   d. Calcium antagonist - Nifedipine (Procardia), 10 mg SL.
2. Hypertensive crisis - Nitroprusside (Nipride) is an arterial and venous vasodilator. It is an excellent drug for hypertensive encephalopathy and malignant hypertension, but the following must be noted:
   a. Constant monitoring of BP is necessary.
   b. Start infusion at a low dosage; many patients are very sensitive to this drug.

c. Always administer via an infusion pump.

d. Infusion is light sensitive and must be wrapped in foil; discard after 24 hours.

e. Titrate for a diastolic pressure of 100 mm Hg; lowering the pressure further may result in a serious decrease in tissue perfusion or shock.

f. If the BP falls too rapidly, turn off infusion and place the patient in a Trendelenburg position. Effects of the drug are dissipated within minutes.

g. In treatment of aortic dissection, propranolol must be administered first to prevent a possible increase in the intravascular shearing forces. Mix 100 mg (2 ampules) in 500 ml D5W and regulate at 0.5–8 µg/Kg/min (average dose, 3 µg/Kg/min). Titrate the rate according to the diastolic pressure.

3. Diazoxide (Hyperstat) - An arterial dilator that is particularly effective in hypertensive encephalopathy and malignant hypertension. Dosage is 100 mg by IV bolus which can be repeated every 10 minutes up to a total of 300 mg. Monitor BP closely. Have a dopamine or levarterenol drip on hand in case of a rapid fall in BP. The side effects include reflex tachycardia, sodium retention, and hyperglycemia. Chemstrip urine for glucose. Because of inability to control dose with bolus approach, nitroprusside is usually favored over diazoxide.

4. Trimethaphan (Arfonad) - Decreases cardiac output and is the drug of choice in aortic dissection. The dosage is 250 mg in 500 ml D5W, starting at 0.25 mg/min (30 ml/hr). Average dose ranges from 0.3–6 mg/min. For maximum effect, elevate the head of the bed.

5. Labetalol (Normodyne, Trandate) - Acts to decrease afterload and drops BP with little change in heart rate and cardiac output. The dosage is 20 mg IV over 2 minutes, with repeat boluses of 40–80 mg every 10 minutes prn up to a total of 300 mg. To administer as an IV drip, mix 200 mg in 200 ml D5W and regulate at a rate of 2 mg/min. It is contraindicated in patients with pheochromocytoma, overt CHF, heart block over first degree, and severe bradycardia.

ED Discharge Planning

Patients with hypertensive crisis, severe hypertension that does not respond well to treatment, and hypertension complicated by organ failure should be admitted. An obstetrician should be consulted for patients with toxemia of pregnancy.

Nonpharmacologic interventions may be employed in patients at significant risk for hypertension (positive family history of hypertension or coronary artery disease) or for preeclampsia, as well as for patients with diagnosed hypertension. In some cases a nonpharmacologic regimen alone may control the BP. Patient discharge instructions should include:

1. Restriction of sodium intake. Instruct patient and family to eliminate high-sodium foods and reduce use of table salt which most North Americans use in great excess. Refer patient to dietician.
2. Weight control and low cholesterol diet to reduce cardiac risk factors.
3. Stress reduction - Counselling, biofeedback, and relaxation techniques may be an adjunct to therapy.
4. Medication compliance - Probably the most important information to convey to the patient is that high BP is a disease that can be controlled but generally not cured. Lack of symptoms does not mean the disease is cured or that medication can be stopped. If feasible, someone in the patient's family can learn to monitor the patient's BP. Readings that fall outside a given parameter can be reported to the family physician.
5. Intake of potassium-rich foods if diuretics are being used.

SELECTED CARDIAC ARRHYTHMIAS

SUPRAVENTRICULAR TACHYCARDIA

The SVTs are a varied group of accelerated rhythms in which the focus of rapid electrical activity is in the atria or the AV junctional node. Some of these arrhythmias (PSVTs) can affect otherwise healthy people, while others (atrial fibrillation and multifocal atrial tachycardia) commonly affect patients with underlying disease. SVTs include PSVT, atrial flutter, atrial fibrillation, and multifocal atrial tachycardia (MAT). The initial approach to any patient with a SVT is outlined in Figure 1.2. It should include assessment for signs of hemodynamic compromise (hypotension, loss of consciousness, angina, congestive failure, ST-T wave changes on ECG), followed by analysis of the rhythm by ECG, possibly with the help of carotid sinus massage.

PAROXYSMAL SUPRAVENTRICULAR TACHYCARDIA

Description

PSVT is an atrial arrhythmia characterized by extremely regular rhythm, usually with narrow QRS complexes, at rates of 160–250. Its onset and termination are often abrupt. P waves may or may not be seen or may be retrograde. The patient often reports palpitations. Other presentations can include hypotension, diaphoresis, chest pain, and other signs of hemodynamic compromise. Syncope, when it occurs, happens most often when the episode of tachycardia spontaneously breaks and a transient sinus arrest follows.

Etiology

PSVT usually results from reentry (circus movement) conduction in the AV node. It can also result from congenital anomalies (e.g., mitral valve prolapse) or from accessory conduction pathways (preexcitation syndromes such as Wolff-Parkinson-White or Lown-Ganong-Levine) or "concealed" pathways that only conduct retrograde from ventricles to atria. Rarely, these rhythms are seen with hyperthyroidism, arteriosclerotic heart disease, and digitalis toxicity. PSVT with 2:1 block suggests digitalis toxicity. PSVT is usually the result of reentrant cycles initiated by atrial extrasystoles.

Intervention

PSVT is often easily broken by the steps listed below, which should be tried sequentially:

1. Vagal maneuvers - Carotid sinus massage should cause PSVT to revert to sinus rhythm. It should be used with caution in elderly patients. Valsalva or diving reflexes (elicited by immersing the patient's face in cold water) can be tried if carotid sinus massage fails and the patient is hemodynamically well compensated.
2. Verapamil - A dose of 5–10 mg is given IV over 3–5 minutes. It will break almost all SVTs and will slow atrial flutter or fibrillation, but it will rarely convert them to sinus rhythm. The onset of activity is within 1–2 minutes, and the drug is effective in 90% of cases. The dose may be repeated once. Use caution if the patient is taking digoxin or propranolol; these drugs are contraindicated in patients with an accessory pathway. Verapamil has replaced cardioversion as the treatment of choice, because the drug is so reliable. Although verapamil is a negative inotrope, it may be given to patients in CHF if the failure is rate related.
3. Cardioversion - If the patient is severely compromised (hypotension, angina), cardioversion is indicated. Cardioversion can also be used as a last resort if all other treatments fail. Small amounts (20 J) often suffice. Cardioversion is contraindicated in digitalis toxicity. (See Chapter 16 for further details.)
4. Edrophonium (Tensilon) - A 1-mg test dose is recommended, then 5–10 mg are given by slow IV push. The peak effect should be in 3 minutes. Edrophonium can produce nausea, hypotension, and vomiting. Often, carotid sinus massage is more successful after edrophonium has been given.
5. Digoxin - If there is no evidence that digoxin toxicity is the cause of the arrhythmia, digoxin at 0.5 mg IV can be given. Digoxin is contrain-

dicated if the patient has a known accessory pathway and atrial fibrillation, because digoxin can allow conduction through the accessory pathway while slowing conduction through the AV node, resulting in ventricular tachycardia or fibrillation.
6. Propranolol (Inderal) - A dose of 5–10 mg is given IV over 5 minutes. This is effective 50% of the time. Be very cautious when giving propranolol if verapamil was recently given, as the two drugs together can precipitate high-grade AV block or CHF. Propranolol is contraindicated in patients with asthma, hypotension, or known CHF.

See Appendix D for the use of emergency medicine drugs.

ATRIAL FLUTTER

Description

Atrial flutter presents with an atrial rate of 250–350 with varying degrees of AV block (usually 2:1). P waves (called F waves in atrial flutter) are often inverted with a saw-toothed appearance. Carotid sinus massage will abruptly change the ventricular response in atrial flutter by producing transient 3:1 or 4:1 block (at the same time the flutter waves become easier to see). A ventricular rate of exactly 150/min suggests the possibility of atrial flutter with an atrial rate of 300/min and 2:1 block.

Etiology

Atrial flutter can rarely occur paroxysmally in generally healthy people. It is seen in association with mitral valve prolapse, rheumatic valvular disease, cor pulmonale and pulmonary emboli, arteriosclerotic heart disease, alcohol intoxication, and thyrotoxicosis.

Intervention

The goal of treatment is to slow the ventricular rate and convert the rhythm to sinus or, possibly, atrial fibrillation. If the patient shows signs of decreased cardiac output, synchronized cardioversion is indicated after carotid massage. Control of ventricular response rate with medications is preferable if the patient often goes in and out of atrial flutter. Pharmacologic therapy is outlined below:

1. Verapamil, 5–10 mg as a slow IV push, can be given as initial therapy. A small number of patients will convert to sinus (30% of patients given verapamil for atrial flutter will convert to sinus rhythm; the rest will slow their ventricular response rate).

2. Digoxin, 0.5 mg IV, can be given initially but may take 30 minutes to take effect. Most patients will slow eventually. Some will convert to sinus rhythm; a small percentage will convert to atrial fibrillation.

Maintenance medications for patients not converted are digoxin or propranolol or both to control rate. For those patients who have been converted to sinus rhythm, digoxin or quinidine or both can be used as prophylaxis against further episodes of atrial flutter.

ATRIAL FIBRILLATION

Description

Atrial fibrillation is one of the most common arrhythmias, consisting of an irregular ventricular response (140–200/min in untreated cases), an absence of P waves, and a wormy baseline. QRS complexes are usually narrow except where there is underlying bundle branch block or in the Ashman phenomenon, where a wide aberrantly conducted QRS complex occurs after a particularly long RR interval. Ashman beats resemble (but are not) PVCs.

Atrial fibrillation is usually seen in patients with CHF and long-standing arteriosclerotic heart disease or valvular disease (usually mitral), with cardiomyopathy, and occasionally with thyrotoxicosis. Patients often present in congestive failure due to a combination of their underlying disease, the rapid ventricular rate, and the loss of the atrial "kick," which can add 25% to the cardiac output of noncompliant ventricles.

Intervention

Therapy is aimed at controlling the ventricular response rate. Conversion to sinus rhythm is often short-lived, particularly in patients with large left atria, patients in atrial fibrillation for more than 6 months, and patients with mitral regurgitation. Therapy consists of:

1. Digoxin, 0.5 mg IV, can be given initially with subsequent doses of 0.250 or 0.125 mg given IV every few hours until ventricular rate is under 100. If the patient is already on digoxin, use smaller initial doses and monitor for signs of digitalis toxicity. If and when the patient converts to a regular rhythm, the ECG should be carefully evaluated to confirm that the patient is in sinus rhythm.
2. Propranolol, 1 mg IV, can be given every 5 minutes until the rate slows or verapamil, 5–10 mg given by slow IV push, can be administered to slow down patients not in CHF. These two agents should not be given together.

3. Procainamide, 10–15 mg/Kg given IV at a rate not to exceed 100 mg every 5 minutes, may be used for chemical cardioversion. Sudden hypotension may be a side effect.
4. Electrical cardioversion is very effective. Emergency cardioversion should be employed for patients with acute MIs or hemodynamic compromise. Cardioversion in the ED is not recommended if the patient has been in atrial fibrillation for 48 hours or longer, because of the risk of sudden embolus.

MULTIFOCAL ATRIAL TACHYCARDIA

Definition

MAT is an irregular rhythm that looks superficially like atrial fibrillation. It is characterized by the following:

1. Atrial rate >100/min
2. Presence of P waves with irregular P-P (and PR) intervals
3. P waves of at least three different morphologies

Etiology

MAT is a rhythm of elderly and ill patients, all of whom have other severe disease, such as pulmonary disease, CHF, septicemia, and electrolyte disturbances. Many patients with MAT are taking bronchodilators that may perpetuate the arrhythmia.

Intervention

Therapy is exclusively aimed at treating the underlying disease. Digoxin is not recommended.

SINUS ARREST AND SINUS BLOCK

Sinoatrial (SA) arrest (Fig. 1.9) - A sporadic failure of the sinus node, which results in the absence of a sinus impulse. The P-P interval is prolonged. SA arrest is seen with digitalis, vagal stimulation, and myocardial disease. Treatment, when necessary, consists of discontinuing digitalis or administering atropine (0.6–2.0 mg IV). Pacemaker placement can be considered for symptomatic SA arrest.

SA exit block - Regular sinus impulse formation occurs without atrial or ventricular depolarization because the impulse is blocked from reaching these areas. The P-P interval is usually prolonged to some multiple of the regular intervals. SA exit block can be seen with acute MI, hyperkalemia, digitalis administration, or quinidine administration.

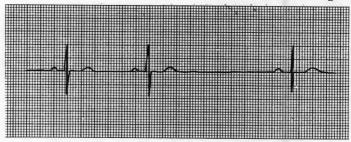

Figure 1.9. Sinoatrial arrest. (From Pousada L, Osborn HH. Emergency medicine for the house officer. Baltimore: Williams & Wilkins, 1986:42.)

ATRIOVENTRICULAR BLOCK

AV block is a general term referring to impaired conduction in the atria adjacent to the AV node, in the AV junction itself, in the adjacent His bundle, or in the more distal conduction system.

FIRST-DEGREE AV BLOCK (FIG. 1.10)

When the PR interval is longer than 0.20 seconds and all atrial beats are followed by ventricular beats, first-degree AV block exists. This is usually the result of impaired conduction in the AV junction. First-degree block can be caused by a disease or physiologic process affecting the myocardium. It may indicate underlying disease, increased vagal tone in a healthy individual, drug effect, or metabolic disturbance. No treatment is required.

SECOND-DEGREE AV BLOCK

When not all atrial impulses are conducted to the ventricles, second-degree AV block exists. This entity is subdivided into Mobitz type I (Wenckebach) block (Fig. 1.11) and Mobitz type II block (Fig. 1.12).

Mobitz type I (Wenckebach) block is usually due to impaired conduction in the AV junction proximal to the His bundle. The PR interval increases progressively until one atrial impulse is completely blocked and the anticipated QRS does not occur. The PR interval after the pause is within the normal range, and the cycle subsequently repeats itself. The dropped beat may occur after every second atrial impulse (2:1 Mobitz type I block, which simulates Mobitz type II block) or may occur less frequently (3:1, 6:1, etc.). The QRS duration is usually normal.

Mobitz I (Wenckebach) block is most often seen in acute inferior wall MI, presumably because the AV node is supplied by a branch of the right coronary artery. Mobitz type I (Wenckebach) block is usually a temporary

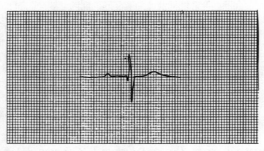

Figure 1.10.   First-degree AV block. (From Pousada L, Osborn HH. Emergency medicine for the house officer. Baltimore: Williams & Wilkins, 1986:44.)

condition that requires monitoring but no treatment unless hemodynamic compromise occurs or the block increases.

Mobitz type II block is usually due to more distal His bundle or trifascicular (intraventricular) block. The PR interval is fixed, with dropped beats (P waves not followed by QRS) occurring in regular (2:1, 3:1, etc.) or irregular ratios. The QRS duration is often increased.

Mobitz type II block is potentially serious. Regardless of a stable BP, any dropped beats with fixed PR interval need to be brought immediately to the physician's attention. The greatest danger associated with this rhythm is its often benign appearance. It can occur with acute anterior wall infarction or myocarditis and chronically as a result of degenerative or congenital myocardial disease. Most patients with Mobitz type II block will eventually develop complete heart block.

VENTRICULAR ARRHYTHMIAS

PREMATURE VENTRICULAR COMPLEXES (FIG. 1.13)

The presence of PVCs indicates the need for medical evaluation. PVCs are commonly seen in conjunction with myocardial ischemia, digitalis toxicity, CHF, and electrolyte imbalance. In a patient with an acute MI, PVCs represent a serious danger. Unless contraindicated by CHF or heart block, PVCs in a patient with an acute MI should be treated prophylactically with lidocaine (for further details, see "Myocardial ischemia and Infarction," presented earlier).

PVCs occur prematurely and may be unifocal (of consistent shape) or multifocal (of more than one shape), with a wide (>0.12 seconds), bizarre QRS, T wave deflected in the opposite direction from the QRS complex, and usually a compensatory pause. PVCs not only decrease stroke volume and possibly cardiac output but warn of potentially lethal ventricular arrhythmias. Of particular concern are PVCs that are:

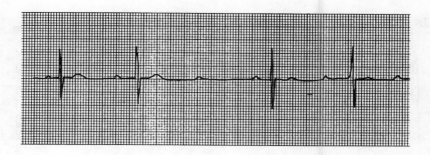

Figure 1.11. Second-degree AV block. Mobitz type I (Wenckebach). (From Pousada L. Osborn HH. Emergency medicine for the house officer. Baltimore: Williams & Wilkins, 1986:45.)

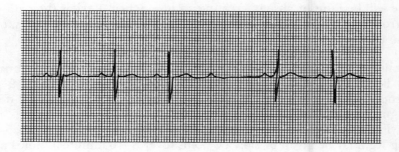

Figure 1.12. Second-degree AV block. Mobitz type II. (From Pousada L. Osborn HH. Emergency medicine for the house officer. Baltimore: Williams & Wilkins, 1986:46.)

1. Multifocal (multiformal)
2. Consecutive PVCs (couplets or salvos)
3. PVCs occurring on or near the previous T wave (R-on-T phenomenon)
4. Bigeminy, i.e., with every other beat being a PVC

Intervention

Notify the physician. Administer oxygen. Standard treatment consists of a lidocaine bolus of 1 mg/Kg followed by a lidocaine drip (2 gm lidocaine/500 ml D5W) at 2–4 mg/min. If PVCs persist, lidocaine can be repeated up to 3 mg/Kg with a drip of 3–4 mg/min. (See Figure 1.4 for ventricular ectopy algorithm.) If PVCs are frequent (6 or more/min), the patient may experience a decrease in cardiac output. Monitor the patient for signs of decreased tissue perfusion, including drop in BP, altered level

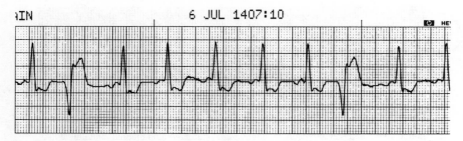

Figure 1.13.   Premature ventricular complexes.

of consciousness, and chest pain. The effect of PVCs on stroke volume can be easily determined by taking the patient's pulse. During the PVCs, pulse will be faint or absent, creating a pulse deficit. Review the patient's electrolytes. Hypokalemia, particularly in conjunction with digitalis, may cause PVCs.

Procainamide - Treatment of choice if patient is sensitive or unresponsive to lidocaine. Loading dose, 20 mg/min, followed by a drip (2 gm procainamide in 500 ml D5W) at 1– 4 mg/min. Maximum total dose, 1 gm. Monitor the patient closely for hypotension.

Bretylium - If PVCs fail to respond to first-line treatment, bretylium, 5–10 mg/Kg, may be given by slow IV bolus (over 8–10 minutes). Bolus may be repeated every 15–30 minutes up to a total of 30 mg/Kg, followed by an IV drip of 1–2 mg/min (1000 mg bretylium in 250 or 500 ml D5W). The drug may cause nausea and vomiting as well as transient BP alterations.

VENTRICULAR TACHYCARDIA (FIG. 1.14)

Defined as three or more consecutive PVCs, ventricular tachycardia may cause a patient response ranging from slight BP alteration to unconsciousness with absent pulse. One of the major determinants of patient response is a heart rate that can range from 100 to 250/min.

Intervention

Assess the patient's hemodynamic response including level of consciousness, BP, and presence of chest pain.

1. Stable patient - Start oxygen, administer lidocaine according to hospital's protocol, and notify physician.
2. Hemodynamically unstable patient - A patient with a BP of <90 mm Hg, chest pain, or decreased level of consciousness should be treated

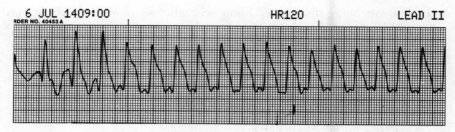

Figure 1.14. Ventricular tachycardia.

as unstable ventricular tachycardia. Start oxygen, call for assistance, notify the physician and prepare to synchronize cardiovert the patient, starting with 50 J. A successively higher number of joules are employed until conversion is accomplished. Lidocaine or other effective antiarrhythmic should be started by bolus and drip to prevent recurrence. (See Figure 1.5 for ventricular tachycardia algorithm.)
3. Patients with pulseless ventricular tachycardia should be treated as if they have ventricular fibrillation and be given a precordial thump and immediately defibrillated with 200 J. Follow the ventricular fibrillation algorithm (Fig. 1.5) for pulseless ventricular tachycardia.
4. Torsade de pointes - A form of ventricular tachycardia that is associated with conditions that prolong the QT interval including myocardial ischemia, drugs such as quinidine and procainamide, and electrolyte imbalance. The QRS interval of high-risk patients should be monitored. Standard treatment for ventricular tachycardia is usually most effective in torsade de pointes. Treatment includes isoproterenol drip, which increases heart rate and shortens the repolarization time, and temporary overdrive cardiac pacing.

The primary nursing concern in care of a patient with cardiac arrhythmias is:

1. Cardiac output alteration - Decreased cardiac output is particularly seen in frequent PVCs, rapid supraventricular arrhythmias, bradycardias, and heart blocks. Nursing assessment of patients at risk for decreased cardiac output is the primary nursing intervention.
2. Identification of patients at risk for arrhythmias - Initiate appropriate monitoring for patient with signs or history of myocardial ischemia, syncope, respiratory distress, drug toxicity, etc.

ED Discharge Planning

Patients with newly developed or unstable arrhythmias or patients who are hemodynamically unstable need admission to a monitored unit or

ICU. Patients being discharged home with chronic or stable arrhythmias will need information on:

1. Medication action, side effects, etc.
2. Returning to the ED for dizziness, fainting, chest pain, etc.

VASCULAR DISORDERS

AORTIC ANEURYSM

An atherosclerotic aneurysm is an outpouching or dilation of an arterial wall. With increasing size, pressure within the aneurysm may cause spontaneous rupture. Immediate exsanguination and death may occur; however, initially there is often an interval of several hours during which self-limited leaking takes place. Although aneurysms of peripheral arteries are seen, aortic aneurysms are most common. The aneurysm usually involves one or all three layers of the artery wall.

Aneurysms of the thoracic aorta are frequently asymptomatic. Large thoracic aneurysms may cause chronic chest pain due to bony erosion of the sternum or vertebrae. Hoarseness may result from impingement on the recurrent laryngeal nerve. Bronchial compression may result in coughing.

Dissection of the thoracic aorta may result in formation of a false channel. This has been called a "dissecting aneurysm," but it is technically not an aneurysm, since it does not involve all three wall layers. Aortic dissection is a splitting of the arterial wall, which usually arises from an intimal tear in the ascending aorta. A major causative factor is systemic hypertension. Although dissection may be asymptomatic, it is usually heralded by severe chest pain of sudden onset that radiates to the back and is "tearing" in quality. Central nervous system symptoms may result, and shock is common although often delayed.

The overwhelming majority of aneurysms of the abdominal aorta are caused by atherosclerosis. Aneurysms of the segment of aorta between the diaphragm and the renal arteries are rare and are usually associated with similar changes throughout the aorta. Symptoms are rare unless rupture occurs. The risk of rupture is small until the diameter exceeds 6 cm. Acute onset of severe local tenderness radiating to the back suggests rupture.

Assessment

History
Because most aortic aneurysms are asymptomatic, patients presenting to

the ED will not give a history of chronic pain. Most patients will describe sudden onset of pain accompanied often by syncope or faintness resulting from blood loss. If the aneurysm tamponades for a period of time, the pain may lessen or faintness may disappear temporarily, but symptoms will reappear, and the patient will progress to frank shock when bleeding resumes.

A history of uncontrolled hypertension, recent episode of blunt chest trauma (e.g., a steering wheel injury), Marfan's syndrome, and chest pain or the sudden onset of shock are suggestive of aortic dissection, and the patient should be categorized as emergent.

Physical Findings

General - Note if the patient is in shock or appears diaphoretic or cyanotic.

Vital signs - Monitor for signs of shock, including tachycardia and hypotension. Take BP in both arms.

Lungs - Listen for rales.

Heart - Auscultate for gallops or the murmur of aortic insufficiency (dissection of proximal aorta).

Abdomen - An intact abdominal aneurysm can be felt as a periumbilical pulsatile mass that is not tender. A ruptured aneurysm that has tamponaded can be felt as a pulsatile mass that is exquisitely tender.

Extremities - Compare arterial pulses bilaterally throughout the body. Femoral pulses are diminished in some patients. Note peripheral vasoconstriction and cyanosis.

Neurologic signs - Note any focal deficits caused by loss of regional arterial supply. Paraplegia may result from severe hypotension and decreased blood supply to the spinal cord.

Diagnostic Tests

CBC - A spun Hct should be obtained. However, the rapidity of the course often causes the Hct to be misleading with regard to actual blood volume.

Foley catheter - A urinary catheter should be placed to monitor renal perfusion via urine production.

ECG - An ECG may show signs of acute ischemia or infarction if there is sufficient loss of blood volume or compromise of the coronary vessels secondary to thoracic dissection.

X-rays - A portable chest film may demonstrate dilatation of the thoracic aorta or a widened mediastinum. A cross-table lateral abdominal film may reveal calcification in the aneurysmal wall.

Aortogram - An aortogram may show dilatation or dissection of the aorta, but it is useful only in the stable patient. Check the arterial puncture site and peripheral pulses after the aortogram.

Sonography - A sonogram can document the presence and size of the aneurysm in the stable patient.
CAT scan - May be helpful in establishing the diagnosis.

Intervention

The goal of treatment is to prevent rupture, stabilize the patient, and prepare for possible surgery.

Unruptured aortic aneurysm - Depending on the size, the patient should be advised of the need for either early or eventual surgery. Outpatient follow-up should include careful monitoring of the size and growth of the aneurysm.
Dissecting aorta - Dissection is either distal or proximal:

1. Distal dissection: medical. Vigorous therapy produces the best results (see "Hypertension" in this chapter for details of management).
2. Proximal dissection: surgery usually offers the best results. Surgery is indicated if the patient develops secondary aortic insufficiency, obstructs a major vascular pathway, shows evidence of impending rupture as suggested by intrapleural bleeding, or despite aggressive antihypertensive therapy has further extension as suggested by continued pain or an expanding mediastinal shadow.

Ruptured aneurysm - Rupture requires immediate surgery. See "Shock" presented earlier in this chapter for management and stabilization prior to surgery. When bleeding has resulted in shock, the mortality approaches 80%, even with prompt surgical repair. Patients for whom surgery is delayed or pending will be treated with antihypertensives, and fluid and electrolyte balance will be carefully monitored. Take measures to decrease the patient's physical and psychologic strain and exertion (i.e., deep coughing, pain, Valsalva maneuver) which increase BP. Narcotics and tranquilizers may be ordered for the same purpose. Continuous cardiac monitoring and frequent (every 2–15 minutes) BP determinations are indicated. An increased systolic BP, widening pulse pressure, decreased level of consciousness, and oliguria warn of a worsening condition.

THROMBOPHLEBITIS

Thrombophlebitis is a common disorder of veins in which there is formation of a thrombus (clot) in association with vein inflammation. Factors that commonly predispose to formation of venous thrombi include immobilization (either postsurgical or posttraumatic), CHF, stroke, veins damaged by chronic or previous thrombus formation, estrogen administration (viz. oral contraceptives), systemic lupus erythematosus, or such hypercoagulable states as sickle cell, leukemia, myeloma, or intraabdominal carcinomas. Septic thrombophlebitis is most common in drug addicts or patients who in hospitals or clinics have had contaminated IV lines placed.

Thrombophlebitis may develop in superficial or deep veins anywhere in the body. Septic thrombophlebitis is most common in superficial veins of the arms and, sometimes, the legs. Venous thrombi of the deep veins of the thighs (the ileofemoral system) and of the pelvis may embolize, with potentially fatal complications. Deep venous thrombosis is often clinically silent.

Assessment

History
The patient will commonly present with a complaint of pain, edema, and reddened extremity. Patients suspected of having thrombophlebitis should be questioned as to recent local trauma or skin infections. The absence or presence of fever, shortness of breath, or chest pain should be noted. A history of recent immobilization (even several hours of sitting) or underlying systemic disease should be elicited. All women of childbearing age should be questioned as to use of oral contraceptives. Any previous episode of thrombophlebitis should be noted. A history of IV drug abuse is important.

Physical Findings
Vital signs - Check for fever, tachycardia, or increased respiratory rate.
Lungs - Listen for bilateral breath sounds or a pleural rub.
Abdomen - Note the presence of any masses.
Extremities - Note swelling, erythema, tenderness, or warmth. Look for any involvement of superficial veins or possibility of deep venous thrombosis. Check for a positive Homan's sign (pain on passive dorsiflexion of foot). Check for signs of local trauma or infection, and always look between the toes. Delayed cooling after being uncovered may occur in an affected leg. Swelling may be subtle; measure and compare the two legs.

Diagnostic Tests
Doppler (noninvasive venous plethysmography) - Screening procedure for impaired blood flow. It has few risks but is not highly reliable.
Venogram - Is the most reliable diagnostic test but has risks including initiation of thrombosis and dye reaction.
Laboratory tests - CBC, ESR, and coagulation studies including platelet count, PT, and PTT should be obtained.

Intervention

1. Immobilization and rest - Bed rest with elevation of the extremity for 7–10 days is recommended. Patients with small, superficial thrombophlebitis may be treated as outpatients. Moist heat and antiinflammatory agents are used to treat the pain and inflammation.
2. Anticoagulation - The treatment of deep vein thrombosis is anticoagulation, initially with heparin, as described in Chapter 2 on "Pulmonary Embolus." Anticoagulation with heparin may be initiated in the ED, but only if there will be several hours delay before the patient is evaluated by ward staff.

ED Discharging Planning

Patients thought likely to have deep vein thrombosis or septic thrombophlebitis should be admitted for further diagnosis and anticoagulant or antibiotic therapy. Patients who do not require hospitalization should be reevaluated as outpatients, and their discharge instructions should include:

1. Limitation of activity for a specific period of time
2. Avoidance of constricting clothing (girdles, garters) and leg crossing
3. Avoidance of oral contraceptives and smoking
4. Use of antiembolism stockings, if patient is ambulatory
5. Maintaining good fluid intake
6. Use and precautions for ordered medication
7. Prescription to see a physician for continued leg discomfort and swelling and to return to the ED for respiratory difficulty or chest pain

SUGGESTED READINGS

Cardiopulmonary Arrest

Albarran-Sotelo R, et al. Textbook of advanced cardiac life support. Dallas, Texas: American Heart Association, 1987.

Jones S, Bagg AM. L-E-A-D drugs for cardiac arrest. Nursing 1988;18:34–41.

Persons CB. Transcutaneous pacing. Focus Crit Care 1987;14:13–19.

Rice V. Acid-base derangements in the patient with cardiac arrest. Focus Crit Care 1987;14:53–61.

Rosequist CC. Current standards and guidelines for cardiopulmonary resuscitation and emergency cardiac care. Heart Lung 1987;16:408–418.

Standards and guidelines for cardiopulmonary resuscitation (CPR) and emergency cardiac care (ECC). JAMA 1986;255:2905–2984.

Shock

Bouzoukis JK. Shock. Primary Care 1986;13:193–205.

Ellrodt AG. Sepsis and septic shock. Emerg Clin North Am1986;4: 809–837.

Frankl WS. Cardiogenic shock and low output syndrome. In: Chung EK, ed. Cardiac emergency care. Philadelphia: Lea & Febiger, 1985:41–55.

Gravenstein JS, Paulus DA. Clinical monitoring practice. 2nd ed. Philadelphia: JB Lippincott, 1987:43–104.

Hammond B. Cardiogenic shock: a review. J Emerg Nurs 1983;9:201–205.

Syncope

Kapoor WN, et al. Prolonged electrocardiographic monitoring in patients with syncope. Am J Med 1987;82:20–26.

Kapoor WN, Karpf M, Wieand S, Peterson JR, Levey GS. A prospective evaluation and follow-up of patients with syncope. N Engl J Med 1983;309:197–204.

Lipsitz LA. Syncope in the elderly. Ann Intern Med 1983;99:92–105.

Schultz KE. Vertigo and syncope. In: Rosen P, Baker FJ, Barkin RM, Braen GR, Dailey RH, Levy RC, eds. Emergency medicine. 2nd ed. St Louis: CV Mosby, 1988:1773–1802.

Simon RP. Syncope, seizures, and other causes of episodic loss of consciousness. In: Mills J, Ho T, Salber PR, Trunkey DD, eds. Current emergency diagnosis and treatment. 2nd ed. Los Altos, California: Lange Medical Publications, 1985:97–109.

Chest Pain

Donat WE. Chest pain: cardiac and noncardiac causes. Clin Chest Med 1987;8:241–251.

Forshee T. Chest pain. Nursing 1986;16:34–41.

Hedges JR, Kobernick MS. Detection of myocardial ischemia in the emergency department patient with chest discomfort. Emerg Med Clin North Am 1988;6:317–340.

Neff J. Standardized care plans—chest pain (nontraumatic). J Emerg Nurs 1986; 12:327–330.

Smith CE. Assessing chest pain quickly and accurately. Nursing 1988;18:52–59.

Myocardial Ischemia and Infarction

Jaffe AS. Acute myocardial infarction: state of the art. Circulation 1986;74:120–123.

Lewis VC. Monitoring the patient with acute myocardial infarction. Nurs Clin North Am 1987;22:15–32.

Riegel BJ. The role of nursing in limiting myocardial infarct size. Heart Lung 1985;14:247–254.

Robison JS. Acute right ventricular infarction: recognition, evaluation, and treatment. Crit Care Nurs 1987;7:42–53.

Schakenbach LH. Prinzmetal's angina: current perceptions and treatments. Crit Care Nurs 1987;7:90–99.

Zeller FP, Spinler SA. Alteplase: a tissue plasminogen activator for acute myocardial infarction. Drug Intell Clin Pharm 1988;22:6–14.

Congestive Heart Failure

Depman ST, Wendel CH. Congestive heart failure and pulmonary edema. Primary Care 1986;13:17–75.

Kleinhenz TJ. The inside story on preload and afterload. Nursing 1985;15:50–55.

Lanros NE. Assessment & intervention in emergency nursing. 2nd ed. Bowie, Maryland:

Prentice-Hall Publishing, 1983:213–222.

Smith MS. Realistic management of congestive heart failure. Emerg Med 1987:111–121.

Van Parys E. Assessing the failing state of the heart. Nursing 1987;17:42–49.

Hypertension

Feldstein JS. Hypertensive emergencies. Primary Care 1986;13:109–117.

Hall WD. Isolated systolic hypertension in the elderly. Mod Concepts Cardiovasc Dis 1987;56:29–33.

Jackson RE. Hypertension in the emergency department. Emerg Med Clin North Am 1988;6:173–196.

McRae RP, Liebson PR. Hypertensive crisis. Med Clin North Am 1986;70:749–767.

Selected Cardiac Arrhythmias

Hoffman JR. Emergency department management of life- threatening arrhythmias. Emerg Med Clin North Am 1986;4:761–771.

Karnes N. Differentiation of aberrant ventricular conduction from ventricular ectopic beats. Crit Care Nurs 1987;7:56–66.

Lazarus M, Nolasco V, Luckett C. Cardiac arrhythmias: diagnosis and treatment. Crit Care Nurs 1988;8:57–65.

Ordonez RV. Monitoring the patient with supraventricular dysrhythmias. Nurs Clin North Am 1987;22:49–59.

Ornato JP. Management of paroxysmal supraventricular tachycardia. Circulation 1986;74:108–109.

Reyes AV. Monitoring and treating life-threatening ventricular arrhythmias. Nurs Clin North Am 1987;22:61–76.

Vascular Disorders

DeSanctis RW, Doroghazi RM, Austen WG, Buckley MJ. Aortic dissection. N Engl J Med 1987;317:1060–1067.

Doyle JE. Treatment modalities in peripheral vascular disease. Nurs Clin North Am 1986;21:241–253.

Fahey VA. An in-depth look at deep vein thrombosis. Nursing 1989;19:86–93.

Raviola CA, Trunkey DD. Vascular emergencies. In: Mill J, Ho MT, Salber PR, Trunkey DD, eds. Current emergency diagnosis & treatment. 2nd ed. Los Altos, California: Lange Medical Publications, 1985:399–416.

Weiland AP, Walker WE. Thoracic aneurysms. Crit Care Q 1986;9:20–31.

Chapter 2

RESPIRATORY EMERGENCIES

ACUTE RESPIRATORY FAILURE

Description

Acute respiratory failure can be defined as an acute drop in blood pO_2 to 50 mm Hg or below or an acute increase in pCO_2 to 50 mm Hg* or above and can be defined as follows:

1. Hypercapnic respiratory failure, i.e., pCO_2 is elevated with a normal or reduced pO_2, usually due to hypoventilation
   a. Normal lungs but abnormal respiratory control due to neuromuscular disease or chest wall abnormality
   b. Intrinsic lung disease, with inadequate CO_2 elimination (e.g., emphysema, chronic bronchitis, asthma)
2. Nonhypercapnic respiratory failure, i.e., pO_2 is usually reduced and pCO_2 is normal or reduced, usually due to oxygenation failure
   a. Diffusion impairment (e.g., interstitial lung disease)
   b. Ventilation/perfusion mismatching (e.g., CHF, pneumonia, asthma, pulmonary embolus
   c. Hemoglobin abnormalities, where pO_2 is normal (e.g., anemia, carbon monoxide poisoning)
   d. Abnormal tissue oxygen uptake (e.g., cyanide poisoning)

Assessment

History
Common causes of acute respiratory failure include:

---

*See "Appendix A" for definition of common abbreviations used in the text.

51

Infection - Ask about sputum production (amount, color, and length of time), as well as fever, pleuritic chest pain, etc.

Pulmonary disease - Determine whether there is a history of asthma, bronchitis, or emphysema. Note a smoking history.

Heart disease - Ask about previous hypertension, CHF, or MI.

Trauma - Note any history of trauma sufficient to cause ventilatory impairment (e.g., multiple rib fractures, penetrating chest wounds, head trauma, laryngeal injury.)

Exposures - Note any history of exposure to fumes or of smoke inhalation.

Drugs or medications - Determine whether the patient is an alcohol or drug abuser or on any medications that may provoke bronchospasm (e.g., beta blockers).

Allergies - Note any drug or food allergies.

Physical Findings

General - Respiratory distress may be displayed by tachypnea, diaphoresis, flaring nares, and retraction of sternocleidomastoid and intercostal muscles. There may be a change in mental status, with restlessness, agitation, confusion, lethargy, stupor, or coma.

Vital signs - BP, temperature, and heart rate should be determined along with respiratory rate. A rectal temperature should be obtained when the patient is sufficiently stable.

Skin - Look for rashes, ecchymoses, urticaria, or petechiae. Cyanosis is not an invariable finding and may only be seen with a pO_2 under 40 mm Hg and normal hemoglobin quantity and function.

HEENT - Look for signs of trauma. Check pupil size and response. Note facial burns or soot and singed hairs. Drooling may be a sign of upper airway obstruction.

Neck - Listen for stridor due to upper airway obstruction (foreign body, epiglottitis, fractured larynx, etc.). Look for rigidity, adenopathy, masses, displaced trachea, and neck vein distention.

Lungs - Note dullness to percussion, hyperresonance, increased fremitus, rales, rhonchi, wheezes, and decreased or absent breath sounds.

Heart - Listen for murmurs or gallops.

Neurologic signs - Complete a Glascow coma scale.

Diagnostic Tests

ABGs - A blood gas analysis must be obtained immediately. Repeat blood gas analyses should be obtained 15 minutes after any change in oxygenation or ventilation. In order to improve the accuracy of ABG determinations, see that the patient has been receiving the prescribed O_2 concentration for 10–15 minutes and that the patient has not been suctioned (condition permitting) for 15 minutes prior to drawing the arterial sample. Note the O_2 concentration (F_IO_2) and time on the laboratory slip. Draw blood in a heparinized syringe and send to the laboratory stat in an ice-filled bag.

CBC - Check Hct and WBC with differential.

SMA - Check bicarbonate for metabolic compensation of chronic respiratory insufficiency or for acute metabolic acidosis with hyperventilation and acute fatigue.

CO level - This should be determined on all victims of toxic fumes or smoke inhalation.

Toxicologies - Serum and urine drug levels should be checked as clinically indicated.

Sputum - The patient may not have sufficient strength to cough. Sputum specimens may be obtained by nasotracheal or endotracheal suctioning with a suction trap. Specimens may be sent for culture and sensitivity and Gram stain for rapid testing for bacteria.

X-rays - A chest film is necessary. If upper airway obstruction is suspected, a stat lateral neck film should be obtained (see "Upper Airway Obstruction" in this chapter).

Intervention

1. General considerations - Ventilate immediately. Indications for intubation include:
   a. Coma or stupor with risk of aspiration
   b. Apnea or obviously inadequate respirations
   c. Inability to clear secretions
   d. Upper airway obstruction
   e. Poor or deteriorating blood gases (a pO_2 under 60 despite a high F_IO_2 via face mask, a pCO_2 over 60 and rising, or a pH under 7.20)
   f. Severe chest wall trauma (i.e., flail chest)
      The majority of patients with airway obstruction or inadequate ventilation may be managed by clearing the airway and ventilating with a bag/mask device until an endotracheal tube is passed to secure the airway. The endotracheal tube needs to be well secured; restraint of patient's arms may be required. If cervical spine trauma is suspected, a lateral cervical spine film visualizing all seven vertebrae is obtained. If cervical spine injury is confirmed, nasotracheal intubation or cricothyrotomy is preferable to endotracheal intubation.
2. Administer oxygen immediately - Use the lowest F_IO_2 necessary. Any increase in pO_2 carries the risk of causing respiratory depression in patients with chronic hypercapnia. In addition, administration of more than 60% oxygen can result in direct damage to the alveolar-capillary membrane within 12–24 hours. Administer oxygen via a face mask. This may be difficult because confused or agitated patients will often

remove face masks. Nasal prongs are often better tolerated, but the F_IO_2 is unpredictable. Rebreathing masks deliver high F_IO_2 but may cause CO_2 retention.

3. Provide airway care. This includes:
   a. Elevation of head of bed
   b. Suctioning, i.e., give a high O_2 concentration before and after suctioning
   c. Deep breathing and coughing
   d. Humidification
4. Bronchodilators - Use for bronchospasm (see "Chronic Obstructive Pulmonary Disease" in this chapter for further details).
5. Monitor ABGs - Ventilate the patient to normalize the pH. A pO_2 of at least 50–60 mm Hg is desired; do not attempt to normalize the pCO_2 in chronic CO_2 retainers. Because patients who have been in respiratory distress for several hours have retained bicarbonate to compensate for respiratory acidosis, rapid lowering of pCO_2 may lead to dangerous alkalosis. See Chapter 6 for a review of acid-base balance.
6. Fluid administration - Administer fluids with a microdrip or an IV pump. Overhydration may result in CHF. Monitor the patient for increase in heart and respiratory rate, wheezing, crackles (rales), and decreased pulmonary gas exchange as seen on ABG.

ED Discharge Planning

The majority of patients with acute respiratory failure will require admission, and most will require intensive care. The patient's mental status may improve dramatically with correction of hypoxemia and acid-base imbalance. Provide the patient with a brief explanation of what has and what will happen. Tell patient and family about admission to the ICU and/or respiratory care unit. Provide as calm and supportive an environment as possible.

UPPER AIRWAY OBSTRUCTION

Etiology

Etiologies of acute obstruction include:

1. Infection - Acute epiglottitis (usually caused by *Haemophilus influenzae*, with rapid onset of hoarseness, dysphagia, sore throat, and fever), peritonsillar abscess, retropharyngeal abscess, or Ludwig's angina

2. Aspiration of a foreign object, usually food
3. Trauma - Blunt, penetrating, or thermal injury to airway
4. Anaphylaxis
5. Smoke inhalation

Etiologies of subacute or chronic obstruction include:

1. Infection - Tonsillar hypertrophy
2. Posttraumatic stricture - Previous external trauma, intubation, or tracheostomy
3. Tumors of larynx and trachea
4. External masses - Goiter, lymphadenopathy
5. Pickwickian and sleep apnea syndromes

Assessment

History
If the patient is capable of giving a history, the following should be elicited:

1. Duration and nature of symptoms such as hoarseness, dysphagia, dyspnea, sore throat, and wheezing
2. Presence of fever
3. Aspiration of foreign object
4. History of trauma to neck or throat
5. History of allergies or recent ingestion of new medicine
6. History of chronic throat infections or pulmonary disease
7. History of exposure to fire and smoke

Physical Findings
Vital signs - Check respiratory rate, pulse, and rectal temperature.
General - Check for cyanosis. Observe for excessive salivation. Note obesity.
HEENT - Examine for signs of burn injury; examine floor of mouth, teeth, and pharynx for infection.
Neck - Check for a midline trachea. Note use of accessory muscles of respiration. Listen for inspiratory stridor, a high-pitched wheezing sound heard best over the trachea, which is the single most important physical finding in upper airway obstruction. However, it is important to remember that stridor may be absent even in severe cases. Severe trauma to the anterior neck and larynx may present with flattening of neck contour, crepitus, and dysphonia.
Lungs - Check for bilateral breath sounds. Listen for wheezing and crackling.

Note: Great care must be exercised in examining the oropharynx of a patient with suspected epiglottitis, as this may provoke complete airway closure. Have emergency airway management equipment including a cricothyrotomy on hand prior to the physician's examination of patient. Often it is better to call in an ENT specialist and get a stat lateral neck x-ray first.

Diagnostic Tests

ABGs - A blood gas analysis is useful to document CO_2 retention and the presence or absence of hypoxia.

X-rays - A soft tissue lateral neck film can often demonstrate a mass, a foreign body, or edema of the pharynx and epiglottis. If x-rays are taken outside the ED, the patient must be accompanied by medical and/or nursing staff, and as indicated, a cricothyrotomy set should be brought with the patient.

Pulmonary function tests - Chronic obstruction may not be so evident; patients may need an outpatient workup to establish the diagnosis.

Intervention

1. Ask the patient if he or she is choking. Examine the posterior oropharynx for foreign body, and with the patient in a lateral position, sweep the mouth in an attempt to remove any visualized objects. Perform the Heimlich maneuver for foreign body aspiration. Patients will be in acute distress, typically with their hand at their throat. If the patient is able to speak and cough, there is a partial obstruction with adequate air exchange, and the Heimlich maneuver is not indicated. For a full obstruction stand behind the patient, clasp your arms around his or her chest with your fists joined, and press into the subxiphoid area with a succession of forceful thrusts. If the patient is pregnant, do chest thrusts.

2. Oxygenation - Severely dypsneic patients may require intubation regardless of the cause. Oxygen should be administered. Have suction available; vomiting is not uncommon.

3. Laryngoscopy and removal of the object by use of a long grasping forcep (Magill) is standard ED treatment. Local or light general anesthesia will be used, and the patient will be placed in a Trendelenburg position. Have emergency equipment and suction close at hand. Bronchoscopy with the patient under general anesthesia may be necessary to visualize and remove the foreign body. If the object cannot be removed or ventilatory support becomes necessary, endotracheal intubation or a cricothyrotomy is indicated.

4. Aminophylline IV drip and isoproterenol or metaproterenol nebulizer may be used to treat laryngeal spasm.

ED Discharge Planning

All patients with respiratory difficulty, aspiration, epiglottitis, or laryngeal edema and those who require intubation or cricothyrotomy need to be admitted. Patients who are discharged following treatment for foreign body aspiration should be accompanied by a friend or relative. Discharge instructions should include:

1. 12 hours of home observation
2. Return to the ED for any respiratory distress, difficulty swallowing, or fever

PNEUMOTHORAX

A pneumothorax may occur spontaneously or as a result of trauma. Air enters the pleural cavity, and as the pressure in the pleural cavity exceeds atmospheric pressure, the lung collapses.

Spontaneous pneumothorax - This condition is probably due to the spontaneous rupture of subpleural blebs. Spontaneous pneumothorax occurs 5 times more often in males than in females, and recurrence on the same side is common. In patients with emphysema, rupture of superficial bullae may occur. Asthmatics may develop mediastinal emphysema, which can then track into the pleural cavity. Other causes of spontaneous pneumothorax include infections (pneumonia, tuberculosis, fungal infections, lung abcesses), some connective tissue disorders (e.g., scleroderma), connective tissue defects (e.g., Marfan's syndrome), neoplasms (either primary or metastatic), sarcoidosis, fibrotic lung disease, and endometriosis.

Traumatic pneumothorax - Surprisingly, a vigorous cough or exertion involving the Valsalva maneuver can cause collapse. Any injury causing perforation of the chest wall, trachea, or bronchial tree or the barometric pressure variations experienced by divers can result in collapse.

Iatrogenic pneumothorax - Pneumothoraces are often caused by various procedures (e.g., endotracheal intubation, bronchoscopy, thoracentesis) or by the use of mechanical ventilators. Any central line insertion or attempt can result in collapse, particularly with the subclavian approach. A chest x-ray must be obtained soon after any central line attempt in the ED.

Assessment

History
Nearly 100% of patients with pneumothorax will complain of chest pain, either crushing or pleuritic. Roughly 60% will complain of dyspnea.

Physical Findings
Vital signs - Look for tachycardia, tachypnea, and hypotension.
Neck - Tracheal deviation to the unaffected side is associated with a tension pneumothorax. Check for distended neck veins.
Lungs - Inspect any site of injury. Examine for evidence of rib fractures (local tenderness or crepitus) or a flail segment (paradoxical motion). The collapsed side will have diminished breath sounds and decreased chest wall movement.

Diagnostic Tests
X-rays - A chest x-ray should always be obtained if collapse is suspected. End-expiratory films are preferred because lung volume is then smallest and the pneumothorax will be easier to see.
ABGs - Because of ventilation/perfusion mismatching, patients with collapse will initially demonstrate some degree of hypoxia on blood gas analysis. After several hours, perfusion of the affected lung decreases with resultant improvement in ventilation/perfusion ratios and some resolution of hypoxia.

Intervention

1. Provide for airway and oxygenation - Administer oxygen by cannula or mask. Have suction equipment and bag/mask device on standby. Position the patient in the mid-Fowler's position if BP permits.
2. Tension pneumothorax is an extreme emergency. A large amount of air is trapped in the pleural cavity, which causes lung collapse and displacement of the heart and great vessels. The two main problems are hypoxia and hypotension. Hypotension may be the result of increased intrathoracic pressure with decreased venous return or of shifting of mediastinal structures with kinking of major vessels. Emergency treatment involves the insertion of a needle or IV catheter, in the second intercostal space in the midclavicular line, directly into the pleural cavity to relieve the pressure. More definitive treatment requires chest tube thoracotomy (usually inserted in the fifth intercostal space in the midaxillary line).
3. Open pneumothorax - Caused by a penetrating chest wound, this condition is also referred to as a "sucking" chest wound. While waiting for the definitive surgical treatment, place an airtight dressing (e.g., petrolatum gauze) directly over the open chest wound, hopefully converting

an open pneumothorax to a closed one. Theoretically, even a plastic wrapping paper or a plastic bag could be used in the field. A chest tube should be inserted later. If the penetrating object is still in place, cover or surround it with petroleum gauze and support it in place until the patient is evaluated by a physician.

4. Closed pneumothorax - There is no external wound. Air in pleural cavity is the result of a rupture of small blebs on the visceral pleura and is most commonly seen in otherwise healthy young men and in older patients with chronic pulmonary disease. The treatment of spontaneous pneumothorax varies, depending on the magnitude, presence of other disorders, and history of previous pneumothorax. In healthy patients who are tolerating a pneumothorax whose magnitude is roughly 25% or less, hospitalization for bed rest and serial chest films may be sufficient. About 1% of normal lung volume will be reabsorbed daily. Tube thoracotomy is the treatment of choice in patients with pulmonary or other serious disease, pneumothoraces of more than 25%, recurrent pneumothorax, and all pneumothoraces associated with trauma.

5. Thoracotomy - Chest tubes will usually be inserted in the ED and connected to water-seal drainage. Chest tubes are sutured in place, and the puncture site is covered with an airtight dressing. Obtain a chest x-ray immediately thereafter, to check tube placement and assess lung reexpansion. Keep tubing and drainage system below the level of the chest. Observe color and amount of drainage and mark this on the drainage container during each shift. Chest tubes should be "milked" or stripped every hour if drainage is thick (i.e., blood clots or mucus).

ED Discharge Planning

Virtually all patients with pneumothorax should be admitted after appropriate therapy is instituted in the ED. Healthy patients with small pneumothoraces usually need to be observed for a day or two in the hospital with repeat chest films.

Since the rate of recurrence is high, patients with spontaneous pneumothorax should be instructed to return to the ED for chest pain, respiratory difficulty, or signs of infection.

PULMONARY EMBOLUS

Ninety percent of pulmonary emboli develop from deep vein thrombosis, although less than one-third of patients have evidence of phlebitis on physical examination. Most deep vein thromboses begin in the calf but propagate proximally into the deep veins of the thigh. Other emboli can originate from the pelvic veins or from the right side of the heart. Emboli almost never arise from the upper extremities. The thrombus, once dislodged, travels to the narrowest vessel; the lower lobes of the lung are most often affected.

Assessment

History

The patient presents with sudden dyspnea; the degree of distress is variable. Other symptoms include cough, pleuritic chest pain, and apprehension. Hemoptysis and syncope may be noted. In most patients one or more of the following predisposing factors can be identified:

1. Postpartum state
2. Severe CHF
3. Underlying neoplasm
4. Prolonged bed rest
5. History of hip fracture or joint replacement surgery
6. Hematologic abnormalities

The differential diagnosis includes all those diseases that cause chest pain, including acute MI, angina, pneumonia, pleural effusion, pneumothorax, musculoskeletal chest pain, and pericarditis.

Physical Findings

General - Agitation is commonly seen.

Vital signs - Tachypnea is seen in 90%; tachycardia, in 50%; fever, in 50% (usually seen with pulmonary infarction); and hypotension, in 15%. Check for neck distention.

Lungs - Listen for rales, a pleuritic friction rub, or decreased breath sounds unilaterally.

Cardiovascular system - Check for rate and rhythm; listen for a gallop or loud P_2.

Extremities - Check for any evidence of phlebitis, either chronic or acute.

Diagnostic Tests

ABGs - Analysis of ABGs may show hyperventilation with hypoxemia. The pO_2 is usually below 80 mm Hg, and the pCO_2 is below 35 mm Hg due to tachypnea and hyperventilation.

CVP - A central line may be placed in hypotensive patients. Hypotension without increased CVP makes the diagnosis of embolism less likely.

X-rays - A chest x-ray is usually not diagnostic unless a pulmonary infarct has occurred. A normal x-ray does not exclude the diagnosis.

ECG - An ECG is in no way diagnostic of pulmonary embolus but may show signs of ischemia and cardiac arrhythmias. In patients with recurrent small pulmonary emboli the ECG may show signs of right atrial and ventricular enlargement (cor pulmonale) consistent with pulmonary hypertension. The most important use of the ECG is to eliminate cardiac ischemia as a cause of dyspnea or chest pain.

Lung scan - A four-view nuclear perfusion can be performed on an emergency basis but is usually scheduled after admission. A sensitive but nonspecific test, a positive scan may result from CHF, pneumonia, or chronic lung disease. However, a negative scan essentially rules out the diagnosis.

Pulmonary angiography - Highly specific for confirming pulmonary embolism.

Intervention

1. Oxygenation and alteration of tissue perfusion - The degree of hypoxemia is a major determining factor in the patient's clinical state. Administer high-flow humidified oxygen by face mask or nasal cannula. Oxygen concentration and method of delivery can be adjusted when ABG results are available. If BP permits, place the patient in a mid-Fowler's position. A large embolus may result in cerebral ischemia, cardiac arrhythmias, shock, and cardiac arrest. Place the patient on cardiac monitor and check vital signs frequently. Start an IV of D5W to run at a moderate rate. Aggressive use of IV fluid may cause excess preload and prime the patient for heart failure.

2. Anticoagulation - Heparin is the drug of choice initially, with the goal of preventing recurrent emboli. It may be given SC, by intermittent IV bolus, or by IV infusion. Infusion is the method most commonly used and may be associated with a lower rate of complications. The dose is 5000 units as IV bolus, followed by 1000-1750 units/hr (50,000 units heparin in 500 ml D5W) run by IV pump. Patients should be monitored for bleeding. The activated PTT should be measured before the heparin bolus and then 4–6 hours after the start of the infusion. A PTT approximatelty 1.5–2.5 times the patient's control is desired. Patients may be started on heparin therapy in the ED if there is a significant delay before patients are evaluated by unit personnel. Contraindications to anticoagulation include active bleeding, recent bleeding peptic ulcer, recent CVA or bleeding intracranial lesion, recent hip or other major surgery, and recent pericarditis. Long-term therapy includes warfarin (Coumadin) or full-dose SC heparin for 4–6 months after the predisposing factor has resolved. Surgical therapy includes inferior vena cava (IVC) interruption procedures and transvenous IVC filter placement; embolectomy can be performed as a heroic measure in severe cases.

3. Thrombolytic agents (urokinase and streptokinase) are newer treatment modalities that may be useful in massive, hemodynamically significant pulmonary emboli.

ED Discharge Planning

All patients who are diagnosed or suspected of having pulmonary embolism require admission. A significant number of these patients may require admission to the ICU or an intermediate care unit. In addition to regular monitoring and assessment, measures to prevent further embolization should be instituted, including:

1. Bed rest and thigh-high antiembolus stockings
2. Teaching the patient to deep breathe and perform leg exercises in bed
3. Monitoring for signs of thrombophlebitis
4. Elevation of the foot of the bed 10°; but do not "gatch" (raise at knees) the bed

ASTHMA

Asthma is a disease of airway obstruction resulting from bronchospasm, bronchial wall edema, and hypersecretion of mucous glands. Asthma attacks range in severity from slight wheezing to life-threatening respiratory failure. In severe attacks, impaired airflow results in alveolar hypoventilation with hypoxemia and respiratory acidosis.

Status asthmaticus - A life-threatening condition in which an acute asthmatic attack continues in spite of treatment. The patient requires admission to the ICU for aggressive therapy and continuous monitoring.
Pregnant asthmatics - Asthma and the resulting acid-base imbalance and hypoxia may be more damaging to mother and child than the drugs used to treat it. All pregnant asthmatic patients should receive supplemental oxygen. Corticosteroids, beta-2-specific agents (isoetharine), and theophylline are all accepted methods of treatment for the pregnant asthmatic. These patients should be admitted liberally and should be made known to the obstetrical service.

Assessment (Fig. 2.1)

History
Patients will commonly tell the triage nurse they have asthma. Due to the patient's respiratory distress, obtaining a full history may not be possible prior to treatment. An ED history should contain:

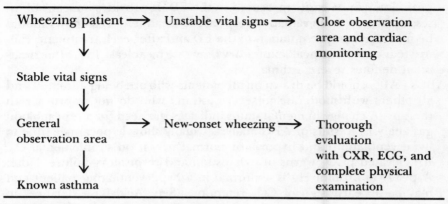

Figure 2.1. Asthma treatment flow sheet.

1. Duration of asthma
2. Maintenance medications, with time of last dose
3. History of steroid use
4. Frequency of hospitalizations and ED visits (including most recent)
5. Precipitating causes of attacks, including that of the current episode
6. Duration of this attack
7. Other medical conditions (especially hypertension, angina or cardiac disease, and pregnancy)

Patients who have retained CO_2 and required intubation in the past and those who have been treated more than once within the week for asthma are high-risk patients who should be observed carefully and aggressively treated. Patients with new-onset wheezing should be carefully evaluated for pneumonia, CHF, pulmonary embolus, foreign body, and allergic reaction before they are labelled asthmatics.

Physical Findings
Vital signs - Obtain a full set of vital signs, including temperature. Tachypnea and tachycardia are common findings. A rectal temperature may be necessary for those who are mouth breathers.
Lungs - Check for bilateral breath sounds. Note degree of wheezing and airflow, as well as use of accessory muscles of respiration. Scant or a sharp decrease in wheezing may indicate very limited air movement and impending respiratory failure.
Extremities - Check for cyanosis, clubbing, or edema.
Neurologic signs - Note any alteration in mental status (e.g., lethargy or agitation).

Diagnostic Tests
Peak expiratory flow rate - A maximal exhalation from total lung capacity,

peak flow can be easily measured in the ED. It provides a means of assessing airflow and evaluating response to treatment. Peak flows should be measured on presentation to the ED and after each treatment. Failure to increase the peak expiratory flow rate by at least 15% after treatment denotes severe asthma.

ABGs - ABG should be drawn on all patients who are being admitted and all others with moderate to severe asthma who do not improve with therapy. A change in mental status indicates the need for a repeat blood gas analysis. Results of ABG analysis usually show hypocapnea (due to hyperventilation) and hypoxia or normal pO_2 if on supplemental O_2. An elevated pCO_2 warns of exhaustion and respiratory failure. Note: A pCO_2 of 40 mm Hg is abnormal in a hyperventilating patient and may be an early sign of CO_2 retention. (See "Acid-Base Balance" in Chapter 6.)

X-rays - Chest films should be done in all patients with new-onset wheezing or fever or when clinical findings are inconsistent with asthma. Asymmetrical breath sounds in an asthmatic may indicate pneumonia or pneumothorax and necessitate a chest x-ray. In general, pregnant patients should not be x-rayed.

ECG - An ECG should be done in all patients with tachycardia over 130, irregular pulse, angina-like chest pain, or a history of cardiac disease.

Theophylline level - A level should be obtained for all those patients on xanthine therapy who claim compliance.

Intervention

1. Oxygen administration - All asthmatics require supplemental O_2. Oxygen may be given by nasal cannula (5–6 liters/min) or Venturi mask (28% or more if necessary). Some patients prefer O_2 by cannula because the mask gives them a suffocating, closed-in feeling. Oxygen must always be used when IV aminophylline is being administered, as a fall in pO_2 can result from medication-induced ventilation/perfusion imbalance. Patients with chronic obstructive lung disease and chronic CO_2 retention should be treated with a low concentration (24% or 1–2 liters/min) and observed very closely. Patients in impending respiratory failure with rising pCO_2 and altered level of consciousness should be intubated and placed on mechanical volume-cycled ventilation. IPPB treatment should never be used for asthmatics.

2. Hydration and mobilization of secretions - Fluids by either the PO or the IV route (1000 ml of D5/0.45% NaCl or D5/0.2% NaCl) initiated early may help to mobilize secretions and mucous plugs. Patients who are vomiting must have an IV line, and the possibility of theophylline toxicity should be considered.

3. Relief of bronchospasm

a. General considerations - Patients who present in extremis and those with a history of CO_2 retention or respiratory failure should receive several therapeutic interventions (inhaled bronchodilators, IV aminophylline, IV steroids, etc.) all at once. For others, recent studies indicate that inhaled bronchodilators are superior to those given SC and IV and have fewer side effects. Moreover, the addition of aminophylline in these patients is no better than inhaled adrenergic agents used alone.

b. Aerosol bronchodilator therapy
   i. Metaproterenol (Alupent) can be used if the patient understands how to use an inhaler or can be taught. The patient can inhale 1 puff (0.65 mg) every 10–20 minutes for three doses. Rounds of metaproterenol inhalation can be used every hour or so if a response is documented. Patients who cannot use a hand-held inhaler can receive metaproterenol 5% given as 0.3 ml (15 mg) in 5 ml sterile water (not NS) via a nebulizer.
   ii. Isoetharine (Bronkosol) is an acceptable alternative given in doses of 0.55 ml diluted 1:3 with saline.
   iii. Albuterol (Proventil, Ventolin) is a long-acting bronchodilator that has greater selectivity for beta-2 receptors than does metaproterenol. It may be given via nebulizer as 0.5–1 ml of a 5% solution in doses of 2.5–5 mg.

c. Epinephrine in a 1:1000 solution is traditionally given in doses of 0.2–0.3 ml SC every 20 minutes (three doses is a round) and may be used every 2 hours throughout the treatment, provided there is some kind of demonstrable response in peak flow or other objective parameter. Epinephrine may be given down the endotracheal tube in an intubated patient in doses of 5–10 ml of the 1:10,000 solution. Since epinephrine has beta-1 (heart) and beta-2 (bronchodilating) activity, patients with angina, tachycardia over 130/min, ischemic changes on the ECG, or arrhythmias should be treated with agents that have specific beta-2 receptors. Terbutaline (Bricanyl) has beta-2 specificity and can be given SC in addition to or instead of epinephrine. The dose is 0.25 mg SC every 45 minutes to a maximum dose of 0.50 mg every 4 hours. The drug may cause a slight drop in BP and rise in heart rate in response to arteriolar dilatation.

d. Aminophylline is often given after treatment with the sympathomimetic agents, although both may be used initially in patients with severe obstruction. The theophylline level should be checked, and those without a significant level should be loaded with aminophylline, while those with inadequate but appreciable levels should be partially loaded. The dose is based on lean body weight, not total body weight, because theophylline does not distribute in fatty tissues. An initial loading dosage of 6 mg/Kg in 100 ml D5W is given over 20–30 minutes. Usual maintenance doses (0.7–0.9 mg/Kg/hr) may be reduced (0.3–0.5 mg/Kg/hr) in elderly patients or those with CHF or liver disease. If theophylline toxicity is suspected (nausea, vomiting, tachycardia, agitation, headache, abdominal cramps, seizures, etc.), a stat theophylline level should be sent. An effective therapeutic level is 10–20 µg/ml, with risk of toxicity increasing at concentrations over 20 µg/ml.

4. Antiinflammatory agents - Steroids should be started early for those patients who do not respond to bronchodilator treatment or have been on maintenance corticosteroids, since the effect from IV administration may take several hours. Usual dosage of hydrocortisone (Solu-Cortef) is 100–200 mg IV every 4–6 hours.

5. Measures to promote comfort and relieve anxiety - Asthmatics who continuously return to the same ED for treatment have the benefit of knowing that they and their response to treatment are known to the ED staff, plus there is comfort in familiar surroundings. Many EDs have a specific room or area designated for asthmatics. Most asthmatics can be treated while sitting in a chair; patients with altered level of consciousness and those whose condition might require intubation need to be placed on a stretcher. To reduce stress and provide reassurance is one of the most valuable treatments that can be offered by the ED staff.

6. Use of sedative drugs - No type of sedation should be administered to ambulatory asthmatics. However, once an asthmatic is intubated, sedation with morphine and diazepam will facilitate ventilation of an agitated and combative patient.

7. Antibiotics are not usually helpful, since most infections that provoke asthma are viral in nature. Antibiotics are indicated for febrile asthmatics with productive coughs or other sources of infections and for those with an infiltrate on chest x-ray.

8. Anticholenergic agents have been used successfully to treat acute asthmatic attacks. Atropine (0.5–1 mg) via the endotracheal tube can be used in intubated patients. Ipratropium bromide (Atrovent) can be used in the ED as an inhaler (and, when the solution becomes available, via a nebulizer.)

Treatment Protocol

	Time in ED (hours)
1. Physical examination; check peak flow (PF), and order theophylline level.	0
2. Start a beta agonist via inhaler, 2 puffs every 10 minutes for 3 doses, or start a beta-2 agent via	½

a nebulizer. Assess the patient and check PF afterwards.

3. Epinephrine, 0.3 ml SC every 20 minutes for 3 doses. Check PF after each dose.   1

4. If there is no satisfactory response with further epinephrine or beta agonist or both, start IV aminophylline with supplemental oxygen. Check PF.   2

5. May repeat epinephrine or beta agonist if patient shows a good response. Check PF.   3

6. If response remains inadequate, obtain a blood gas analysis.

7. Start steroids (hydrocortisone, 100–200 mg IV).

8. Decide whether to admit or (if the patient has responded well) discharge the patient.   4

Note: Very ill patients should have an injection of epinephrine, a nebulizer started, a blood gas drawn, and a line started for IV aminophylline and possible steroids all within the first few minutes of presentation.

ED Discharge Planning

Patients should be treated until peak flow rate is over 300 liters/min. Patients who have not shown significant improvement within 4 hours should be recommended for admission. Patients with the following conditions should be admitted:

1. A pCO_2 over 40 with CO_2 not normally retained
2. Low peak flow (under 250 liters/min) unresponsive to treatment
3. Lactic acidosis
4. Angina, arrhythmias, or ischemia on ECG
5. Pneumonia
6. Theophylline toxicity
7. No significant improvement after aggressive therapy
8. Treatment in the ED 2 or 3 times in 1 week
9. High-risk patients who do not show significant improvement, i.e., pregnant asthmatics, those on chronic steroid therapy, or those with a history of intubation or CO_2 retention.

ED Discharge Instructions

All asthmatics discharged from the ED should have their medications carefully checked, be given adequate prescriptions, and be given or advised to seek appointments for an outpatient visit within the week. Patients should be given a brief note for their usual health care provider, summarizing their ED visit. Discharge instructions should include:

1. Use of metered-dose inhaler (MDI) - Common use is 2–3 inhalations 3–4 times a day. Disbursement of aerosol particles is improved by spacing inhalations at 5–10-minute intervals with slow, even inspiration and breath holding before expiration. Caution the patient against abuse of the drugs, as tolerance and side effects can develop.
2. Inhalers that contain nonselective beta-adrenergic stimulants such as epinephrine and isoproterenol may cause cardiac complications and arrhythmias.
3. Asthma is a complex disorder that is best evaluated and treated by the patient's regular health care provider. Intermittent ED care is no substitute for comprehensive care. The patient needs to know how diet, exercise, and stress can trigger asthma attacks.
4. Pursed-lip breathing can aid in control of breathing and should be used until breathing is eased.
5. Counselling the patient to seek medical care without delay if usual measures do not result in improvement.

CHRONIC OBSTRUCTIVE PULMONARY DISEASE

Definition

COPD refers to a group of lung disorders characterized by airflow limitation, dyspnea, and activity intolerance. The two most common types of COPD are chronic bronchitis and emphysema or a combination of both. Approximately 50% of patients with COPD have an asthmatic element to their disease. Chronic bronchitis is defined as sputum production on most days for at least 3 months yearly for 2 successive years. Emphysema is an anatomic alteration of the lung, characterized by an abnormal enlargement of airspaces distal to the terminal nonrespiratory bronchiole. The American Lung Association reports that COPD is found primarily in men over 45 years old and that the death rate is over 40,000/yr.

Etiology

Smoking is the greatest risk factor for the development of severe irreversible airway obstruction. When compared with the risk for nonsmokers, the risk is increased 10 times for cigarette smokers and 1.5–3 times for pipe and cigar smokers. Increasing age is associated with an increased incidence of chronic airway obstruction; however, this may reflect the cumulative effects of exposure to other risk factors. Areas of high air pollution show an increased incidence of chronic bronchitis and emphysema. Genetic predisposition and alpha- 1 antitrypsin deficiency may play a small role, particularly when symptoms develop before age 40.

Complications

Patients with COPD are at greater risk for the following:

1. Respiratory infection
2. Arrhythmias
3. Pulmonary emboli
4. Pneumothorax (due to bleb rupture)
5. Myocardial ischemia and/or infarction (with or without left-sided heart failure) secondary to hypoxemia or acidosis

The patient with COPD who presents in the ED in acute respiratory distress may be suffering from an exacerbation of the chronic airway obstruction or a complication of the disease. Regardless of the cause the patient in respiratory distress is rapidly assessed and triaged for emergency medical treatment.

Assessment

History
The following points should be addressed:

1. History of dyspnea, smoking, environmental factors, or occupation
2. Chronic productive cough or any change in sputum
3. Medication (bronchodilators, antibiotics) and effect
4. Onset and duration of present exacerbation or the presence of chest pain

Request the patient's previous medical record for the purpose of locating baseline blood gases, blood gases during exacerbations, the results of pulmonary function tests, the frequency of past ED visits and hospitalization, and methods of treatment used in the past.

Physical Findings
General - Note diaphoresis, tremor, cyanosis, or confusion.
Vital signs - Check for tachypnea, tachycardia, pulsus paradoxus, and fever.
HEENT - Note pursed-lip breathing.
Neck - Palpate for a midline trachea. Listen for stridor (upper airway obstruction). Note jugular venous distention (cor pulmonale).
Lungs - Observe chest configuration ("barrel chest" of emphysema or kyphoscoliosis causing restrictive lung disease). Note use of accessory muscles of respiration. Listen for wheezing, diminished breath sounds, increased inspiratory-to-expiratory phase, and rales or rhonchi.
Extremities - Note clubbing, cyanosis, or pedal edema.

Diagnostic Tests

Blood gas - Significant hypoxia, hypercapnea, and acidosis need to be identified and treated quickly. An acid-base nomogram (see Fig. 6.2) can be used to determine whether an acidosis or alkalosis is primarily respiratory or metabolic and acute or chronic. Repeat blood gas analyses should be obtained with every change in the patient's status or change in drug or oxygen therapy. Take measures to protect the patient from repeated arterial punctures; perform an Allen test; and consider an arterial catheter. (See "Acid-Base Balance" in Chapter 6.)

CBC - A Hct will aid in estimating the patient's oxygen-carrying capacity. The WBC and differential count provide markers of infection.

SMA - A serum bicarbonate may aid in distinguishing acute from chronic acidosis.

Sputum - Observe the nature of sputum; a Gram stain acid-fast smear and a culture and sensitivity are often ordered.

ECG - Look for acute changes indicating possible myocardial ischemia or infarction, as well as signs of chronic right atrial and ventricular hypertrophy from pulmonary hypertension. Common findings in chronic lung disease include large, peaked P waves in leads II, III, and aVF (p-pulmonale) and tall R waves and ST depression with T wave inversion in right-sided chest leads (cor pulmonale).

Intervention

1. Oxygenation - The first priority is cautious administration of oxygen. The goal is to increase the pO_2 to roughly 60, a level at which tissue oxygen delivery will increase greatly on the oxyhemoglobin dissociation curve. Either a nasal cannula or a Venturi mask can be used. Excessive oxygen in patients who chronically retain CO_2 may result in progressive hypercapnea with acidosis, caused by reduction of the hypoxic stimulus to breathe. Patients usually respond to an increase in F_IO_2 with an improvement in pO_2 and clinical status. The patient needs to be frequently assessed for vital signs, breathing pattern, and level of consciousness. Serial blood gas determinations should be followed to ensure that hypercapnea is not progressive.

2. Treatment of bronchospasm - Unlike asthmatics, patients with COPD have less immediate response to bronchodilators. All bronchodilators have significant toxicity, and great efforts should be made to avoid these toxicities, because the efficacy of these agents is often limited.

   a. Theophylline - Used to control bronchospasm, it also has a positive effect on mucociliary clearance and respiratory muscle function. Metabolism of theophylline is variable. Clearance is increased in smokers and decreased in patients with liver dysfunction, CHF, sepsis, and the elderly. Theophylline levels above 20 µg/liter may cause gastrointestinal irritation, cardiac arrhythmias, agitation, seizures, and other central nervous system manifestation.

b. Catecholamines - Epinephrine can be given as 0.3 ml SC. Spray pumps (metaproterenol or isoproterenol) can be used, as may a metaproterenol nebulizer (0.3 ml in 5 ml sterile water).

c. Corticosteroids - Many studies indicate that corticosteroids can be beneficial to a significant portion of patients with COPD and acute respiratory failure. Hydrocortisone (Solu-Cortef), 100–200 mg IV, can be given every 4–6 hours. Because the effect does not begin until about 6 hours after administration, ED patients who require steroids will generally need admission.

3. Antibiotics - Unlike asthmatics, patients with COPD often have exacerbations provoked by bacterial infections. Infections should be aggressively treated. Ampicillin, erythromycin, tetracyclines, and trimethoprim-sulfamethoxazole (Septra, Bactrim) are often used because of their broad-spectrum coverage.

ED Discharge Planning and Instructions

The following patients should be admitted:

1. All patients with COPD and pneumonia
2. Patients with significant deterioration of baseline blood gas
3. Patients who do not respond clinically to 4 hours of aggressive ED therapy or who state at the end of this time that they do not feel subjectively improved

Patients with COPD often have repeated hospital admissions and ED treatment that could be avoided by planned home care and evaluation. To start with, the patient needs regular medical and health care maintenance evaluations that may be accomplished in part by a referral to a home care or visiting nurse. In order to decrease future exacerbations the patient needs to be taught:

1. Medication use and precautions
2. To seek prompt treatment for respiratory distress and infections
3. To avoid bronchial irritants, e.g., smoking, powder, sprays
4. Breathing retraining techniques, i.e., pursed-lip breathing, diaphragmatic breathing, relaxation techniques, counted breathing
5. Maintain a balanced diet with small frequent feedings

Only the rudiments of the needed instructions can be accomplished in the ED. Patient learning may be slow due to anxiety, effects of medication (theophylline), and chronic hypoxia, so be sure to include the patient's family when you are giving instructions at discharge.

PNEUMONIA

Pneumonia, an acute inflammation of the lung parenchyma, is most likely to occur when the normal defense mechanisms are decreased. A variety of factors may cause pneumonia, including bacteria, viruses, fungi, chemicals, and dust.

Pneumococcal Gram-positive bacterial pneumonia - The patient has a sudden onset of cough with purulent sputum, with or without hemoptysis, fever, shaking chills, chest pain (pleuritic or constant), and dyspnea. It is usually seen in middle-aged to older patients (except in sickle cell disease patients) and may be associated with such underlying disorders as alcoholism, diabetes, chronic lung disease, drug abuse, CHF, or renal disease. The chest film usually shows lobar consolidation.

Mycoplasma - The patient has a gradual onset of dry to scantily productive cough with headache, myalgias, malaise, arthralgias, and pharyngitis. It is usually seen in younger patients. The chest film may show faint patchy infiltrates that are usually more impressive than the patient's clinical findings.

Mixed flora/anaerobes (aspiration) - The patient presents with copiously productive cough of purulent and often foul-smelling sputum. It is seen in the setting of alcohol or drug abuse or in seizure disorders. The patient may not always recall an episode of depressed consciousness with or without vomiting. The chest film will show infiltrates, depending on the patient's position at the time of aspiration.

Gram-negative bacteria - Community-acquired Gram-negative pneumonias are usually seen in abnormal hosts who have been colonized (e.g., alcoholics, patients who are leukopenic from chemotherapy). The patient will appear very ill. The chest film may show dense lobar consolidation with a bulging fissure (classically seen with *Klebsiella*).

Legionnaire's disease (*Legionella pneumophila*) - This is another cause of community-acquired pneumonia. The patient often presents with cough, neurologic signs, nausea, vomiting, and diarrhea. Patchy alveolar infiltrates are seen on chest x-ray, and hyponatremia may be seen on blood chemistry.

Viral pneumonia - The chest film usually shows bilateral diffuse interstitial infiltrates. A common form of pneumonia with symptoms similar to influenza, including fever, headache, and dry cough.

Staphylococcal pneumonia - Patients look very toxic. Staphylococcal pneumonia may follow pneumonia due to influenza virus. Pneumatoceles may be seen on chest x-ray.

Tuberculosis - Seen in malnourished or immunosuppressed patients and visitors from underdeveloped countries. TB infiltrates may be associated with cavities and are often seen in the apices or superior segments of the lower lobes (reactivated foci). If TB is suspected, an acid-fast stain of the sputum should be performed.

Pneumocystis carinii - This infection is seen in the immunocompromised host (AIDS patients, cancer patients, etc.). Tachypnea is virtually always present. The cough is usually dry or scantily productive. Infiltrates are extremely variable and may be patchy or segmented.

Assessment

History
The patient must be questioned about the following:

1. Previous upper respiratory tract infections
2. Cough and the presence of sputum or hemoptysis
3. Onset of symptoms (sudden versus gradual)
4. Fever or chills
5. Duration of symptoms
6. Dyspnea
7. Chest pain
8. Underlying diseases (asthma, chronic lung disease, tuberculosis, sickle cell, diabetes), and a history of smoking
9. Risk factors for AIDS (IV drug abuse, homosexuality, previous blood transfusions, multiple sexual partners)

Physical Findings
General - Note if the patient appears toxic or comfortable.
Vital signs - Note respiratory rate and effort. Always check a rectal temperature.
Neck - Check for a midline trachea or enlarged nodes.
Lungs - Listen for crackling (rales), egophony, and bilateral breath sounds. Percuss for dullness.
Extremities - Look for cyanosis or track marks.

Diagnostic Tests
CBC - WBC will be elevated in bacterial pneumonia.
Sputum - Obtain specimen for culture and sensitivity, acid-fast stain, and Gram stain.
X-rays - The pattern of infiltration and consolidation will aid in the diagnosis because the distribution pattern varies with the organism.
ABGs - Oxygen tension should always be measured in patients with pneumonia who look ill. An early alveolar-arterial (A-a) gradient can be an early and sensitive indicator of *Pneumocystis carinii* pneumonia.

Intervention

1. Antibiotic therapy - Pneumonia in the ambulatory, otherwise healthy, nontoxic young adult can be treated on an outpatient basis. If pneumococcal pneumonia is suspected on the basis of Gram stain, procaine penicillin, 1.2 million units IM, can be given to establish therapeutic blood levels, followed by penicillin VK, 500 mg PO qid for 2 weeks. Patients allergic to penicillin may be treated with erythromycin, 500 mg PO qid for 2 weeks. If mycoplasma or Legionnaire's pneumonia is suspected, erythromycin (same oral dose) is the drug of choice.
2. Increase fluid intake - Start an IV line for the patient who cannot maintain adequate oral intake and if IV antibiotics are prescribed.

ED Discharge Planning

Admission Criteria
1. Patients with pneumonia and low host resistance, i.e., elderly, chronically ill, immunosuppressed
2. Patients suspected of having pneumonia caused by highly virulent organisms such as Gram-negatives or mixed flora in aspiration, staphylococcus, or neumocystis
3. Patients with newly diagnosed or highly suspected TB
4. Patients who appear toxic or are unable to take oral medications

ED Discharge Instructions
Patients with pneumonia who are discharged home on antibiotic therapy should be told to return to the ED if the fever persists or nausea and vomiting occur. Discharge instructions should include:

1. Increased fluid intake to 2000 ml/day
2. Limited activity or bed rest
3. Deep breathing and coughing to clear airway
4. Antipyretics
5. Obtaining medical clearance before returning to work

SUGGESTED READINGS

Acute Respiratory Failure

Ahrens T. Concepts in the assessment of oxygenation. Focus Crit Care 1987;14:36–44.

Bernard GR, Bradley RB. Adult respiratory distress syndrome: diagnosis and management. Heart Lung 1986;15:250–255.

Bradley RB. Adult respiratory distress syndrome. Focus Crit Care 1987; 14:48–59.

Carrieri VK, Murdaugh C, Janson-Bjerklie S. A framework for assessing pulmonary disease categories. Focus Crit Care 1984;11:10–16.

Hochbaum SR. Emergency airway management. Emerg Med Clin North Am 1986; 4:411–425.

Upper Airway Obstruction

Anonymous. On recognizing epiglottitis in adults. Emerg Med 1987:55–58.

Block AJ, et al. Clinical conference in pulmonary disease: factors influencing upper airway closure. Chest 1984;86: 114–122.

Dennison RD. Managing the patient with upper airway obstruction. Nursing 1987; 17:34–41.

Weaver TE, Millman RP. Broken sleep. Am J Nurs 1986;86: 146–150.

Pneumothorax

Dalber DL, Krome RL. Thoracotomy. Emerg Med Clin North Am 1986;4:441–457.

Marini JJ. Respiratory medicine for the house officer. 2nd ed. Baltimore: Williams & Wilkins, 1987:62–69.

Jenkins JL, Loscalzo J. Manual of emergency medicine. Boston: Little, Brown, 1986: 271–281.

Pulmonary Embolus

Fahey VA. Life-threatening pulmonary embolism. Crit Care Q 1985;8:81–88.

Gerdes L. Recognizing the multisystemic effects of embolism. Nursing 1987;17:34–41.

Moser KM. The therapeutic focus in pulmonary embolism. Emerg Med 1987:67–83.

Roberts SL. Pulmonary tissue perfusion altered: emboli. Heart Lung 1987;16:128–138.

Velenzuela TD. Pulmonary embolism. Emerg Med Clin North Am 1988;6:253–266.

West JW. Pulmonary embolism. Med Clin North Am 1986;70:877–894.

Asthma

Abundis J. Hazards of metered-dose bronchodilator inhalers. J Emerg Nurs 1985; 11:262–264.

Drugs for asthma. Med Lett Drug Ther 1987;29:11–16.

Goodnough SK. Helping your asthmatic patient breathe easier. Nursing 1987;17:32C–32F.

Petty TL. Drug strategies for airflow obstruction. Am J Nurs 1987;87:180–187.

Chronic Obstructive Pulmonary Disease

Hahn K. Slow-teaching the COPD patient. Nursing 1987; 17:34–42.

Keyes FN. Dynamics of ventilation. In: Fincke MK, Lanros NE, eds. Emergency nursing. Rockville, Maryland: Aspen Publishers, 1986:1–17.

Pneumonia

Cavalier JP. Major respiratory and medical problems. In: Fincke MK, Lanros NE, eds. Emergency nursing. Rockville, Maryland: Aspen Publishers, 1986:43–70.

Coleman DA. Pneumonia: where nursing care really counts. RN 1986:22–29.

Stratton CW. Bacterial pneumonias—an overview with emphasis on pathogenesis, diagnosis and treatment. Heart Lung 1986;15: 226–244.

Chapter 3

NEUROLOGIC EMERGENCIES

COMA—THE UNCONSCIOUS PATIENT

Coma is not a disease but is a sustained state of unconsciousness in which the patient is relatively unresponsive to sensory stimuli. The ED* nurse's main goal in caring for an unconscious patient is to maintain vital functions and to protect the patient from injury. Nursing diagnosis for this patient may include:

1. Ineffective airway clearance
2. Ineffective breathing pattern
3. Alteration in fluid balance
4. Potential for injury

Causes of unconsciousness can be categorized according to the following outline:

1. Systemic disorders
   a. Metabolic disorders including hypoglycemia and hyperglycemia, hypotension, acidosis, encephalophy, hypoxia, and postictal states
   b. Intoxications including ethanol abuse, medical or illicit drug abuse, and carbon monoxide poisoning
   c. Infections including sepsis and pneumonia
   d. Aberrations of temperature (hypothermia and hyperthermia)
2. Intracerebral disease
   a. Mass with edema or herniation including tumor, abcess, hematomas, and intracerebral hemorrhage
   b. Infections including meningitis and encephalitis
   c. Vasculitis and cerebritis

---

*See "Appendix A" for definition of common abbreviations used in the text.

3. Psychiatric disorders
   a. Hysteria
   b. Catatonia

Assessment

History

Even a brief history from the ambulance personnel or family can be extremely useful in focusing assessment and initial interventions. Important factors for quick determination are:

1. History of diabetes or seizure disorder
2. History of alcohol or drug abuse
3. History of hypertension or stroke
4. History of kidney, lung, liver, or heart disease
5. History of prior overdose or suicide attempt

Any history of medications or illicit drug use can be very helpful. In the absence of any history, a description of the patient's environment may be helpful (e.g., hot or cold apartment). Friends or family members may be able to describe the mode of onset of coma (headache, fever, seizures, etc.) or possible causes of coma (e.g., recent trauma).

Physical Findings

Vital signs - Frequently monitor respiratory rate and pattern, pulse rate and regularity, BP, and temperature.

HEENT - Note any evidence of trauma. Observe extraocular movements, and check for the presence of the doll's eye reflex (see "Head Trauma" in Chapter 4 for a description). Note pupil size, equality, and reactivity. Check for hemotympanum or otorrhea. Note CSF rhinorrhea. (Test for glucose with a Dextrostix.) Note the quality of breath (ketones, ammonia, alcohol, etc.). Examine the oral cavity for bite marks consistent with a seizure.

Lungs - Listen for bilateral breath sounds. Check for rales.

Heart - Note rhythm and rate, as well as clarity of heart sounds.

Extremities - Note cyanosis or edema. Look for track marks or blisters (barbiturates).

Skin - Note the presence of jaundice, spider angiomata, or rashes.

Neurologic signs - The neurologic assessment must be repeated frequently to determine any change or progression. Note any spontaneous motor movements and the presence or absence of reaction to noxious stimuli. Particularly note decorticate or decerebrate posturing. Use of the Glasgow coma scale helps to avoid some of the ambiguity in terminology used to describe altered levels of consciousness.

Acute Neurologic Syndromes
Uncal or lateral herniation can be seen when an expanding lesion of the temporal lobe causes herniation of the uncus through the tentorial notch. The resulting compression of the oculomotor nerve and brainstem can result in ischemia and hemorrhage. Signs of uncal herniation include:

1. Ipsilateral pupil dilation, sluggish to nonreactive
2. Coma
3. Altered respiratory pattern, i.e., Cheyne-Stokes, respiration, central hyperpnea, ataxia
4. Hemiplegia
5. Decorticate and decerebrate posturing

Central herniation can be seen with medially placed supratentorial expanding lesions. The downward displacement causes a rostral-caudal progression of symptoms. The approximate level of dysfunction in central herniation is listed in Table 3.1.

Infratentorial mass lesions include midbrain, pontine, and cerebellar masses. Signs vary according to the area most involved. The most characteristic signs are:

1. Abnormal breathing pattern
2. Pupils small to midsized and fixed
3. Decorticate or decerebrate posturing

Table 3.1.
Appropriate Level of Dysfunction in Central Herniation[a]

CNS level	Consciousness	Pupils	Doll's eyes	Tone	Respiration
Diencephalon	Lethargy or stupor	Small, reactive	Present	Decortidate	Normal or Cheyne-Stokes
Midbrain	Coma	Midsize, fixed	Absent	Decerebrate	Hyperpnea
Pons	Coma	Midsize, fixed	Absent	Flaccid	Cheyne-Stokes Hyperventilation
Medulla	Coma	Midsize, fixed	Absent	Flaccid	Ataxic (gasping)

[a]Adapted from Nelson JR. The comatose patient. In: Sharpe JC, Marx FW, eds. The management of medical emergencies. New York, McGraw-Hill, 1969.

4. Dysconjugate gaze
5. Cranial nerve palsies

Diagnostic Tests

Laboratory tests - Do a Dextrostix for serum glucose immediately, and check electrolytes including calcium, creatinine, CBC, and PT.

Urinalysis - Check a Chemstrip for glucose, ketones, and blood.

Serum alcohol and drug levels - These can be obtained as needed (see "Drug Overdose: A General Approach" in Chapter 7).

Lumbar puncture - A spinal tap will aid in diagnosis of meningeal infection and may need to be performed immediately. The physician will assess the patient for signs of increased intracranial pressure prior to performing the tap. Serious complications including brainstem compression and herniation can result if a spinal tap is performed on a patient with significantly increased intracranial pressure.

CAT scan - A stat CAT scan of the head should be obtained in any patient who is suspected of having increased intracranial pressure, has coma following head trauma, has coma of unclear etiology, or has focal neurologic signs without metabolic disorder.

INTERVENTION

1. Ensure a patent airway - Inspect the airway and suction, if needed. Remove dentures, if loose. Risk of aspiration of secretions is lessened if the patient can be positioned on his or her side or in a mid-Fowler's position. Consider the possibility of head or neck injury before positioning the patient. An oral airway may aid in maintaining a patent airway and facilitating suctioning.
2. Ensure adequate respirations - Observe the breathing pattern. Poor air exchange and periods of apnea indicate the need for oxygen administration and possible intubation.
3. Fluid administration - Monitor intake and output. Fluid intake, blood administration, and/or vasopressors may be indicated to treat hypotension (see "Shock" in Chapter 1). If the patient shows signs of neurologic injury, the physician may elect to limit fluid intake.
4. Monitor cardiac rate and rhythm.
5. Glucose - A dose of 1 ampule of D5OW as an IV push is indicated if the Dextrostix shows a normal or low serum glucose.
6. Naloxone (Narcan) - A dose of 5 ampules as an IV push is indicated if narcotic abuse is suspected. (See "Drug Overdose: A General Approach" in Chapter 7.)
7. Seizures - Early treatment of seizures will reduce the risk of hypoxia and brain damage (see "Seizures" in this chapter). Institute safety measures and provide for continuous observation.

ED Discharge Planning

Admission Criteria
With few exceptions, patients who present with coma will require admission. Unstable patients will need an ICU bed. Exceptions include the following:

1. Hysterics or patients with other psychiatric disease (who should be evaluated by a psychiatrist in the ED)
2. Hypoglycemic insulin-dependent diabetics who recover promptly and have no other etiology for hypolycemic coma
3. Postictal patients with known seizure disorders

ED Discharge Instructions

Make indicated referrals, i.e., visiting nurse and diet counselling, and give specific discharge instructions concerning:

1. Medications prescribed
2. Activity and safety measures
3. Medical follow-up, clinic appointments

SEIZURES

Definitions

Generalized seizures are marked by a sudden loss of consciousness associated with major motor activity reflecting simultaneous discharge of nearly all neurons of the central nervous system. There is tonic rigidity with concurrent loss of consciousness, apnea, and cyanosis lasting 20–60 seconds, followed by clonic jerking and often, but not necessarily, by tongue biting, eye deviation, and urinary incontinence. There is subsequent flaccidity and coma. When consciousness returns, there is often postictal confusion, headache, and sleepiness. A prodrome may precede a generalized seizure. True seizures, as opposed to hysterical seizures, are marked by the development of Babinski's sign and dilated pupils.

Focal (partial) seizures are marked by seizure activity originating in one part of the body, occasionally with somatosensory disturbances. These imply a focal lesion but may be associated with metabolic imbalances. A patient in the midst of a seizure requires immediate attention. Providing for a patent airway and protection from injury take top priority; the physical assessment and history can be obtained once the patient's condition has stabilized.

The majority of patients who develop seizures before the age of 20 years have *idiopathic* (without identifiable cause) *epilepsy*. Seizures may also be caused by a number of other conditions including drug and/or alcohol abuse or withdrawal, head trauma, brain tumors, and metabolic disorders.

Assessment

History
Important points to cover include age of onset, types of seizures, frequency of seizures, present medication regimen, compliance with medications, and relationship of seizures to alcohol or other drug ingestion.

Physical Findings
General - Check for signs of urinary or fecal incontinence.
Vital signs - Low-grade fever may occur with seizures but should not persist more than 4 hours. Pulse and BP will gradually return to baseline values.
HEENT - Check for head trauma, skull fracture, Battle's sign, raccoon eyes, hemotympanum, or tongue laceration.

Diagnostic Tests
Laboratory tests - Do a stat Dextrostix for serum glucose (hypoglycemia may trigger a seizure), and send a specimen for SMA and CBC.
Toxicology or anticonvulsant drug levels - Identify drugs, if known, including patient's current anticonvulsant medication.
CAT scan - A stat CAT scan is indicated for patients with focal seizures not due to a metabolic disorder. The presence of increased intracranial pressure and a history of recent head trauma are strong indicators for a CAT scan.

Intervention

1. Airway maintenance - The nursing diagnoses of ineffective airway clearance and ineffective breathing pattern both apply to the patient having a seizure. Have a padded tongue blade and an airway close at hand. During a seizure the tongue blade should be inserted between the patient's teeth to prevent injury to tongue or teeth. Do not attempt to force open clenched teeth. Suction to prevent aspiration, and following seizure, place the patient in a side-lying position to facilitate drainage of secretions. When seizures occur in rapid succession (status epilepticus), administration of high-flow oxygen and use of an oropharyngeal or nasopharyngeal airway and a bag/mask device are indicated to prevent severe hypoxia.

2. Protection from injury - If the patient is standing when aura or seizure starts, assist the patient to a stretcher or the floor, if necessary. Guide movements to prevent injury but do not restrain. Stay with the patient during seizure.
3. Anticonvulsant medications - Start an IV line for administration of anticonvulsant drugs.
   a. Phenobarbital - 65–130 mg as slow IV push can be administered every 5–10 minutes to a maximum of 1 gm. Complications include respiratory depression and hypotension.
   b. Phenytoin (Dilantin) - An IV loading dose is 18 mg/Kg given at a rate of 30 mg/min. Dilantin must be diluted in normal saline, as it will precipitate with any solution containing dextrose. The patient must be placed on a cardiac monitor and watched for widened QRS, bradycardia, hypotension, and respiratory depression.
   c. Diazepam (Valium) - Given to treat acute seizures and status epilepticus at a dosage of 5–10 mg as IV push with repeat administration every 10–20 minutes, it may cause hypotension and respiratory depression. Monitor breathing rate and depth and have intubation equipment on standby. Another benzodiazepine, lorazepam (Ativan), which has a longer duration of action than diazepam, may be used to treat acute seizures. In order to prevent recurrence of seizure activity, phenobarbital or phenytoin is commonly given with diazepam. A diazepam drip (50 mg in 500 ml D5W) or IV paraldehyde can be used to control status epilepticus in a patient who has received maximum dosage of phenytoin and phenobarbital. Paraldehyde (5 mg in 500 ml D5W) can be given as a constant infusion and titrated to control seizures; side effects include pulmonary edema or hemorrhage. If all else fails, general anesthesia can be used to control status epilepticus. For management of alcohol withdrawal seizures, see "Alcohol Abuse and Withdrawal" in Chapter 7.

ED Discharge Planning

Patients with new-onset seizure disorder, status epilepticus, or a concomitant illness are commonly admitted, but for those who are not admitted, the following discharge guidelines pertain:

1. Patient should remain on bed rest for at least 1 hour after receiving IV phenytoin.
2. Assess the patient's ability to ambulate.
3. Review medications with emphasis on compliance.
4. Discuss safety measures with the patient and/or family, including driving, use of machinery, and participation in sports.

5. Make indicated referrals for follow-up medical care, a visiting nurse, and social services.
6. Encourage the patient to wear a medical alert identification bracelet or necklace and to contact the Epilepsy Foundation of America for information on seizure disorders and community support groups.

CEREBRAL ISCHEMIA AND STROKE

Cerebrovascular ischemia results from a deficiency in cerebral blood supply, and the resulting neurologic deficit varies considerably from a mild transient interruption to a major stroke.

Transient ischemic attack (TIA) is a loss of neurologic function caused by ischemia, is abrupt in onset, lasts from a few minutes to not more than 24 hours, and clears without residual signs. Symptoms vary according to the arteries involved and include hemiplegia, speech and visual disturbances, dizziness, and confusion.

Reversible ischemic neurologic deficit (RIND) is a loss of neurologic function secondary to ischemia, which lasts for more than 24 hours but ultimately resolves completely. Along the scale of increasing neurologic deficit from TIA to a completed stroke are crescendo TIAs, RIND, and strokes in evolution.

Cerebrovascular accident (CVA, stroke) is a thrombotic, embolic, or hemorrhagic event causing a permanent loss of neurologic function, often with a major degree of disability.

Etiology

Emboli are usually atheromatous plaques from an extracranial site in the internal carotid artery. However, thrombotic emboli from the heart may also occur, especially in the setting of predisposing conditions (e.g., atrial fibrillation, CHF, ventricular aneurysm). Bacterial endocarditis must always be considered in an IV drug abuser with an acute embolic stroke.

True thombosis of the intracranial arteries is a rare occurrence. What is termed "thrombotic stroke" is, in fact, a prolonged and progressive atherosclerotic narrowing of the artery lumen, causing inadequate blood flow to an area of the brain.

Hemorrhage always results in some degree of cerebral infarction and usually occurs in the setting of long-standing systemic arterial hypertension. A small percentage of intracerebral hemorrhage is secondary to arteriovenous malformations, berry aneurysms, or bleeding into a brain tumor.

Assessment

History
Obtain information relating to onset and nature of neurologic deficit. Past medical history should include medication taken, diabetes, cardiovascular disease, and hypertension.

Physical Findings
Vital signs - Heart rate is usually normal; note if the rhythm is irregular. BP is usually increased, occasionally to very high levels. The rate and pattern of respiration is very important and should be assessed accurately. Abnormal respiratory patterns (Cheyne-Stokes, central neurogenic hyperventilation, ataxic breathing, apnea) occur most frequently in brainstem events and can presage acute respiratory failure. The temperature should be normal; if it is elevated, consider infection.
Head - Examine the head carefully to exclude trauma, because significant head trauma may be the result of a fall with loss of consciousness.
Lungs - Auscultate breath sounds and listen for rales.
Neurologic signs - Assess level of consciousness and orientation. Complete the Glascow coma scale, and evaluate pupil size and reaction and motor activity. Check all cranial nerves. Assess reflexes and motor and sensory function. Test for Babinski responses. Evaluate the gag reflex, ability to swallow, and communication impairments (aphasia). Report signs of increased intracranial pressure, including decline in level of consciousness, decreased pulse pressure, and slowing of the heart rate.

Diagnostic Tests
SMA - A Dextrostix for serum glucose should be done immediately.
ABGs - An ABG analysis should be obtained in patients with abnormal respiratory patterns or decreased level of consciousness.
ECG - An ECG must be done to rule out arrhythmia and silent MI.
CAT scan - A CAT scan should be considered if the diagnosis of simple stroke is in doubt.

Intervention

1. Airway clearance and breathing pattern - Decreased level of consciousness and ineffective gag or cough reflex indicate the need for airway protection. If BP permits, place the responsive stroke patient in a mid-Fowler's position. An orophyngeal airway may be required prior to intubation. Intubation will help maintain adequate tidal volume and prevent aspiration. Place a nasogastric tube to decompress the stomach and prevent aspiration.
2. Potential for further neurologic dysfunction - Vasospasm can create

changes in cerebral blood flow following a stroke. Edema formation may cause an increase in intracranial pressure and cerebral edema. Maintaining the BP in the high normal range will act to provide adequate cerebral blood flow. Treatment of hypertension associated with a stroke may not be necessary in the ED unless the pressure is extremely high (systolic over 220 or diastolic over 130). In most cases, the hypertension resolves by itself, and treatment may lead to profound hypotension due to vasomotor instability. Severe hypertension associated with a subarachnoid hemorrhage requires treatment. The drug of choice is nitroprusside, 0.5–8 µg/Kg/min, via IV infusion pump. Other factors that have a detrimental effect on cerebral blood flow are abnormal pO_2 and pCO_2, hyperthermia, an IV line in the internal jugular, emotional stress, suctioning, and neck flexion. Related nursing intervention includes:

a. Frequent assessment of vital and neurologic signs.
b. Monitoring of fluid intake and output; commonly fluids are restricted to 1.5–2 liters/24 hr. Avoid use of hypotonic solution. Start IV with D5/0.45 NaCl.
c. Positioning the patient in either flat or mid-Fowler's position as directed by the physician.
d. Suctioning for no longer than 15 seconds.
e. Observing the patient for seizure activity and protecting the patient from injury.
f. Approaching the patient in a calm, reassuring manner.
3. Patients with depressed consciousness should be given D50W, 1–2 ampules IV, if serum glucose Dextrostix is in the normal or low range. Precede glucose therapy with thiamine, 100 mg IM, in patients with a history of alcohol abuse. Naloxone (Narcan), 2 mg in IV bolus, may also be prescribed.

ED Discharge Planning and Instructions

All patients diagnosed with acute stroke occurring within 3 days of presentation require hospitalization for observation (to watch for compromise of vital functions secondary to intracranial edema). Admission of patients with TIAs is controversial. Many physicians elect to admit all patients with a first ischemic event. Patients who are not admitted may be started on aspirin therapy (325 mg PO daily) and followed as outpatients. Discharge instructions should include:

1. Medication information
2. Restriction of activity for a specified period
3. Referral for outpatient follow-up or to private physician
4. Instruction to return to the ED in the event of the return of symptoms

SPINAL CORD COMPRESSION

Spinal cord compression may be the result of tumor (primary or meta-static), epidural abscess, hematoma, arteriovenous malformation, cervical or thoracic disc protrusion or subluxation (rheumatoid arthritis), or fracture or dislocation of the spine.

Assessment

History
Patients will often complain of back pain associated with tingling or numbness and weakness in the lower extremities. Pain is often intensified by coughing, straining, or lying flat in bed. Localized or radicular (root) pain indicates compression of a spinal nerve root. A change in urinary frequency (either an increase or a decrease) may be described, as well as constipation.

Physical Findings
Neck - Palpate for masses or adenopathy.

Back - Tenderness over the spine on palpation or percussion may be present at the level of the lesion.

Abdomen - An enlarged bladder may be percussed if urinary retention is present.

Neurologic signs - Early findings include loss or alteration of pinprick sensation in the legs without demarcation of a distinct neurologic level. Later findings include demarcation of a distinct sensory level on testing of pinprick, temperature, and vibration in the lower extremities. There may be weakness and hyporeflexia, areflexia at the level of the compression. Below the level of compression hyperreflexia and a positive Babinski sign may be noted.

Diagnostic Tests
CBC - Check the hematocrit and WBC with differential.

X-rays - A chest film will screen for lung tumors. Spinal films may reveal bony erosion (tumor), vertebral collapse or subluxation, or calcification (meningioma).

Lumbar puncture - A spinal tap should not be performed if cord compression is suspected.

Myelogram - This will provide CSF for analysis and aid in identifying the site of cord compression.

CAT scan - The CAT scan is becoming the method of choice for identifying spinal cord lesions.

Intervention

1. Initial management includes immobilization and rapid obtaining of x-rays. A neurologist or neurosurgeon should be consulted immediately. Acute spinal cord compression is a neurologic emergency.
2. Alteration in breathing pattern - Patients with cervical compression are at risk for respiratory depression with decreased rate and volume. Gastric distention can also reduce diaphragmatic excursion.
3. Medical intervention to relieve compression - Dexamethasone (Decadron), 10 mg IV, is given as a bolus. Some authorities recommend mannitol along with steroids. Definitive therapy depends on the etiology. Neurosurgical decompression or radiotherapy or both may be performed after admission. A fracture or dislocation of the cervical spine may require cervical tongs and traction.
4. Measures to relieve pain and anxiety - Prescribed analgesics and positioning will provide the patient with increased comfort. Reassure the family that definitive therapy will relieve pain.

ED Discharge Planning

All cases of acute spinal cord compression require admission. Patients with cervical or high thoracic deficits should be admitted to an intermediate or specialized neurologic/neurosurgery unit.

HEADACHE

Headache is one of the most common human maladies. It may range from mild to sharp and severe. Most persons occasionally experience headaches, but in a small percentage of cases it is a symptom of a neurologic emergency.

Etiology

Etiologies of headache include:

1. Vascular—migraine, cluster, toxic (e.g., fever, alcohol, hypoxia)
2. Muscle contraction (tension)
3. Traction and inflammatory—head trauma, subarachnoid hemorrhage, CVA, tumor, hypertension, meningitis, diseases of the eye, intracranial thrombophlebitis, temporal arteritis
4. Neuralgia—trigeminal, glossopharyngeal

Assessment

History

The triage nurse needs to collect an adequate history and physical findings to determine whether the condition is of an emergency nature. Patients with history of sudden onset of severe pain, change in mental status, head trauma, neurologic deficits, nuchal rigidity, or extreme elevation of BP should be categorized as emergent.

A subarachnoid hemorrhage (SAH) classically produces what a patient may describe as "the worst headache of my life." However, migraine, cluster, and meningitis headaches can also be very severe. The location of the headache is important. Unilateral headache is seen with classic migraine and temporal arteritus.

Occipital/neck/frontotemporal headaches are seen with tension and hypertension. A frontal/facial headache suggests sinusitis or trigeminal neuralgia. Headaches that are well-localized initially may indicate a mass lesion. Generalized headache can be due to SAH, meningitis, or increased intracranial pressures.

The quality of the headache may vary. Migraines are typically throbbing, whereas tension headaches are often steady or band-like.

Lancinating or boring headaches can be seen with neuralgias or cluster headaches. Timing of headaches can be a clue to diagnosis. Migraines are usually episodic. A SAH will produce a headache of abrupt onset, usually during activity. Trauma will produce a postconcussive headache. Patients who complain they awaken from sleep because of pain and have a worse headache in the morning may have a mass lesion. A tension headache has a gradual onset, is worse at the end of the day, and may last days or months.

Associated features distinguish particular headaches. A migraine may be preceded by an aura. Nausea and vomiting are associated with a migraine or increased intracranial pressure. Fever and a headache are suggestive of meningitis, sinusitis, SAH, or CVA. A stiff neck is seen with SAH or meningitis. Visual symptoms accompany the headaches of temporal arteritis, various eye diseases, and migraines. Patients with cluster headaches usually complain of retroocular pain with ipsilateral lacrimation and nasal discharge. Temporal arteritis, seen predominantly in the elderly, is accompanied by polymyalgia rheumatica and constitutional symptoms. Patients with migraine often have a positive family history and may be taking birth control pills.

Physical Findings

Vital signs - Look for BP and temperature elevations.

Neurologic signs - Perform a Glasgow coma scale, and check for signs of head trauma, nuchal rigidity, or focal neurologic findings.

Diagnostic Tests

X-rays - Sinus films can be done for acute sinusitis (the common belief that chronic sinusitis gives rise to "sinus headaches" has never been proven).

Lumbar puncture - Patients with suspected meningitis should have an immediate spinal tap unless there are focal neurologic findings. If so, treatment would consist of blood cultures, broad-spectrum antibiotics, and a CAT scan.

CAT scan - Patients with a suspected SAH, mass lesion, or stroke should have a CAT scan before a spinal tap is attempted.

Intervention

1. Emergency measures - Patients with deteriorating neurologic status require intervention to support airway, breathing, and circulation (ABCs). Start IV administration of normotonic solution, and administer oxygen by cannula or mask. Place the patient on seizure precautions.
2. BP regulation - Reassess vital signs at frequent intervals. (See "Hypertension" in Chapter 1 for information on hypertensive encephalopathy.)
3. Provide a quiet environment. Attempt to reduce noise and to control the number of interventions to which the patient is subjected.
4. Specific intervention for migraine consists of:
   a. At the onset of migraine, ergotamine at a dosage 2 mg PO is given to cause cerebral vasoconstriction, followed by 1 mg PO every 30 minutes up to 6 mg/day; or dihydroergotamine at 1 mg IM is given, followed by 1 mg every 1 hour up to 3 mg/day.
   b. Use 100% oxygen for 15 minutes.
   c. For well-established migraines place the patient in a quiet, dark corner and administer codeine, 30 mg PO every 4 hours, or meperidine, 75 mg IM as prescribed. Success has been reported with use of low-dose phenothiazines, such as thorazine, 5–10 mg IV.
   d. Preventative therapy is indicated when there are 3 or more attacks/month. The drug of choice is propranolol, 20 mg PO qid to start. Other drugs include amitriptyline, methysergide, phenelzine, clonidine, and Fiorinal. Birth control pills should be discontinued.
5. Cluster - Vascular headache, which occurs primarily during sleep, is treated with 100% oxygen for 15 minutes. If headache is well established, drug treatment is identical with that used for migraine.
6. Tension - Onset is gradual and may be accompanied by nausea or dizziness. These headaches are also known as muscle contraction headaches. Instruct the patient to use massage, a heating pad, and a mild analgesic (aspirin or acetaminophen). A muscle relaxant (e.g., ben-

zodiazepine) may be prescribed. If the headache is chronic and associated with depression, a psychiatric consult or a referral to mental hygiene counselling is indicated.

ED Discharge Planning

Patients in whom the headache is a symptom of a severe or life-threatening condition require admission. Patients who do not respond to treatment and those requiring further diagnostic evaluation and monitoring should be admitted.

Instructions to patients should include:

1. Information on the actions and precautions concerning medications
2. Direction on the use of ergotamine which should be taken at the onset of pain
3. Relaxation therapy, biofeedback, exercise programs, psychotherapy, and stress reduction measures (warm bath, massage) which may reduce the frequency and severity of attacks
4. Referral of the patient to an outpatient department or private physician for follow-up

SUGGESTED READINGS

Coma—The Unconscious Patient

Henneman EA. Brain resuscitation. Heart Lung 1986;15:3–11.

Hinkle JL. Treating traumatic coma. Am J Nurs 1986;86:551–556.

Scherer P. Assessment: the logic of coma. Am J Nurs 1986;86:542–550.

Seizures

Bean SC. Convulsions. Primary Care 1986;13:77–83.

Callanan M. Epilepsy: putting the patient back in control. RN 1988:48–56.

Friedman D. Taking the scare out of caring for seizure patients. Nursing 1988;18:52–56.

Santilli N, Sierzant TL. Advances in the treatment of epilepsy. J Neurosci Nurs 1987; 19:141–155.

Stern L. Could you have foreseen this seizure? RN 1984:43–44.

Cerebral Ischemia and Stroke

Dean JM, Rogers MC. Cerebrovascular disease. In: Shoemaker WC, Thompson WL, Holbrook PR. Textbook of critical care. Philadelphia: WB Saunders, 1984:961–968.

Goetter W. Nursing diagnosis and interventions with the acute stroke patient. Nurs Clin North Am 1986;21:309–319.

Grotta JC. Current medical and surgical therapy for cerebrovascular disease. N Engl J Med 1987;317:1505–1516.

Hahn K. Left vs right, what difference side makes in stroke. Nursing 1987;17:44–47.

Wald ME. Cerebral thrombosis: assessment and nursing management of the acute phase. J Neurosci Nurs 1986;18:36–38.

Spinal Cord Compression

Arsenault L. Metastatic cancer and the nervous system. Focus Crit Care 1984;11:39–47.

Chernecky CC, Ramsey PW, Kline PM. Spinal cord compression. In: Critical nursing of the client with cancer. Norwalk: Appleton-Century-Crofts, 1984:195–201.

Wilkowski J. Spinal cord compression: an oncologic emergency. J Emerg Nurs 1986; 12:9–12.

Headache

Jenkins JL, Loscalzo J. Manual of emergency medicine: diagnosis and treatment. Boston: Little, Brown, 1986:135–141.

Saper JR. Headaches. In: Rakel RE, ed. Conn's current therapy. Philadelphia: WB Saunders, 1989:796–802.

Chapter 4

TRAUMA

MULTIPLE TRAUMA

The patient with multiple injuries calls upon the ED* staff and trauma team (if one exists) to function at peak efficiency with a rapid, well-organized approach.

Trauma is the third leading cause of death in the United States and is the leading cause of death in children.

Trauma care must be both rapid and definitive. It is estimated that 10–50% of trauma deaths may be preventable with improved response time and prompt vigorous treatment.

Assessment

The ED nurse is commonly responsible for the initial assessment and triage of the trauma victim. When notification of the patient's arrival has been received, the nurse should summon help and then meet the patient at the ambulance entrance. The initial assessment should begin as the patient is brought from the ambulance. An initial assessment is a rapid review of the patient's ABCs (airway, breathing, and circulation).

Physical Findings
Airway - Check for airway patency, presence of respirations, risk of airway
   obstruction from a foreign body, blood, vomitus, etc.
Breathing - Check the rate and quality of respirations and the use of accessory muscles for breathing.
Circulation - Check the circulation by palpating carotid or femoral pulses,
   noting rate, quality, and regularity. Note signs of shock: moist, cool,
   palid skin. Survey the patient quickly for hemorrhage.

---

*See "Appendix A" for definition of common abbreviations used in the text.

Level of consciousness should be included in the initial trauma assessment and can begin with the patient's response to the nurse's questions concerning the presence of pain, detail of the accident, etc.

Patients with absent or inadequate pulse, impaired breathing or who are hemorrhaging require that the nurse begin resuscitative efforts and assemble the ED team. CPR is initiated for absent pulse and/or breathing, and direct pressure is applied to bleeding wounds. After the assessment of ABCs, the nurse should make a head-to-toe assessment, observing for deviations from normal. While this assessment is being conducted, be alert for changes in the ABCs and behavior changes that may indicate hypoxia and shock. A systematic head-to-toe assessment should include:

Head and neck - Ensure a patent airway. Check the patient's pupils (use Glasgow coma scale), and look for oral bleeding, swelling, vomitus, and neck asymmetry that may endanger the airway. Check ear and nose bleeding and drainage. Palpate the head for depressions, bleeding, glass, etc. Carefully palpate the cervical spine for pain, and keep the cervical spine immobilized until cleared by x-ray. Assess for deviation of the trachea from midline.

Chest - Observe for symmetry and motion of the chest wall. Assess for signs of injury: petechiae, bruises, contusions, pain, deformity of ribs, clavicle, and vertebrae, SC emphysema. Auscultate bilaterally for breath sounds.

Abdomen and pelvis - Question the patient about abdominal pain. Gently palpate for tenderness: localized or rebound. Observe for symmetry, bruising, wounds, etc.

Extremities - Examine for position, deformity, and signs of external injury. Question the patient about pain; ask the patient to move each extremity. Assess for presence and quality of peripheral pulses.

History

Information may be obtained from family, friends, or accompanying police. It should include details of the accident: location of patient, force and direction of impact, and patient's condition and treatment delivered at the scene. Ask the patient and/or family about past or current illnesses, use of medication, and allergies.

Trauma is a crisis for both the patient and the family. Separation, pain, powerlessness, and lack of information, in addition to examination and diagnostic procedures, compound the emotional impact of the injury. Patients exhibit a wide range of responses to the crisis, including withdrawal, denial, regression, anger, and emotional behavior. The ED nurse's communication with the patient and family can help to lessen the psychologic effects of trauma. From the time the patient enters the ED, talk with him or her as a person, not as an injury. Providing comfort measures, hand holding, calling the patient by name, and keeping the patient covered and warm have a beneficial effect. Lessening the number of unanticipated events will improve the patient's ability to cope. Keep the patient informed about procedures that will be performed. When telling the patient about an x-ray, be sure to include that he or she will be moved onto a hard table and will be alone in the room for a short period of time. Keep the family up to date on the patient's condition, and attempt to prepare them for the degree of the patient's injury. Let the physician know that family and/or friends are waiting. Make provisions for the family to see the patient, even if briefly, as soon as the situation permits.

Diagnostic Tests

Radiologic examination - The optimum situation is to have x-ray capabilities in the ED so that interruption of assessment and intervention by x-ray are minimal. Use of an x-ray suite outside of the ED necessitates reevaluation of the treatment plan, with ongoing monitoring and support equipment close at hand. Unstable patients must be attended at all times while undergoing radiography.

Cervical spine x-ray - In patients with a high risk of cervical spinal injury a lateral film of the cervical spine, visualizing all seven cervical vertebrae, must be taken as soon as possible. The cervical spine films should be taken with the patient on the stretcher in the ED unless the patient is stable and can be transported easily to the x-ray area.

CBC - Send for a CBC stat, with a sample retained for spinning an immediate Hct in the ED. When evaluating the spun Hct, remember that in the face of acute blood loss the Hct may not fall initially until equilibration has occurred. Also remember that the rate at which the Hct falls is a function of the amount of fluid administered.

Type and hold - A tube of blood, labelled appropriately and signed by the person drawing it, should be sent immediately to the blood bank for type and hold. Should blood transfusion be necessary on an emergent basis "type-specific" blood can be obtained within minutes and is preferable to cross-matched blood.

ECG - A 12-lead ECG should be performed. Patients with blunt chest trauma may sustain a myocardial contusion. All patients should have continuous ECG monitoring.

SMA - Chemistry values need to be closely monitored because altered fluid volumes, IV fluids, GI losses, blood administration, and renal functioning have significant effects on electrolytes. Collect blood sample from site as far from IV as possible and send stat.

Coagulation studies - Include PT, PTT, and platelet count. Coagulopathy is a common complication of multiple trauma and massive transfusions. Studies should be repeated following the transfusion of 6–10 units of blood.

Gastric lavage - A nasogastric tube may be inserted if there is no suspicion of basilar skull fracture. Test the aspirant for blood. Attach to low suction to decompress the stomach and prevent aspiration.

Urine - A routine urinalysis and a stat Chemstrip in the ED for hematuria should be done as soon as possible. If condition permits, have the patient void. A Foley catheter can be inserted if there is no suspicion of urethral injury (blood at the meatus).

Multiple trauma victims are categorized as emergent and require ongoing nursing assessment for the following:

1. Ineffective airway clearance from obstruction and secretions
2. Ineffective breathing pattern from injury, pain, and anxiety
3. Decreased cardiac output from alteration in rate, rhythm, afterload, preload, or conduction
4. Alteration in comfort from physical and psychologic injury
5. Alteration in fluid volume from blood and/or fluid loss and IV fluid administration
6. Impaired tissue perfusion from fluid deficit and vascular damage

Intervention

1. Airway - All trauma patients should receive supplemental oxygen which can be given by nasal prongs or mask. Before cervical spine x-rays are obtained, all methods of airway management must be done with the head in "neutral" position, supported by sandbags about the head and tape over the forehead or by a semirigid cervical collar. Although explaining the importance of neck immobility to the patient is indicated, relying on the patient's voluntary cooperation is not satisfactory. Until spinal injury can be ruled out, the usual method of hyperextension and oral intubation is contraindicated. If airway control is necessary before cervical spine films can be taken, the following approaches can be utilized:

    a. Jaw thrust and/or lift - The tongue may be cleared from the back of the pharynx by bringing the jaw anteriorly either by "lifting" it by lifting the chin or by "thrusting" it forward by pushing from behind the angles of the mandible. This is a temporary maneuver and will require two staff members if the patient is to be ventilated by a bag/mask device or for suctioning. It is not useful to protect the airway from blood or vomitus.

    b. Blind nasotracheal intubation - This is performed without hyperextending the neck by passing a tube blindly through the nose into the trachea. Provide supplemental oxygen and suction as needed.

    c. Cricothyrotomy and/or tracheostomy - If airway protection and control are necessary before spinal films can be obtained or if orofacial anatomy is distorted or obscured by hemorrhage, a direct surgical approach to the airway is indicated. A cricothyrotomy is performed by making a surgical opening through the cricothyroid membrane. The opening can be enlarged to enable the insertion of a small tracheostomy tube. Complications of a tracheostomy performed in the ED under less-than-optimal conditions include bleeding and injury to muscles, thyroid gland, and neck vessels. Cervical spine precautions, if in effect, may further complicate the procedure. After the procedure, secure the tube with tracheostomy tape, dress the wound, inflate the cuff, and ascultate the lungs.

2. Breathing - Many processes may interfere with ventilation despite a satisfactory airway. As previously mentioned, all trauma patients should have supplemental oxygen. Nursing assessment of breathing includes determination of rate, presence of an abnormal breathing pattern (tachypnea, Cheyne-Stokes respiration, etc.), respiratory effort, and lung sounds, in conjunction with results of ABG analysis. Patients should be on continuous cardiac monitoring, since arrhythmias, including PVCs and bradycardia, may be indicative of hypoxia. Injuries that may compromise breathing and reduce gas exchange include:

   a. Tracheobronchial tear - This may result from either penetrating or blunt (deceleration or crush) injury. In its most serious form it is manifested by subcutaneous air in the neck or upper chest, as well as ventilatory insufficiency with massive pneumothorax and a persistent air leak from the lung. Anticipate that this patient may require immediate transport to the OR for bronchoscopy and surgical repair.

   b. Tension pneumothorax - This arises when air accumulates in the pleural space at greater than atmospheric pressure (see "Pneumothorax" in Chapter 2 for a further discussion). The physician may elect to decompress the pleural cavity quickly by inserting a needle or small catheter into the involved hemithorax. The needle may be connected to IV tubing, and the tubing may be placed under water until a formal tube thoracostomy can be performed.

   c. Open pneumothorax and/or sucking chect wound - When an opening is created in the chest wall, air may move in and out, producing a "sucking" wound. If all the air does not escape, a tension pneumothorax may develop. If the opening is sufficiently large, e.g., as occurs from a close-range shotgun blast, air during respiration may move through the chest wall opening rather than through the normal upper airway. Examination reveals a patient with a penetrating chest wound, with the sound of air being sucked into the chest during inspiration and respiratory distress. Immediate therapeutic intervention consists of covering the opening with an occlusive Vaseline gauze dressing. Frequent monitoring of the airway, breathing, and circulation is needed. As soon as possible a tube thoracostomy should be performed to reexpand the lung.

d. Flail chest - A flail chest exists when a significant portion of the chest wall is functionally detached. This occurs with multiple rib fractures or detachment of the sternum. During inspiration, the "flail" segment moves "paradoxically" inward as the normal chest wall expands outward. The segment, which may be located in the posterior as well as the anterior chest, is commonly accompanied by pulmonary contusion and may result in hypoventilation. After locating of the flail segment, assess the patient for the presence of rapid, shallow respirations, cyanosis, and tachycardia. In addition to providing for high oxygen concentration, pulmonary toilet, and pain management, therapeutic intervention centers around measures to stabilize the chest wall. If ventilatory insufficiency exists, medical management may include endotracheal intubation and placement on a volume ventilator (internal splinting) until the flail segment stabilizes and the patient can ventilate adequately without assistance. Nursing care of a patient with flail chest will be directed toward promoting airway clearance, maximizing gas exchange and pain control.

3. Circulation and fluid balance - Assessment for adequacy of cardiac output and tissue perfusion includes frequent monitoring of the following:

a. Cardiac rate and rhythm - Some degree of tachycardia is to be expected as a response to physical and emotional stress. Heart rates over 120/min will have a negative effect on cardiac output and may indicate circulatory shock. Bradycardia may be seen in patients who take medications such as digoxin or propranolol (Inderal) but may be indicative of severe hypoxia and impending cardiopulmonary failure.

b. BP - The patient's BP should be evaluated in light of the patient's normal pressure and in conjunction with hourly urine, skin condition, and mental status evaluation. In patients with multiple trauma, shock is most often hypovolemic in nature. A loss in blood volume of more than 30% (blood volume is approximately 7% of the body weight in kilograms or 5 liters in a 70-Kg man) may be manifested by a drop in BP and by tachycardia, tachypnea, flat neck veins, low central venous pressure, metabolic acidosis, and/or decreased urine output. When external hemorrhage is present, direct pressure should be applied. Clamps or tourniquets should be avoided in the ED.

4. MAST suit - The MAST suit is an inflatable suit that, when placed on the patient and inflated, is believed to increase peripheral resistance, thereby causing an increase in cardiac output and BP. The suit also acts to minimize bleeding and stabilize fractures (see Chapter 16 for

further details). Use of the MAST suit is contraindicated in pulmonary edema, pregnancy, and evisceration of abdominal contents. Once the desired effect of increased BP and stabilization of vital functions has been achieved, the MAST suit can be slowly deflated. This should be done first with gradual deflation of the abdominal compartment, and then, if the patient's BP remains stable, the leg sections may be deflated one at a time. If the BP falls by 5–10 mm Hg or more, the garment should be reinflated.

5. Fluid administration - Two large-bore (12–14-gauge) IV lines should routinely be started. Take the opportunity to draw blood for type and hold, when the IV is started. Crystalloid solutions, either NS or Ringer's lactate, are the usual choice. If the patient shows signs of hypovolemia, the initial fluid should be 2000 cc rapidly administered. This may be followed by colloid solutions or blood. Type-specific blood should be available within 5 minutes, when needed. Warming of rapidly administered blood and IV fluids is indicated to prevent hypothermia and cardiac arrhythmias. See "Shock" in Chapter 1 for detail of management of hypovolemic shock. An accurate intake and output record is essential. Although shock in the trauma victim usually occurs as a result of volume loss, some patients suffering blunt or penetrating chest trauma may present with hypotension and congestion of the central circulation as manifested by elevated venous pressure and distended neck veins. This situation may be the result of pericardial tamponade or tension pneumothorax.

   a. Tension pneumothorax - (See the earlier discussion of "Tension Pneumothorax" in Chapter 2.)

   b. Pericardial tamponade - Tamponade develops when there is rapid accumulation of blood or effusion within the confines of the pericardial sac, resulting in compression of the heart and decreased cardiac output. (See "Pericarditis" in Chapter 9 for a further discussion of tamponade.) Pericardial tamponade should be suspected in patients with a history of steering wheel percussion, bruised sternum or severe left chest injury, and fractures. Assess the patient for decreased cardiac output including distended neck veins, decreased BP, and diminished heart sounds (Beck's triad) and pulsus paradoxus (fall in BP of 10 mm Hg or more during inspiration). Therapeutic intervention includes fluid and oxygen administration, a high Fowler's position if the patient's condition permits, and a pericardiocentesis. To perform a pericardiocentesis the physician will insert a large-bore needle (with the patient under local anesthesia) between the xiphoid and the lower costal margin, directing the needle toward the midclavicle. Fluid and/or blood is obtained once the parietal pericardium is entered. To locate the pericardial surface and avoid entering or injuring the myocardium, the pericardiocentesis needle is connected to the V lead of an ECG by an alligator clip. When the myocardium is touched, the ECG shows a current of injury pattern. If the tamponade is severe or recurring and pericardiocentesis is required, a chest exploration and repair should be considered.

c. Myocardial infarction - Infarction may precede or result from trauma, and the patient may present in cardiogenic shock. See "Shock" and "Myocardial Infarction" in Chapter 1 for discussions of cardiogenic shock.

6. Infection - One of the major causes of death in trauma patients is sepsis. The number and speed with which invasive procedures are performed puts the patient at risk of infection. The ED nurse is in a position to monitor and set standards for infection control practices. A broad-spectrum antibiotic may be started while the patient is in the ED, and tetanus therapy may be given according to the patient's history.

ED Discharge Planning

After all injuries are initially identified and vital functions are stabilized, the trauma patient requires frequent reassessment and planned intervention. The level of care and frequency of observation required will determine whether the patient is admitted to a surgical care unit or intensive care area.

HEAD TRAUMA

Head trauma accounts for approximately one-fourth of all trauma deaths. Head injury can result from direct or indirect impact that causes the brain to move forward, rebound backward, or rotate against the rigid, irregular surface of the skull. Most frequently seen in motor vehicle accidents, head trauma is also a common finding following falls, seizures, intoxication, and physical assault. Patients may present with serious brain injury without any physical signs of head injury (e.g., a child who has been shaken violently).

Classifications

1. Concussion - Concussion implies head injury without a significant anatomical brain lesion. Temporary loss of consciousness can occur, as can amnesia. The patient may complain of headache, dizziness, or nausea, but the patient should be without any neurologic deficits.
2. Contusion - Contusion implies a more significant degree of trauma.

Part of the brain is bruised, and focal neurologic deficits may be seen.
3. Intracranial hemorrhage
   a. Epidural hematoma - Epidural bleeding is usually due to a tear in the miningeal artery or, less commonly, in a large sinus, causing bleeding between the skull and the dura mater. The typical course is unconsciousness, followed by a lucid period lasting a few hours to days, followed by a secondary depression of consciousness. In 75% of cases a fracture is found on skull series. Epidural hematoma is uncommonly associated with seizures.
   b. Subdural hematoma - Subdural hematoma is caused by rupture of small vessels bridging the subdural space, which causes immediate, direct pressure on the brain. It occurs more commonly in the elderly (due to cerebral atrophy, which stretches the veins) and in patients on anticoagulants. The clinical course is often slower in onset than that of an epidural hematoma, and patients may or may not regain consciousness with a lucid interval.
   c. Subarachnoid hemorrhage - Subarachnoid bleeding can result in bloody CSF, but because of the possibility of brainstem herniation, lumbar puncture is ofen omitted. The clinical picture frequently includes headache, nuchal rigidity, deteriorating level of consciousness, seizures, and hemiparesis.
4. Brain hemorrhage or laceration - Intracerebral bleeding is often related to cerebral contusions and laceration. The increasing intracranial pressure results in a deteriorating level of consciousness and ipsilateral dilated pupil. Further alterations in vital signs, respirations, and pupil response will be seen if increased pressure results in tentorial herniation.
5. Impalement or missile injury - Degree and type of injury depend on the direction, size, shape, and velocity of the missile or bullet.

Assessment

As soon as the patient's basic ABCs (airway, breathing and circulation) are secured, the ED nurse should carefully assess the level of consciousness of any patient with potential head injury. Continue to assess the patient for signs of concomitant injury (see under "Multiple Trauma"). All examinations of a patient with suspected head injury must be done with the head and neck in fixed neutral position until cervical spine x-rays are taken and read.

History
Observers on the scene, ambulance personnel, and the patient (if conscious) should be questioned as to the causes of head trauma. It is particularly important to inquire about any loss of consciousness or seizure activ-

ity. Recent use of drugs or alcohol should be documented whenever possible. A past medical history that includes chronic illnesses, medication, and allergies should be obtained. Asking the conscious patient about events surrounding the accident may be helpful in eliciting memory deficits.

Physical Findings

Vital signs - Frequent reassessment of vital signs is essential in patients with head trauma. Check the patient's respiratory rate and pattern. An altered respiratory pattern may be indicative of brain injury. Tachycardia, particularly when seen with hypotension, is characteristic of hypovolemia and may indicate hemorrhage outside the nervous system. A combination of hypertension and bradycardia (Cushing's sign) is associated with increasing intracranial pressure. Temperature should be a regular part of the assessment of patients with altered mental status. Loss of thermoregulation (especially hyperthermia) may be seen as a late sign of increased intracranial pressure and must be controlled because it increases the metabolic rate.

Glasgow coma scale (GCS) - The GCS scores a patient's neurologic function. The system rates the best response in three areas as follows:

Glasgow Coma Scale (GCS)

1. Best verbal response
   None 1
   Incomprehensive sounds 2
   Inappropriate words 3
   Confused 4
   Oriented 5
2. Eyes open
   None 1
   To pain 2
   To speech 3
   Spontaneously 4
3. Best motor response
   None 1
   Abnormal extension*...2
   Abnormal flexion⁺...3
   Withdrawal...4
   Localized..5
   Obeys commands 6
Total score (maximum)..15

*Abnormal flexion - decorticate rigidity and/or posture.
⁺Abnormal extension - decerebrate rigidity and/or posture.

Patients with a GCS of ≥11 generally do well; patients with a score of ≤7 often do poorly.

Neurologic assessment - A full and careful neurologic examination is indicated, with frequent reassessment for potential changes. In addition to those already mentioned, the following should be included in assessment of a patient with head trauma:

Pupillary reactions - Pupils normally round, equal, and reactive to light average 2–4 mm in diameter and are an excellent indicator of cerebral dysfunction. Changes in pupil size and reaction to light may indicate a dangerous increase in intracranial pressure and must be brought to the immediate attention of the physician.

Motor and sensory dysfunction - Progressive muscle weakness and loss of temperature and sensory awareness should all be brought to the physician's attention.

Drainage from ear or nose - Bloody drainage can be tested for CSF by eliciting a halo sign. When fluid is placed on filter paper, a dark stain surrounded by a lighter ring or halo indicates the presence of CSF. Clear drainage should be tested for glucose with a Dextrostix. A positive test indicates a CSF leak.

Battle's sign - Ecchymosis of the mastoid process of the temporal bone and ecchymosis of the periorbital areas, called raccoon's eyes, are indicative of basal skull fractures.

Diagnostic Tests

Radiologic examination - Stat portable cervical spine x-rays should be obtained if there is any question of cervical trauma.

CAT scan - A CAT scan may be obtained on a stat basis for patients showing the following results:

1. A GCS score that falls by 2 or more points while the patient is in the ED
2. Signs of herniation
3. Multiple injuries in a patient who cannot be transferred
4. Unstable spinal injuries
5. Penetrating skull trauma
6. Focal neurologic deficits

(Transporting the head-injured patient for CAT scan presents a potential risk. The CAT scan suite must be set up so that emergency treatment can be instituted, if necessary. Frequent assessment for deterioration in neurologic status must be incorporated into the CAT scan process.)

CBC - A stat spun Hct and a platelet count are indicated. A significant

drop in Hct is an indication of injury and bleeding outside the CNS.
SMA - Check serum electrolytes. A stat Dextrostix for blood sugar is indicated for all patients with altered level of consciousness.
ABGs - A blood gas analysis is obtained if there is any question as to respiratory compromise or electrolyte imbalance.
Serum alcohol and drug levels - These levels should be determined, if clinically indicated.

Intervention

1. Airway - Stabilization of airway is the first priority in the treatment of patients with head injury. In patients who have potential cervical spinal injury, head and neck immobilization has to be maintained until x-ray clearance has been obtained (discussed elsewhere in this chapter). Inability to effectively clear the airway may result in anoxia, hypercapnea, and aspiration. Suction the patient as necessary and provide supplemental oxygen. Suctioning through the nares should not be done until a basal skull and dural tear have been ruled out.
2. Head trauma victims are categorized as emergent. They require frequent nursing assessment for the presence of the following:
   a. Ineffective airway clearance from secretions and vomitus
   b. Ineffective breathing pattern
   c. Alteration in comfort from physical and psychologic injury
   d. Alteration in sensory perception and thought process due to injury and environmental stressors
   e. Impaired cerebral tissue perfusion from brain swelling
3. Fluid administration - An IV line should be started; the internal jugular should be avoided, as its use may impair venous return. Hypotonic crystalloid (one- quarter to one-half NS) should be administered slowly unless the patient is in shock and requires volume replacement. Patients with head trauma should be kept on the "dry" side in order to prevent edema. Fluids should be delivered via a microdrip or IV pump to prevent excess fluid administration. It is necessary to maintain an intake and output record.
4. Seizures - Provide as much rest and quiet as the situation permits. Observe the patient for seizures, and institute seizure precautions (injury, airway, and aspiration protection). Seizures may be treated with phenytoin (Dilantin), 15 mg/Kg total dose, with no more than 50 mg/min given. Dilantin can only be administered in NS, and rapid administration may cause hypotension. Patients should have constant ECG and BP monitoring while receiving IV phenytoin.
5. Medication - Patients with altered mental status should receive 1 ampule (25 gm) of 50% dextrose and 1 ampule (2 mg) of naloxone (Narcan). Thiamine, 100 mg IM should be administered before glu-

cose is given to patients with a history of alcohol abuse. Sedation or neuromuscular paralysis with agents such as pancuronium may be necessary in order to obtain an x-ray or CAT scan, but it should be used with caution.

6. Control of cerebral edema - Brain edema causes increased intracranial pressure, which decreases cerebral perfusion and results in ischemia and further damage to cerebral tissue. The development of herniation is a true emergency, and members of the neurosurgery staff should be contacted stat. Treatment protocol to decrease cerebral edema in severe head injury includes the following steps:
   a. Limit fluid intake.
   b. Administer mannitol, 1–2 gm/Kg (always place a Foley catheter).
   c. Administrater dexamethasone, 4–10 mg IV (with Maalox and Tagamet to prevent gastric irritation).
   d. Hyperventilate the patient to maintain pCO_2 at 25–30 mm Hg. (Mild hypocapnea causes vasoconstriction and reduces intracranial pressure).
   e. Elevate the head of the bed to 30°.
   The nurse needs to be aware of what aspects of care cause an elevation of intracranial pressure, so nursing care can be modified accordingly. The following increase intracranial pressure and, therefore, should be avoided:
   a. Stimulation of pain response (frequently performed to assess level of consciousness)
   b. Elevated temperature
   c. Valsalva maneuver
   d. Suctioning
   e. Extreme flexion or rotation of head and neck
   f. Loud noises
   g. Impairment of cerebral venous return (i.e., with IV lines)
7. Scalp wounds - After the wound has been shaved and well irrigated, it should be closed with two layers of sutures. Prophylaxis with diphtheria-tetanus vaccine should be given as needed.
8. Infection - Antibiotic prophylaxis may be used with patients with a fracture through the nose or sinus, since meningitis is a possible complication.

ED Discharge Planning and Instructions

Patients with loss of consciousness of 5 minutes or more are generally admitted for 24-hour observation. Patients with more severe head trauma require frequent assessment of neurologic and vital signs for prevention, early recognition, and prompt treatment of complications. It should be noted that patients with head injury may require prolonged rehabilitation and the post-ED care plan should address:

1. Motor dysfunction and impaired mobility
2. Intellectual and sensory impairment
3. Nutritional needs
4. Skin integrity
5. Alteration in bladder and bowel elimination
6. Personality changes and communication problems
7. Family support

Patients who have suffered minor head injury may be discharged to a family member and/or a friend. The patient needs to be observed for 24 hours for possible aftermath of head trauma. A family member or friend should be given written instructions on what to look for and should return the patient to the ED should the patient show any of the following:

1. Behavior changes, i.e., confusion, irritability, or difficulty awakening from sleep (patient should be checked every 2 hours)
2. Prolonged or severe headache
3. Nausea and vomiting lasting over 2 hours

Instruct the patient not to drive a car, operate machinery, or drink alcohol for a minimum of 24 hours.

SPINAL CORD INJURY

Spinal cord injury (SCI) usually occurs in healthy young males and is most often associated with auto accidents, falls, personal assaults, football, and water sports. About 10–15% of patients with severe head injury from falls or vehicular accidents will have an associated cervical spinal injury. All trauma victims should be approached with a high index of suspicion concerning SCI. Patients with suspected SCI should be transported on a splint board, with a firm collar and sandbags.

Neurologic Syndromes

1. Complete lesions are those with no evidence of motor or sensory function. These patients have an extremely poor prognosis for significant return of useful motor function.
2. Partial lesions are those with any evidence of motor or sensory function. These patients may have return of significant motor function.
   a. Quadriplegia - Patients presenting with quadriplegia should have

careful attention paid to their vital signs, especially temperature and BP. Because of sudden changes in sympathetic-parasympathetic control mechanisms, spinal shock (secondary to peripheral vasodilation) and inability to regulate central core temperature may result. In high cervical lesions, severe bradycardia and even cardiac standstill can result.

b. Paraplegia - Although the systemic manifestations of spinal cord injury are less frequent, the patient still needs to be monitored for BP and temperature fluctuations.

c. Conus medullaris syndrome - Sacral anesthesia, paraparesis or paraplegia, and bladder and/or bowel dysfunction are all hallmarks of this lesion.

d. Central cord syndrome - This lesion is characterized by loss of bilateral upper extremity function with relative preservation of lower extremity motor function in patients with cervical cord injuries. This lesion results from disruption of tissue at the center of the cord and the peripheral tissue containing the corticospinal tracts to the lower extremities is spared.

Assessment

A basic trauma assessment should be immediately initiated. Airway stabilization takes precedence and should be performed in such a way as to prevent further injury to the spine (see "Multiple Trauma" in this chapter). Obtain a history of the accident, and question the patient about neck and back pain, numbness, tingling, and sensation in extremities. Consider alcohol or drug intoxication.

Physical Findings

Vital signs - Frequent BP and heart rate determinations are required. Patients with SCI can be hypotensive due to the effect of injury on the sympathetic nervous system. Other indicators of circulatory perfusion, including level of consciousness and urinary output, need to be regularly assessed.

Breathing - With high cervical spinal fractures some compromise of respirations is common, since the phrenic nerve arises at C3–5. Frequent monitoring of rate, tidal volume, ABGs, abdominal breathing, and ability to cough and clear the airway will aid in determining whether ventilatory support is necessary.

Signs of cervical injury - Signs of cervical injury include:

a. Flaccid areflexia (quadriplegia, paraplegia, bilateral upper extremity weakness)

b. Flaccid rectal sphincter

c. Flexion in upper extremities with absent extension
d. Decreased sensation below clavicles
e. Diaphragmatic breathing
f. Priapism

Diagnostic Tests

X-ray - Patients who cannot be moved must have portable lateral spine films. Patients should not be moved until the cervical spine x-rays are read. All seven cervical vertebrae must be visualized, which may require a member of the ED staff to use manual traction to pull the patient's arms toward his or her feet. If the patient can be moved, AP and lateral as well as an open mouth view of the cervical spine should be obtained. In an emergency the patient can be turned by "log rolling."

Intervention

1. After cervical spine x-ray and airway stabilization, immediate efforts are made to reduce and stabilize the bony injury. This may be accomplished by placement of Gardner-Wells tongs with 5–10 pounds of cervical traction. Later placement of external halo brace stabilization is becoming increasingly popular, as this allows for mobilization of the patient.
2. Patients with thoracic and lumbar injuries may require operative stabilization following ED evaluation and treatment.
3. Airway - With cervical spinal injury the patients may not be able to clear their airway, and periodic suctioning may be necessary. A nasogastric tube should be inserted to avoid vomiting with possible aspiration. Since ventilatory support is frequently required, suction, intubation equipment, oxygen, and a bag/mask device must be close at hand. When intubation is attempted, the neck must not be hyperextended. Occasionally, a surgical airway must be placed by using cricothyrotomy and a cuffed tracheostomy tube.
4. Cardiovascular instability - Due to loss of sympathetic innervation the effects of the vagus are dominant. Bradycardia and hypotension may require treatment with atropine, 0.5–1 mg IV, and a vasopressor such as dopamine. Patients with loss of sensory and motor control below the level of injury will:
   a. Have decreased ability to regulate body temperature and should be covered to prevent excess heat loss.
   b. Have loss of bladder control with catheterization necessary to prevent distention.
   c. Require "log rolling" or lifting by three or more staff members for turning and moving from stretcher to bed.

ED Discharge Planning

Patients with spinal fractures and SCI will be admitted, and those with cervical SCI will need intensive or specialized neurologic care because of the high potential for respiratory and circulatory insufficiency. Prevention of complications and establishing short-term rehabilitation goals should begin with admission of the patient.

Families of patients with possible SCI are under particular stress during the initial evaluation period. Frequently, diagnostic procedures and clinical examination are lengthy, and prognosis is uncertain. Provide families with clear but brief explanations of what is known of the patient's condition up to that point. Most important is to provide an opportunity for the family to see or speak with the patient and to help them to be supportive to the patient and to each other.

Stable patients with SCI may be transferred to a specialty center if one exists. Unstable patients and those with other serious injuries must be admitted and stabilized before transfer is attempted.

CHEST TRAUMA

The majority of serious chest injuries due to blunt trauma occur in motor vehicle accidents and falls. Gunshot wounds and stabbings account for the majority of penetrating chest injuries.

Assessment

Blunt and penetrating chest injuries are categorized as emergent. Assessment of the patient's ABCs (airway, breathing, and circulation) is started immediately (see "Multiple Trauma" in this chapter).

Physical Findings
Vital signs - Note BP, regularity, rate, and quality of pulse. A rapid, thready pulse and a low or declining BP may be indicative of shock. When obtaining a history, include usual BP reading and the use of antihypertensive and cardiac medications.
Neck - Check to see that the trachea is in midline position. Observe for neck vein distention, and palpate for fine air bubbles, which denotes SC emphysema.
Chest - Examine for areas of bruising, signs of steering wheel impact, penetrating wounds, bleeding, asymmetry of chest movement, and paradoxical motion of a section of the chest wall (flail chest). With paradoxical motion the detached segment moves inward during inspiration while the rest of the chest expands. Palpate for bony crepitation and

SC emphysema. Auscultate for bilateral breath sounds and muffled heart sounds (cardiac tamponade).

Pain - Question the patient as to the presence of pain at the site of chest injury. An increase of pain with inspiration, becoming more severe with each breath, accompanied by dyspnea or cyanosis may be indicative of a tension pneumothorax.

Complications

Blunt Trauma

Rib fractures - Patients with simple rib fractures (single rib involvement with no underlying injury) have minor injuries and can be treated effectively with rest, local heat, and analgesics. Elderly patients or those with underlying lung disease, multiple rib fractures, pulmonary contusion and hemopneumothorax are more prone to develop complications. These patients should be admitted and treated with vigorous chest physiotherapy, with or without chest tubes. Fractures of the first to third ribs denote that considerable force has been exerted, and they are often associated with other serious intrathoracic injuries, such as major vessel injury. Patients with fracture of the lower (tenth to twelfth) ribs frequently have concurrent liver, spleen, or kidney injury.

Flail chest - Fractures of a series of ribs in more than one location will cause a "flail chest" with a section of ribs having paradoxical motion and respiratory insufficiency. Detachment of the sternum from the ribs can create a "flail sternum" (see "Multiple Trauma" in this chapter).

Pulmonary contusion - Commonly associated with multiple rib fractures and/or flail chest, this is a potentially lethal injury because the resulting contusion can lead to hypoxia, atelectasis, retained secretions, and hypercapnia. Development of rapid, shallow respirations and tachycardia warn of impending respiratory failure. Principles for treatment of flail chest and pulmonary contusion include:

1. Maintaining adequate ventilation and gas exchange by pain control and encouraging deep breathing and coughing.
2. Stabilization of the flail segment by mechanical volume ventilation and PEEP if the patient's pO_2 is low (<60 mm Hg) or the pCO_2 is elevated (>55 mm Hg) on room air.
3. Maintaining careful intake and output. Overhydration worsens the effects of pulmonary contusion and hastens development of shock lung.

Myocardial contusion - This rare but potentially lethal complication should be suspected in any patient with blunt (steering wheel and bicycle handlebar) injury who has severe tenderness of the anterior chest or a sternal fracture. The patient may present with dyspnea, chest pain, and tachycardia. Diagnosis and intervention are similar to those of a myocardial infarction and include:

1. Admission to an ICU
2. Cardiac monitoring for development of arrhythmias
3. Frequent BP determinations, as hypotension and shock may develop if cardiac output declines
4. Administering oxygen and providing for the patient's comfort by pain control and positioning in mid-Fowler's

Ruptured aorta - Rupture of the thoracic aorta is most commonly seen in motor vehicle accidents, with the mechanism of injury being high-speed acceleration-deceleration. A high index of suspicion based on the type and severity of the accident is crucial for an early diagnosis. A widened mediastinum on x-ray, signs of cardiac tamponade, and hypotension are common findings. Rapid initiation of IV fluids and surgical intervention are indicated.

Penetrating Trauma

Simple pneumothorax - As a result of either blunt or penetrating trauma, air may enter the pleural space and cause a pneumothorax. Patients with a 20% or greater pneumothorax will present with pleuritic chest pain, diminished breath sounds and hyperresonance on the affected side, tachycardia, and dyspnea. Administer oxygen, position for maximum ventilation, monitor vital signs, and prepare for closed thoracotomy. A chest tube, size 28–32 French, is commonly inserted in the fourth or fifth intercostal space in the midaxillary line.

Sucking chest wound - A sucking chest wound as from a shotgun wound causes free entry of air into the pleural cavity. If there is no free egress of air out of the chest, increasing positive pressure causes a pneumothorax as well as a shift of mediastinal structures. A patient who is symptomatic needs immediate treatment. As the intrathoracic pressure increases, the patient will develop severe respiratory distress, tachycardia, and cyanosis. Shift or displacement of the trachea to the unaffected side can be seen. Immediate treatment is necessary to prevent a drop in cardiac output and cardiac arrest. Immediate closure of the chest wound by a sterile Vaseline dressing and chest tube insertion are essential.

Hemothorax - Varying amounts of blood may collect in the pleural space from trauma to the chest wall or intrathoracic structures. Massive hemothorax is defined as the loss of between 1.5 and 3 liters of blood in the pleural space and is likely to require surgical intervention. In addition to showing signs of cardiorespiratory distress the patient may develop signs of shock. In addition to the placement of chest tubes, therapeutic intervention includes:

1. Fluid replacement with Ringer's lactate or NS. If blood loss is signifi-

cant, packed cells may be administered and autotransfusion may be considered.

2. Oxygen administration with endotracheal intubation if adequate breathing pattern and gas exchange cannot be maintained.
3. Frequent monitoring of chest tube drainage. In addition to measuring output at least every hour, any sudden increase or stoppage of thoracostomy drainage needs immediate evaluation. Chest tubes should be gently "stripped" or "milked" every 1–2 hours to remove clots that may have formed. The chest drainage device may be connected to wall suction to hasten drainage and reexpansion.

Pericardial tamponade - Although this most commonly results from penetrating injury, blunt trauma may occasionally produce tamponade. (See "Pericarditis" in Chapter 9 and "Pericardial Tamponade" in this chapter for a further discussion.)

Open Chest Thoracotomy
ED thoracotomy is a potentially lifesaving procedure. Patients with penetrating trauma and at least some signs of life at the scene may benefit from emergency thoracotomy. Patients with blunt thoracic trauma generally do not benefit unless they arrive in the ED with obtainable vital signs that then deteriorate. To be prepared to perform open chest thoracotomy the ED will need to have a thoracotomy tray, a knife or saw for cutting cartilage and sternum, and internal defibrillator paddles.

Lower Thoracic Injuries
All penetrating wounds below the nipple should be considered to be thoracoabdominal injuries, and intraabdominal trauma must be considered. Esophageal and tracheobronchial injuries, although not common, should be suspected in lower thoracic trauma.

ED Discharge Planning

All but the most superficial penetrating thoracic injuries and simple rib fractures should be admitted. This should include:

1. Any injury complicated by pneumothorax or hemothorax
2. Multiple rib fractures or "flail chest"
3. Simple rib fractures in an aged patient or one with a history of chronic obstructive lung disease
4. All thoracoabdominal traumatic wounds
5. Severe deceleration injuries

In planning care for a patient with thoracic trauma the following nursing diagnoses should be considered:

1. Ineffective airway clearance
2. Alteration in breathing pattern
3. Impaired gas exchange
4. Fluid volume deficit
5. Decreased cardiac output
6. Alteration in comfort and pain

ED Discharge Instructions
For patients who do not require admission, ED discharge instructions should include:

1. Rest with no lifting or strenuous activity
2. Use of analgesics for pain relief
3. Symptoms to be alert for: sudden pain, shortness of breath, dyspnea, and signs of infection
4. Directions for follow-up care with a private physician or clinic appointment

INTRAABDOMINAL TRAUMA

Description

The abdomen is considered to extend from the fifth intercostal space to the buttock creases. Therefore, a stab wound to the lower chest must also be considered a penetrating wound of the abdomen. Intraabdominal injuries may be due to either blunt or penetrating trauma and may result in extensive blood loss and hypovolemic shock.

High deceleration injuries are the most common causes of pelvic fractures. Fractures of the posterior half of the bony pelvis, including the sacrum, sacroiliac joint, and acetabulum, are often associated with life-threatening hemorrhage, due to their proximity to pelvic vessels. The urinary bladder and urethra are the most frequently injured organs in pelvic fractures. Whereas 70% of pelvic fractures are uncomplicated, the remainder suffer from continued blood loss, multiple organ injuries, and significant morbidity and mortality.

Assessment

A basic trauma assessment should be initiated on arrival in the ED. Note altered level of consciousness or appearance of shock.

History
The time of injury, as well as initial vital signs, physical findings, and treat-

ment in the field should be obtained. In penetrating trauma, information relating to the kind of penetrating object (length of knife, caliber, velocity of bullets, etc.) may be very useful in estimating extent of injury. In blunt trauma, useful information includes distance of fall, position in motor vehicle, use of seat belts, and velocity of injuring force.

Physical Findings

Vital signs - Frequent checks for hypotension, tachycardia, and tachypnea are indicated until the patient is fully examined and deemed stable.

Abdomen - Observe for signs of penetrating injury or ecchymoses or abrasions associated with blunt injury. Clinical manifestations of intra-abdominal injury may include tenderness, guarding or splinting of abdominal wall on palpation, decreased or absent bowel sounds, and pain referred to the shoulder due to phrenic nerve irritation.

Musculoskeletal signs - Tenderness or pain is elicited on compression of the iliac crests and symphysis pubis and with movement of the hips in a fractured pelvis. Inspect for areas of abrasion, contusion, swelling, hematomas, and changes in skin color. Palpate extremities for pain, displacement, crepitus, movement, and decreased or absent pulses. Absent pulses in the setting of trauma constitutes a surgical emergency.

Diagnostic Tests

CBC - Check serial spun Hcts and monitor for a dropping Hct.

Amylase - A high serum amylase suggests pancreatic injury.

Urinalysis - Chemstrip in the ED and send to the laboratory for routine study.

Nasogastric tube - Observe aspirant for blood.

X-rays - Chest, abdominal, and pelvic films are taken to detect free air under the diaphragm, a foreign body, and bony fractures of the pelvis or lower ribs.

IVP - Indicated for gross hematuria and, when possible, prior to surgery to ensure the presence of two functioning kidneys.

Other commonly performed diagnostic tests include a GI series, CAT scan, angiography, and cystogram to detect bladder injury. Foley catheterization is indicated unless there are signs of pelvic fracture or urethral injury. Blood at the meatus is an absolute contraindication to blind insertion of a catheter. A retrograde urethrogram must be done to rule out urethral injury before catheterization in these cases.

Intervention

1. Fluid administration - Potential for hypovolemic shock due to blood loss. The prominent injuries that cause life-threatening hemorrhage are ruptured spleen, liver, or aorta and pelvic fracture with vascular

injury. Assess for signs of shock, and start two large-bore (12- or 14-gauge) IV lines and begin lactated Ringer's solution. Send blood for type and cross-match. If signs of shock are present or the Hct has dropped, blood administration should be started with type-specific blood until cross-matched blood is available. Place IV solution and blood on blood warmer and pump when administering large volumes rapidly. The packed red cells run more rapidly if mixed with 100–200 ml of crystalloid. Transfuse hypotensive patients immediately; it is not unusual for a severely injured patient to require 20–40 units of blood. Apply the MAST suit and inflate leg and abdominal compartments. Besides aiding in treatment of hypotension, the MAST suit temporarily stabilizes the pelvis to reduce further hemorrhage from severe fractures. All x-rays, including IVP and cystogram, can be performed through the trousers. The MAST suit inflated to a pressure of 40–50 mm Hg may be left in place on hemodynamically unstable patients for 12–24 hours. However, they should be deflated every 1–2 hours to permit blood flow to the extremities. (For further details on the use of the MAST suit, see Chapter 16.)

2. Tissue perfusion - Monitoring of BP along with clinical signs of perfusion (level of consciousness, skin temperature, good urine output, absence of cyanosis, capillary refill time of 2 seconds or less) will aid in evaluating the status of fluid and blood replacement. Inability to maintain a BP of 100 mm Hg, a pulse rate of 100/min or more, and a urine output of <30 ml/hr is an indication that fluid replacement is inadequate. Insert a Foley catheter if signs of urethral injury and pelvic fracture are absent. Do not force the catheter. A urology consult is indicated if there is resistance to a Foley insertion. Use a urimeter to monitor hourly urine output.

3. Peritoneal lavage - Diagnostic peritoneal lavage is performed on patients with blunt trauma, in those with penetrating wounds who do not meet the criterion for immediate surgery, and in unconscious patients with multiple trauma. Verify that the bladder and stomach are empty to prevent injury during the procedure. After use of a local anesthetic a peritoneal dialysis or similar type catheter is inserted into the abdomen. One liter of NS is infused into the catheter, and the fluid is aspirated. The fluid is examined for blood; a count of >50–100,000/mm^3 is considered positive. A positive peritoneal lavage is considered an indication for exploratory laparotomy. Stab wounds to the abdomen that appear superficial may be explored in the ED. Emergent exploratory laparotomy is indicated for the following: patients who do not respond to fluid therapy, gunshot wounds, impaled foreign objects, evisceration, physical signs of peritonitis, open pelvic fractures, and blood in the rectum or stomach.

4. Infection - Antibiotics should be started preoperatively for intra-

abdominal contamination. Tetanus therapy should be given for open wounds according to the patient's immunization history.

5. Alteration in comfort - Because narcotics may mask significant diagnostic findings, they are withheld until the patient is fully assessed and the BP is stabilized. Plan patient care and diagnostic procedures to avoid unnecessary movement. Stabilization of pelvic fractures with the MAST suit, a spine board, skeletal traction, or external fixation will decrease pain and pelvic bleeding.

6. Pelvic arteriograms - Indicated in patient with pelvic fractures with severe and prolonged bleeding. Arteriography is useful for both diagnosis and therapy (embolization of the bleeding vessel).

ED Discharge Planning and Instructions

All patients with abdominal injuries, pelvic fractures, or positive physical or laboratory findings should be admitted. Patients with severe pelvic fractures, those who are hemodynamically unstable, and those requiring emergency surgery should be admitted to the ICU for continuous monitoring.

Patients with pelvic fractures will require weeks of bed rest unless an external fixation is done. External fixation and early mobilization may reduce the incidence of complications of immobility, pain, and respiratory distress syndrome from thromboembolism.

Patients with blunt abdominal trauma who show no signs of injury but fall into a high-risk group (elderly, pregnant, history of chronic illness) should be admitted for 24 hours of observation. Patients who are discharged should be reevaluated in 24–48 hours, and discharge instructions should include:

1. No lifting or strenuous activity for a specified time
2. Return to the ED for increased pain, nausea, vomiting, difficult or painful urination, blood in urine or stool, and elevated temperature
3. Use of analgesics

BURNS

According to the Centers for Disease Control statistics, an average of 4,897 persons died in residential fires each year during the period 1978–1984. Fire death rates were highest for young children (under 4 years of age) and the elderly (over 65 years of age). Prevention education should be aimed at increasing the use and testing of home smoke alarms, safe use of home heaters, teaching children not to play with matches, and discouraging people from smoking in bed.

Assessment

Immediate priorities are the same as for any trauma patient: Establish a patent airway, assess for breathing pattern and adequate circulation, and institute treatment as needed. The burn victim may also present with trauma or other serious medical emergency. Resuscitation and treatment of life-threatening injuries take precedence over burn care.

History
The conscious patient should be questioned about the circumstances of the burn injury. A thorough history will aid in the presentation, detection, and treatment of the numerous complications that are a common component of burn injury. Since examination of the airway may initially be negative, ask the patient if he or she was in an open or closed space, the duration of exposure, and the kind of material burning in the fire (e.g., chemicals, plastics). Any history of medical intervention at the scene should be obtained from the patient or the ambulance crew. Past medical history, allergies, previous immunizations (specifically tetanus), and alcohol or drug dependencies are relevant to treatment. Higher mortality and morbidity rates are seen in older burn patients who have chronic illness (e.g., cardiopulmonary, diabetes).

Physical Findings
Vital signs - Observe for signs of airway compromise (laryngeal edema can occur quite early, particularly following a fire in a closed space). Initially take vital signs every 15 minutes. Place BP cuff on nonburned arm; if necessary use a sterile barrier or towel under the cuff. Do not leave the cuff in place between BP determinations. If auscultation is difficult due to edema, a Doppler monitor may be used to obtain a systolic pressure. Monitor carefully for hypotension. Shock secondary to burns is usually a late finding, and a patient with hypotension should be examined for other medical or surgical conditions.

Head and neck - Examine the upper airway for signs of thermal injury, including burns around the mouth and nose, singed nasal hairs, carbonaceous sputum, and hemoptysis. Ask the patient to talk whenever vital signs are taken in order to assess for hoarseness. Listen for stridor or protracted coughing. If airway injury is suspected, the epiglottis and cords should be inspected via direct or indirect laryngoscopy.

Lungs - Listen for rales, rhonchi, or wheezes. Inspect the chest wall for signs of trauma as well as edema or circumferential burn pattern that can lead to chest constriction and decrease air exchange.

Heart - Continuous ECG monitoring is indicated. Although tachycardia is expected, rates above 120/min, frequent atrial premature contractions, and the presence of PVCs may warn of hypoxia.

Skin - Completely undress all seriously burned patients to determine the severity and extent of all burns.

Burn Classification and Assessment (Fig. 4.1)

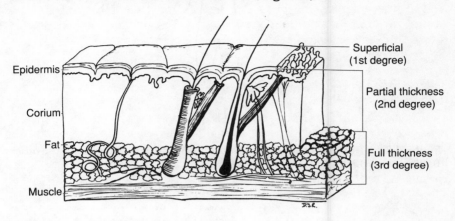

Figure 4.1. Levels of burn injury.

Superficial partial-thickness (first-degree) burn - Involves only the epidermal layers and is typified by a sunburn.

Partial thickness (second-degree) burn - A superficial second-degree burn involves destruction of both the epidermis and the upper dermal layers of the skin. The burn appears pink and is exquisitely tender to the touch, with blistering and oozing typical. A deep second-degree burn that involves the deeper dermal structures will appear dark red to waxy white, is poorly vascularized, and has less sensitivity to pain.

Full-thickness (third-degree) burn - Involves destruction of all skin layers including the SC fat. It appears dry and leathery and may be white or charred with thread-like coagulated veins often visible. It is not painful, and the involved area is without sensation. The term fourth-degree burn is sometimes used to describe involvement of muscle, tendon, or bone. Underestimation of deep partial-thickness and full-thickness burns is not unusual due to the variety and similarity of wound appearances.

Extent of burn - Size is classified as the percentage of total BSA involved. Burned areas of various depths should be listed separately with the percentage of BSA involved. The BSA can be estimated by using the "rule of nines" (see Fig. 4.2) or be determined more accurately by using the Lund-Browder chart (see Fig. 4.3).

Rule of Nines - The "rule of nines" divides the body into areas corresponding to 9% (or multiples of 9%) of the BSA. The perineum is counted as 1%. Smaller burns are evaluated by comparing the

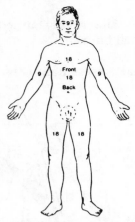

Figure 4.2. "Rule of nines." (From Munster AM. Burn care for the house officer. Baltimore: Williams & Wilkins, 1980.)

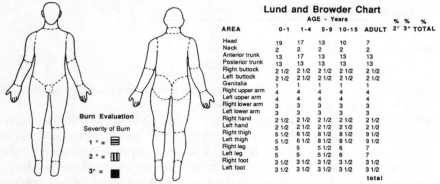

Lund and Browder Chart

AREA	AGE - Years					% 2°	% 3°	% TOTAL
	0-1	1-4	5-9	10-15	ADULT			
Head	19	17	13	10	7			
Neck	2	2	2	2	2			
Anterior trunk	13	17	13	13	13			
Posterior trunk	13	13	13	13	13			
Right buttock	2 1/2	2 1/2	2 1/2	2 1/2	2 1/2			
Left buttock	2 1/2	2 1/2	2 1/2	2 1/2	2 1/2			
Genitalia	1	1	1	1	1			
Right upper arm	4	4	4	4	4			
Left upper arm	4	4	4	4	4			
Right lower arm	3	3	3	3	3			
Left lower arm	3	3	3	3	3			
Right hand	2 1/2	2 1/2	2 1/2	2 1/2	2 1/2			
Left hand	2 1/2	2 1/2	2 1/2	2 1/2	2 1/2			
Right thigh	5 1/2	6 1/2	8 1/2	8 1/2	9 1/2			
Left thigh	5 1/2	6 1/2	8 1/2	8 1/2	9 1/2			
Right leg	5	5	5 1/2	6	7			
Left leg	5	5	5 1/2	6	7			
Right foot	3 1/2	3 1/2	3 1/2	3 1/2	3 1/2			
Left foot	3 1/2	3 1/2	3 1/2	3 1/2	3 1/2			
								total

Burn Evaluation

Severity of Burn

1 ° =

2 ° =

3° =

Figure 4.3. Lund-Browder chart. (From Munster AM. Burn care for the house officer. Baltimore: Williams & Wilkins, 1980.)

burned area to the palm of the patient's hand (roughly equivalent to 1% of BSA). Although the "rule of nines" is easy to use, it does not take age and body proportion into consideration and therefore should not be used for children under 15 years of age.

In *electrical burns*, the major tissue damage will be muscle necrosis, neural injury, and vascular coagulation along the path of the current. True extent of the damage may only be evident on surgical exploration. Although not always obvious, electrical current injury leaves an entrance and exit site.

Victims of *lightning injury* may be successfully resuscitated if CPR is promptly initiated. Due to the effect of lightning on cell metabolism, CPR should be continued for a prolonged period of time.

Chemicals produce tissue injury by protein coagulation rather than by heat. Most *chemical burns* should be treated by flushing the wound with copious amounts of water. Be sure to remove the patient's clothes which may retain some of the chemical. If there is chemical contact with a large surface area, a shower can be used. Dry chemicals should be brushed from the skin before flushing, as heat is produced by the reaction of water and alkali powder. In order to prevent absorption, gasoline and other similar petroleum products should be washed from the skin with a soap solution.

Tar is best removed after it has been flushed with cool water. Peal tar off the skin; any difficult areas can be dissolved with mineral oil.

Diagnostic Tests

Baseline studies - Include CBC, SMA, chest x-ray, and ECG.

Carboxyhemoglobin levels - Draw a specimen for carboxyhemoglobin determination for all patients burned in a closed space or exposed to smoke or fumes. The test requires 7 ml of blood in a heparinized tube.

ABGs - A blood gas should be drawn on all patients with airway problems, evidence of respiratory compromise, or cardiac arrhythmias.

Urinalysis - Check for myoglobin and hemoglobin. Both will cause a positive reaction on Chemstrip. A positive Chemstrip with no RBCs on urinalysis implies myoglobin or hemoglobin. A Foley catheter is indicated in all patients requiring IV fluids or with burns to the perineum. Connect a urimeter for hourly urine output measurements.

Nasogastric tube - Patients with burns over 20% of their BSA often develop ileus and should have a nasogastric tube placed. Intubated patients and those being transported to a burn center need to have a nasogastric tube. All patients with severe burns should be kept NPO (despite complaints of thirst) until GI functioning and risk of aspiration are assessed.

Intervention

1. Airway: potential for impaired gas exchange - Immediate resuscitation takes precedence. Assuring an adequate airway is the first step. All patients should receive high-flow, humidified oxygen. Encourage periodic deep breathing and cough, and be prepared if the patient requires suctioning, intubation, mechanical ventilation, and bronchodilator therapy. Inability to intubate is an indication for cricothyrotomy.

2. Administer 100% oxygen to all patients with smoke inhalation until a carboxyhemoglobin level is available. For a further discussion of carbon monoxide poisoning, see Chapter 7.

3. Fluid administration: potential for hypovolemia and reduced perfusion - Any patient with more than 15% of BSA burned should receive IV fluid therapy. Significant burns cause shifts in body fluid volume and increased capillary permeability. Small burns uncomplicated by other factors, such as electrical injury, do not require IV fluid. Electri-

cal burns whose path crosses the chest should have an IV line and continuous ECG monitoring. Although it is not usually possible to weigh the patient in the ED, a near-accurate determination is important, for it provides the basis for calculation of IV fluid. According to the size of the burn, one or two large-bore IV catheters should be inserted. Whenever possible, IV lines should be started in an unburned area. In patients with a large burn area (more than 40%) or those with underlying cardiopulmonary disease, a jugular or subclavian central venous line may be started. The goal of fluid therapy is to restore hemodynamic stability, as evidenced by a pulse rate below 110/min, a clear sensorium, urine output of 30–50 ml/hr, a CVP under 10 cm H_2O, and a pulmonary wedge pressure in the normal range. Although a number of formulas for calculating IV fluid resuscitation exist, listed are the two most commonly used in EDs.

a. Modified Brooke formula: Give 3 ml Ringer's lactate per Kg body weight per %BSA burned. For the first 24 hours, give half in the first 8 hours and half over the next 16 hours. In the second 24 hours, give 2000 ml D5W, and add plasma as needed.

b. Parkland formula: In the first 24 hours, give 4 ml Ringer's lactate per Kg body weight per %BSA burned. Give half in the first 8 hours and half over the next 16 hours. In the second 24 hours, continue Ringer's lactate as needed. Begin 2000 ml D5W. Add plasma or blood as needed.

Remember that the schedule for fluid replacement begins from the time of injury, not the time of arrival in the ED.

4. Wound care - After initial airway and hemodynamic stabilization has been achieved, the burn wound can be cleaned and dressed. Remove all clothing and jewelry that may retain heat and be difficult to remove later due to edema. Wash or irrigate the wound with room temperature NS. Never use iced saline, as it can cause additional thermal injury. Patients with chemical burns should be placed in a shower or irrigated gently with sterile water (specific neutralizing agents are contraindicated). Hydrofluoric acid burns are treated by injecting 10% calcium gluconate into the burn. Tar can be removed with a Neosporin or a Polysporin cream or ointment that contains an emulsifying agent. Wound cleansing can be accomplished with a diluted solution of povidone-iodine (1:4 parts H_2O), Hibiclens (1:8 parts sterile NS), or a mild soap and water solution. Loose tissue and debris can be removed by using forceps and scissors and irrigation. Blisters are usually left intact, although the finding of vasoactive fluids in the blister fluid may change this recommendation in the near future. All blisters should be evaluated. Partially open blisters or blisters containing cloudy exudate should be removed. After the wound is cleansed and debrided, rinse with sterile NS and apply topical agent. Silver sulfadiazine, an antibacterial that can be applied on freshly burned tissue, is

a common choice. After a topical agent, apply a bulky dressing of opened gauze pads and Kerlex rolls. Elastic net can be used to secure the dressing. Adjacent body surfaces, such as behind the ears, under the breasts, or between the fingers, should be padded to promote healing and prevent adherence. Dressing should be loose enough to permit full range of motion and allow for swelling.

5. Infection - The potential for infection is great. Preventive measures include wound debridement, use of gloves, masks, gowns, and hats, and limiting the number of staff members in contact with the patient. Diphtheria-tetanus is administered according to the patient's history (see "Tetanus" in Chapter 9 for details). Penicillin may be started at this time, but broad-spectrum antibiotics are not indicated.

6. Alteration in comfort - IV narcotics for pain control can be employed as long as the patient is hemodynamically stable. Use of IM injection is not recommended in patients with large burns, because of poor absorption and unequal distribution. Morphine sulfate, 2–4 mg, can be given at frequent intervals. For minor burns, cool saline compresses may be applied to the burn wound to reduce pain. Keep the patient warm, and cover with sterile sheets.

ED Discharge Planning

Admission Criteria
Patients 5–50 years of age

1. Partial-thickness (second-degree) burns covering 15% or more of BSA
2. Deep partial-thickness and/or full-thickness (third- degree) burns covering 7% or more of BSA

Patients under 5 years and over 50 years of age

1. Partial-thickness burns of >10% BSA
2. Deep partial-thickness and/or full-thickness burns of >3% BSA
3. Burns in vital areas (hands, feet, eyes, ears, perineum)
4. High-voltage electrical burns
5. Burn injuries complicated by inhalation injury or major trauma

All patients with major burns should be considered for transfer to a burn center. The referral to the burn center should be made as soon as initial stabilization of the patient's airway and hemodynamic status has been affected.

Patients with minor burns of <5% BSA in adults or 10% in children or elderly without injury to any vital areas can often be treated on an outpatient basis. Each patient's individual circumstances will need to be assessed prior to discharge home.

ED Discharge Instructions
Discharge instructions for patients with minor burns should include:

1. Keeping dressing clean and dry
2. Keeping burned extremity elevated by utilizing a sling or pillows to reduce edema and pain
3. Demonstrating a range of motion exercises for the burned extremity
4. Use of prescription and nonprescription medication
5. Need for increased protein and fluid intake
6. Effect on activities of daily living and return to work and/or school
7. Use of loose fitting clothing
8. Arrangements for reevaluation within 48 hours

WOUND MANAGEMENT—LACERATIONS

Assessment

Assure the adequacy of airway, breathing, and circulation. Obtain a description of the injury, including method of injury, location of wound, when injury occurred, and treatment received prior to arrival in the ED.

Bleeding - Observe for amount of arterial or venous bleeding. If bleeding is extensive, check the patient for signs of shock, and monitor vital signs. Assess for signs of neurovascular compromise (diminished sensation or movement) and the five "Ps": pain, pallor, pulselessness, paresthesia, and paralysis.

Wound - Assess the type of wound:

Abrasion - Scraping of epidermis caused by rubbing against hard, rough surface.

Avulsion - A full-thickness skin loss; underlying muscles, tendons, and nerves may also be injured.

Contusion - A closed injury in which blood extravasates into tissue. Usually caused by blunt trauma.

Laceration - An open cut that may be superficial or deep and may damage underlying structures.

Puncture wound - Penetration of the skin and possibly underlying structures by a sharp, pointed object.

Intervention

1. Bleeding - Apply direct pressure and elevate. If bleeding is extensive, consider fluid replacement and obtain a Hct and coagulation studies.
2. Wound cleansing - Wound cleansing should be done under sterile con-

ditions, with the wound and surrounding skin being scrubbed for approximately 5 minutes. A narrow border around the wound should be shaved, except for eyebrows which are never shaved. The wound should be free of foreign material. Avoid the use of tissue injurious surgical soaps within the wound. Puncture wounds should be soaked for 10–15 minutes in NS and a surgical solution. After wound cleansing irrigate the wound for several minutes with NS. A wound flush system or catheter tip syringe may be used for wound irrigation. Administer tetanus immunization and consider the need for pain relief.

3. Bites - Risk factors for developing wound infection include patient over 50 and delay in treatment of more than 24 hours. Puncture wounds have a higher infection rate. General treatment considerations include irrigation with copious amounts of sterile saline or iodine solution or both, debridement of any devitalized tissue, and inspection for foreign material. Patients with dog bites, cat bites and scratches, and human bites are at risk for infection and cellulitis. Wounds are scrubbed, not usually sutured, and antibiotic prophylaxis is prescribed for high-risk wounds such as bites on hands, puncture wounds, and human bites. Notify the local health department for suspicious animal bites, so that the animal may be secured for assessment of rabies.

ED Discharge Planning

Patients with the following are candidates for admission:

1. Obviously infected lacerations in vital areas such as hands and face
2. Lacerations that involve tendons and nerves or both and for which primary repair is being considered
3. Very deep or extensive lacerations for which adequate wound care and close follow-up are essential

ED Discharge Instructions
1. Keep wound and dressing clean and dry.
2. Keep extremity wound elevated to reduce swelling and discomfort.
3. Review specific medication instructions for antibiotics and analgesics.
4. Have the patient return to the ED for redness, swelling, increased pain, pus, and fever.
5. Give date to return to the ED for wound check and/or suture removal

NEAR-DROWNING

Alcohol and drug abuse appear as prime causes of accidental drowning in adults. Nonaccidental causes range from suicide to assault. Many drowning deaths result from backyard swimming pool accidents. More than a quarter of the victims are capable swimmers. The male-to-female ratio is 3:1, except in bathtub drownings, where females predominate.

Pathophysiology

Most drownings are wet drownings in which variable amounts of water and, possibly, vomitus are aspirated. In dry drowning, no water or liquid is aspirated due to laryngospasm; therefore, disturbances of fluid and acid-base balance are less severe.

In saltwater or seawater drowning, because of hypertonicity of the aspirated water and the osmotic gradient created, fluid is drawn into the alveoli. This transfer of fluid into the lungs may cause pulmonary edema and a degree of hemoconcentration due to the loss of intravascular fluid.

In freshwater drowning, this hypotonic water is quickly (3–4 minutes) absorbed via the pulmonary capillary membrane. The resulting increase in intravascular fluid may lead to a transient hypervolemia. In addition, freshwater promotes the washout of surfactant, leading to eventual alveolar collapse and hypoxemia secondary to pulmonary shunting. Damage to the pulmonary membrane leads to the leakage of plasma proteins into the alveolus and promotes fluid accumulation in the lung. Large amounts of freshwater (>22 ml/Kg can result in electrolyte imbalance, as well as hemolysis, hemoglobinuria, renal failure, and disseminated intravascular coagulation.

The two most important factors in neurologic survival are the length of the hypoxic episode and the temperature of the water. Water temperature has been cited in recent literature as a major determinant of survival. Many cases of full neurologic recovery following submersion for more than 20–40 minutes in cold water have been reported even when the patient has fixed and dilated pupils on arrival at the hospital.

In warm water, a poor outcome is more likely if the following factors are present:

1. Submersion longer than 5 minutes
2. No resuscitation for 10 minutes or more
3. Blood pH of <7.10 on arrival at the hospital

Assessment

Perform an immediate assessment of the ABCs (airway, breathing, and circulation) and the level of consciousness. Hypoxemia may cause the patient to be lethargic, agitated, combative, confused, or semicomatose or in cardiopulmonary arrest.

History

Obtain information on the drowning episode from the ambulance crew or a witness. History should include type of water (freshwater, saltwater, contaminated water), water temperature, length of submersion, time elapsed prior to resuscitation and on-the-scene treatment. Question as to the possible cause, such as alcohol and/or drug ingestion, suicide attempt, seizure disorder, assault, trauma. (With diving accidents, think of cervical spinal injury and head trauma.) Although a full history can be obtained after initial treatment and stabilization, it is valuable to know at this point about any history of cardiopulmonary disease, medications, and allergies.

Physical Findings

Airway/breathing - Inspect airway patency; remove or suction any debris or vomitus. Caution: Do not manipulate the neck until cervical trauma has been ruled out. Note rate, depth, and pattern of respirations as well as the presence of dyspnea and cough. Auscultate lungs for adventitious sounds, such as fine and course crackling (rales and rhonchi) and wheezing. Observe for cyanosis.

Vital signs - Obtain complete vital signs including rectal temperature. Insert a thermocoupler probe for patients who feel cold. Place on cardiac monitor. Monitor BP and CVP for the effects of altered fluid balance.

Level of consciousness - Perform Glascow coma scale; inspect for evidence of head trauma.

Diagnostic Tests

ABGs - Check pH and pO_2.

CBC - Hct will reflect changes in blood volume.

SMA - Electrolytes may be elevated or decreased according to the type of water aspirated. Serial SMA should be obtained during the acute period. BUN and creatinine are obtained to assess renal function.

Urinalysis - Decreased urine output and proteinuria are suggestive of acute renal failure.

X-ray - Chest x-rays are obtained for evidence of aspiration, atelectasis, and pulmonary edema.

ECG - Note changes indicative of ischemia—arrhythmias and ST/T wave changes.

Intervention

1. Immediate resuscitation at scene - Avoid the use of the Heimlich maneuver or water-draining procedure, as these waste precious time and may lead to gastric regurgitation and aspiration.
2. Breathing - Maintain airway patency (protect cervical spine as indicated) and provide high concentration of oxygen with tight-fitting nonrebreather mask. Patients with respiratory insufficiency and/or

pO$_2$ below 60 mm Hg should be intubated and given 100% oxygen. CPAP or PEEP has been shown to significantly improve ventilation/ perfusion ratios. IV aminophylline and inhaled beta-adrenergic agents may be used to treat or prevent bronchospasm. Insert a nasogastric tube to reduce the risk of aspiration.

3. Fluid and electrolyte imbalance - Insert one or two IV lines. For patients not in shock the fluid of choice for freshwater aspiration is dextrose 5%; for saltwater aspiration, the fluid of choice is lactated Ringer's solution. Monitor CVP and urine output to assess fluid status.

4. Acid-base balance - Patients may present with both respiratory and metabolic acidosis. After ensuring adequate ventilation, metabolic acidosis (pH < 7.1) is treated with sodium bicarbonate, 0.5–1 mEq/Kg. Response to treatment can be assessed by monitoring ABG values, respiratory rate, and depth and level of consciousness (see Chapter 6 on acid-base balance).

5. Cardiac arrhythmias - With correction of electrolyte imbalance, hypoxemia, and acidosis, most arrhythmias will resolve. Place patient on continuous ECG monitoring. Should arrhythmias persist, antiarrhythmic therapy may be given.

6. Cerebral resuscitation - Employ standard measures to prevent or control cerebral edema, including hyperventilation; furosemide or mannitol, if indicated; elevation of the head of the bed to a 30° angle; careful monitoring of fluid balance and intracranial pressure monitoring in the ICU. Use of steroids or barbiturates is controversial. In patients with hypothermia, initiate internal and external rewarming (see Chapter 6). Note that CPR must be continued in hypothermic patients until their temperature reaches 89.6°F (32°C) or above.

ED Discharge Planning

Patients with significant near-drowning episodes should be admitted and monitored for at least 24 hours. Alteration in mental status and abnormal chest x-ray or ABGs are positive indications for admission and possible ICU observation.

SUGGESTED READINGS

Multiple Trauma

Beckwith N, Carriere SR. Fluid resuscitation in trauma: an update. J Emerg Nurs 1985; 11:293–299.

Cardona VD. Nursing practice through the cycles of trauma. In: Cardona VD, Hurn PD. Mason PB, Scanlon-Schilpp AM, Veise-Berry SW. Trauma nursing: from resuscitation through rehabilitation. Philadelphia: WB Saunders, 1988:71–101.

Craig MC, Copes WS, Champion HR. Psychosocial considerations in trauma care. Crit Care Nurs Q 1988;11:51–58.

Halpern JS. Patterns of trauma. J Emerg Nurs 1982;8:170–175.

Lenehan GP. Emotional impact of trauma. Nurs Clin North Am 1986;21:729–740.

O'Hara MM. Emergency care of the patient with a traumatic amputation. J Emerg Nurs 1987;13:272–277.

Rodriguez A. Resuscitation, stabilization and evaluation in the admitting area. In: Cowley RA, Conn A, Dunham CM, eds. Trauma care. Philadelphia: JB Lippincott, 1987:62–77.

Stauffer D. The trauma patient who is pregnant. J Emerg Nurs 1986;12:89–93.

Trunkey DD, Sheldon GF, Collins JA. The treatment of shock. In: Zuidema GD, Rutherford RB, Ballinger WF, eds. The management of trauma. 4th ed. Philadelphia: WB Saunders, 1985:105–125.

Head Trauma

Bires BA. Head trauma: Nursing implications from prehospital through emergency department. Crit Care Nurs Q 1987;10:1–18.

Fink ME. Emergency management of the head-injured patient. Emerg Med Clin North Am 1987;5:783–795.

Frazee JG. Head trauma. Emerg Med Clin North Am 1986;4: 859–873.

Gardner D. Acute management of head-injured adult. Nurs Clin North Am 1986;21: 555–562.

Jess LW. Assessing your patient for increased ICP. Nursing 1987;17:34–41.

Hockberger RS, Schwartz B. Blunt head injury: a spectrum of disease. Ann Emerg Med 1986;15:202–207.

Manifold SL. Craniocerebral trauma. Focus Crit Care 1986;13: 22–35.

Spinal Cord Trauma

Bryson BL, et al. Trauma to the aging cervical spine. J Emerg Nurs 1987;13:334–341.

Dillingham TR. Prevention of complications during acute management of the spinal cord-injured patient: first step in the rehabilitation process. Crit Care Nurs Q 1988;11:71-77.

Metcalf JA. Acute phase management of persons with spinal cord injury: a nursing diagnosis perspective. Nurs Clin North Am 1986;21:589–598.

Podolsky S. Efficacy of cervical spine immobilization methods. J Trauma 1983;23:461–463.

Romeo JH. The critical minutes after spinal cord injury. RN 1988;51:61–67.

Walleck CA. Central nervous system II: spinal cord injury. In: Cardona VD, Hurn PD, Mason PB, Scanlon-Schilpp AM, Veise-Berry SW. Trauma nursing: from resuscitation through rehabilitation. Philadelphia: WB Saunders, 1988:419–448.

Chest Trauma

Cunningham JL. Assessment and care of the patient with myocardial contusion. Crit Care Nurs 1987;7:68–75.

Gough JE, Allison EJ, Raju VP. Flail chest: management implications for emergency nurses. J Emerg Nurs 1987;13: 330–333.

Hammond BB. Nursing assessment of blunt cardiac trauma. Nurs Clin North Am 1986; 21:677–684.

Kite JH. Cardiac and great vessel trauma assessment, pathophysiology, and intervention. J Emerg Nurs 1987;13: 346–351.

Lockhart CG. Thoracic trauma. Crit Care Q 1986;9:32–40.

Parker JG. Thoracic trauma nursing assessment and management. Nurs Clin North Am 1986;21:685–692.

Tenzer ML. The spectrum of myocardial contusion: a review. J Trauma 1985;25:620–627.

Intraabdominal Trauma

Burney RE. Peritoneal lavage and other diagnostic procedures in blunt abdominal trauma. Emerg Med Clin North Am 1986; 4:513–525.

Maher AB. Early assessment and management of musculoskeletal injuries. Nurs Clin North Am 1986;21:717–727.

McSwain NE. Mechanism of injuries in blunt trauma. In: McSwain NE, Kerstein MD, ed. Evaluation and management of trauma. Norwalk, Connecticut: Appleton-Century-Crofts, 1987:1–24.

Peter NK. Care of patients with traumatic pelvic fractures. Crit Care Nurs 1988;8:62–85.

Semonin-Holleran R. Critical nursing care for abdominal trauma. Crit Care Nurs 1988; 8:48–56.

Weiskittel P, Sommers MS. The patient with lower urinary tract trauma. Crit Care Nurs 1989;9:53–65.

Burns

Abshagen D. Topical agents and emergency care for minor burn injuries. J Emerg Nurs 1984;10:325–331.

Boswick JA, ed. The art and science of burn care. Rockville, Maryland: Aspen Publishers, 1987.

Demling RH. Fluid resuscitation after major burns. JAMA 1983;250:1438–1440.

Mikhail JN. Acute burn care: an update. J Emerg Nurs 1988;14:9–18.

Robertson K, Cross P, Terry J. The crucial first days. Am J Nurs 1985;85:30–47.

Wound Management—Lacerations

Grossman JA. Minor injuries and disorders: surgical and medical care. Philadelphia: JB Lippincott, 1984.

Sheehy SB, Marvin JA, Jimmerson CL. Manual of clinical trauma care: the first hour. St Louis: CV Mosby, 1989:269–277.

Near-Drowning

Butler S. Out of the water, but not out of the woods. RN 1988;51:26–30.

Gross PL, et al. Environmental hazards. In: Wilkins EW, et al, eds. MGH textbook of emergency medicine. 2nd ed. Baltimore: Williams & Wilkins, 1983:185–187.

Gonzalez-Rothi RJ. Near drowning: consensus and controversies in pulmonary and cerebral resuscitation. Heart Lung 1987;16:474–482.

Graves SA. Drowning and near-drowning. In: Kravis TC, Warner CG, eds. Emergency medicine. Rockville, Maryland: Aspen Publishers, 1987:665–676.

Ornato JP. Special resuscitation situations: near drowning, traumatic injury, electric shock and hypothermia. Circulation 1986;74:23–26.

Chapter 5

GASTROENTEROLOGIC EMERGENCIES

ACUTE ABDOMINAL PAIN

Abdominal pain, a common chief complaint, is a symptom of a wide array of diseases and dysfunction. The triage nurse needs to be alert to the potentially life-threatening causes of abdominal pain, including abdominal aortic aneurysm, ectopic pregnancy, ruptured spleen, and ruptured appendicitis. Careful history taking and physical assessment will act to keep the number of miscategorized patients to a minimum.

Assessment

History
A thorough evaluation of the cause of acute abdominal pain cannot be overemphasized. Obtain a detailed discussion of the present episode of pain, including precise location, onset, duration, quality, severity, provocative or palliative maneuvers, and associated symptoms (fever, vomiting, diarrhea, dysuria, vaginal discharge, bleeding, etc.). In general, the new onset of abdominal pain that lasts longer than 6 hours in an otherwise healthy individual should be considered to have surgical importance. Previous episodes of abdominal pain, whether similar or dissimilar to the current pain, should be noted along with previous workups, diagnoses, and treatments. A detailed menstrual history should be obtained in all females of childbearing age with abdominal pain. List current medications, particularly those with gastric effects, e.g., aspirin and antiinflammatory agents.

Physical Findings
General - Note pallor, cyanosis, jaundice, or shocky appearance. Patient's

position and movement may vary with the nature of the discomfort, e.g., patients with renal colic writhe in pain.

Vital signs - Look for hyperventilation or tachycardia with severe pain or acidosis. Obtain orthostatic BP* and rectal temperature.

Chest - Note movement with respirations. Listen for diminished or adventitious breath sounds.

Abdomen - Observe the movement of the abdominal wall. Note distention, presence of fluid wave (ascites), pulsations, and scars. Auscultate in all four quadrants. In assessing the abdomen, auscultation must precede palpation in order to avoid any interference or alteration of bowel sounds caused by elicited pain or tenderness. Bowel sounds occur at a rate of 3–12 times/min. There is a significant normal variance in rate, pitch, and volume. Palpate lightly, for resistance, masses, and tenderness.

Diagnostic Tests

Laboratory tests - Check CBC with WBC and differential, SMA including calcium, liver function tests, and amylase. A urinalysis with RBC and WBC is essential.

Type and hold - Blood should be sent for typing if GI bleeding is suspected or surgery is contemplated.

ABGs - ABG analysis is necessary if respiratory distress is present or acid-base imbalance is suspected.

ECG - An ECG is needed for patients with a history of heart disease or cardiac risk factors. It is useful in all patients to rule out the possibility of an inferior wall myocardial infarction that may present as abdominal discomfort.

Nasogastric tube - This is indicated for all patients with signs of intestinal obstruction or evidence of GI bleeding.

Paracentesis and peritoneal lavage - This is indicated if hemoperitoneum is suspected.

Culdocentesis - This is indicated if a ruptured ectopic pregnancy is suspected.

X-rays - Upright PA and lateral chest films are taken to rule out free air (perforation) and lower lobe pneumonia. Supine and upright films of the abdomen are routine in every patient suspected of having an acute abdomen. Lateral decubitus films of the abdomen are suitable substitutes for an upright film if the latter is not obtainable.

Contrast studies - Films of the GI or genitourinary tracts may be necessary as indicated by the working diagnosis.

---

*See "Appendix A" for definition of common abbreviations used in the text.

Intervention

1. Provide basic life support as outlined in Chapter 1 under "Cardiopulmonary Arrest" and under "Shock" and in Chapter 2 under "Acute Respiratory Failure."
2. Fluid and electrolyte balance - Keep the patient NPO until a diagnosis is determined. Start an IV of Ringer's lactate or normal saline if the patient is in severe distress, hypotensive, or vomiting. Monitor the patient's intake and output, and check electrolyte results.
3. Comfort measures - Explain to the patient that an analgesic cannot be given until a diagnosis is established. However, this rule is not absolute. A patient in severe abdominal pain can sometimes be made more comfortable with low doses of analgesics, such as meperidine (Demerol), 25 mg IM, without obscuring the results of subsequent examinations. Another alternative for the severely distressed patient is the administration of hydroxyzine (Vistaril), 25–50 mg IM. Morphine is to be avoided, since it may increase pain due to its effect on smooth muscle, slowing peristalsis and stomach emptying. Position the patient in the most comfortable position, usually a mid-Fowler's or side-lying position with the head of the stretcher raised.

Common Gastrointestinal Disorders Associated with Abdominal Pain

Cholecystitis - Most often associated with gallstones, acute cholecystitis causes bouts of biliary colic occurring 30–90 minutes after a meal and subsiding within 1–4 hours. The pain is dull and constant and radiates to the back or right infrascapular region. Nausea, vomiting, and fever are common. Intervention includes:

1. Nasogastric tube decompression with IV hydration
2. Administration of antibiotic (ampicillin or cephalosporin)
3. Preparation for surgery, ideally within 48 hours

Appendicitis - Inflammation of the vermiform appendix reaches its peak incidence in the second and third decades of life. Appendicitis typically begins with diffuse umbilical pain that is not very severe. The pain gradually shifts to the right lower quadrant, causing sharply localized pain. However, atypical pain may remain diffuse and never localize preoperatively. Anorexia usually follows, with nausea in 90% of patients. If vomiting occurs, it occurs after the onset of pain and usually not more than once or twice. Patients suspected of having acute appendicitis are immediately hospitalized or taken to surgery. When the diagnosis is in doubt, but appendicitis is a possibility, the patient must be admitted for observation.

Peptic ulcer - Patients complain of episodes of epigastric distress relieved by antacids or milk. There is usually an exacerbation of these symptoms over the 2–3 days prior to presentation. Sudden onset of severe, midepigastric pain quickly spreading over the entire abdomen with radiation to one or both shoulders may be seen with acute perforation. The pain may be so severe as to cause a syncopal event concomitant with perforation. Penetration may present with boring pain radiating to the back. Bowel sounds are absent or markedly decreased. There is marked guarding or "board-like rigidity." Diffuse rebound and palpable tenderness are noted.

Nasogastric suction and fluid and electrolyte stabilization should be performed prior to immediate surgical repair of a perforation. Oral antacids may be given in the ED to patients with painful ulcers but should not be given to any potential surgical candidate. IV cimetidine may be prescribed. All patients with a penetrating or perforating ulcer should be hospitalized on the surgical service. Patients with bleeding ulcers or with painful ulcers that have proven refractory to outpatient treatment with antacids or oral cimetidine should likewise be admitted.

ED Discharge Planning

Patients who do not respond to treatment, who are unable to tolerate oral fluids, who require a nasogastric tube, or who are being considered for surgical intervention should be admitted.

ED Discharge Instructions
1. Explain the diet, which is usually a slow progression from clear liquid to solid food over a 24-hour period.
2. Review medications prescribed.
3. Give specific instructions for nausea, vomiting, diarrhea, fever, and urinary tract infection.
4. Have the patient return to the ED or the patient's private physician if symptoms continue or increase in severity.

INTESTINAL OBSTRUCTION

Mechanical bowel obstruction can be caused by a variety of conditions, including tumors, intussusception, inflammation, adhesions, radiation therapy, and strangulated hernias.

Paralytic ileus may be caused by acute abnormalities of any structure touching bowel, such as ureteral distention, retroperitoneal hemorrhage or trauma, systemic infections, antidiarrheal agents, electrolyte imbalances, especially hypokalemia, and intestinal ischemia.

Assessment

History

The syndrome of intestinal obstruction is characterized by crampy and paroxysmal pain. Signs and symptoms vary considerably, depending on location and duration of obstruction. Vomiting is profuse and may have a fecal smell. Continuous pain between bouts suggests strangulation with peritonitis. Obstipation, or failure to pass gas or stool from the rectum, is evident only after total evacuation of bowel distal to the obstruction. Question the patient about previous abdominal conditions and surgery, such as neoplasm, Crohn's disease, diverticulosis, or salpingitis. In partial bowel obstruction, such as from impaction, the patient may give a history of having liquid stools.

Physical Findings

Vital signs - Tachycardia and hypotension may indicate severe volume depletion or peritonitis. Fever suggests the possibility of strangulation in patients with mechanical obstruction.

Abdomen - With a mechanical obstruction, bowel sounds come in rushes and are frequently high pitched, tinkling, or musical and separated by quiet periods, while with paralytic ileus, bowel sounds are diminished or absent. There may be distention and tympany. Abdominal tenderness is present diffusely; however, localized tenderness, rebound, and guarding indicate peritonitis and possible strangulation. Previous surgical scars should be noted in addition to external hernias.

Rectal examination - May detect an obstructing mass. The presence of blood on rectal examination suggests a mucosal lesion, such as cancer, intussusception, or infarction.

Diagnostic Tests

SMA - Proximal small bowel obstruction produces great amounts of vomiting, causing loss of water, sodium, chloride, hydrogen ions, and potassium, and results in dehydration, azotemia, hypochloremia, hypokalemia, and metabolic alkalosis. Distal small bowel obstruction may produce large fluid loss, but electrolyte abnormalities are less prominent.

CBC - Hemoconcentration may accompany dehydration. Leukocytosis may be seen with strangulation.

X-rays - Obtain an upright chest x-ray and a KUB view with the patient both flat and upright. Abdominal x-rays may show distention of bowel loops proximal to the obstruction. Free air under the diaphragm indicates perforation. If large bowel obstruction is suspected, emergency barium enema should be performed.

Intervention

1. Hydrate and correct for electrolyte imbalance. Start an IV of Ringer's lactate or D5W. Measure CVP if BP is low. Antibiotics can be administered as prescribed. Electrolyte and acid-base imbalances are assessed and corrected.
2. Insert nasogastric tube and connect to suction.
3. Alter the patient's position for comfort; a mid-Fowler's position will usually be most comfortable. Medication for pain is commonly withheld because it may interfere with evaluation of the patient.

ED Discharge Planning

All patients with intestinal obstruction should be admitted to the surgical service.

GASTROINTESTINAL BLEEDING

The patient with GI bleeding may present to the triage nurse with symptoms that range from mild and vague to life-threatening hemorrhage. Bleeding can occur from any place along the GI tract and is classified as upper or lower tract bleeding. Common causes of upper GI bleeding are peptic ulcer, gastritis, "stress ulcers," esophageal varices, and neoplasms. Common causes of lower GI bleeding include neoplasm, colitis, polyps, diverticulosis, hemorrhoids, and fissures.

Assessment

History
Obtain a history of the suspected bleeding, i.e., time, amount, and stool color. Hematemesis and melena stools always signify upper GI bleeding, whereas bright blood per rectum usually suggests a lower GI bleed. Associated symptoms may also include pain, cramps, vomiting, fatigue, weakness, and syncope. Drug ingestions should be carefully noted, especially aspirin, nonsteroidal antiinflammatory drugs, anticoagulants, and alcohol. If the patient admits to black bowel movements, ask about intake of iron and Pepto-Bismol. Past history should include presence of prior bleeding, ulcer history, prior surgery, history of alcoholism or liver disease, or recent trauma.

Physical Findings

Vital signs - Always check orthostatic pulse and pressure changes. Patients on beta blockers may not mount a tachycardia.

Skin - Observe for color, i.e., pallor and cyanosis, and for signs of liver disease (jaundice, spider angiomata, palmar erythema).

Abdomen - Note bowel sounds (present, diminished, hyperactive, absent), ascites, hepatosplenomegaly, and tenderness.

Rectal examination - Note the color of the stool and the briskness of the reaction to heme testing.

Diagnostic Tests

CBC - Check a spun Hct immediately. Remember that the Hct may initially appear normal and may only decrease after the patient receives fluid.

Laboratory tests - Send for SMA including liver enzymes, amylase, and electrolytes. BUN elevation is often seen in upper GI bleeding. Send a PT and PTT to check for coagulopathy.

Nasogastric tube - All patients should have a large nasogastric or Ewald tube passed and be lavaged until the returns clear and show bilious material. Note whether "coffee grounds" or bright red blood is present. It is not recommended to heme test aspirated contents, as the test is too sensitive and the trauma of insertion will give a false positive. Consult the physician concerning placement of a nasogastric tube if esophageal varices is a possible diagnosis.

Endoscopy - Endoscopy is usually performed once the patient has been stabilized, bleeding has slowed, and the stomach can be emptied to enable good visualization. Emergency endoscopy is recommended for upper tract bleeding that does not cease with conservative management.

Additional procedures - Other diagnostic procedures include the nuclear bleeding scan (very sensitive), angiography, sigmoidoscopy, and barium contrast studies.

Intervention

1. Correct fluid volume deficit - Two large-bore IV lines should be placed, and normal saline or Ringer's lactate, should be administered in large volumes. The transfusion of choice is fresh whole blood, but packed cells and fresh frozen plasma (if needed) are usually used (see "Shock" in Chapter 1 for further details of management). Cirrhotic patients with ascites and those with edema should not receive crystalloid unless absolutely necessary, as it may lead to further edema. D5W and salt-poor albumin are better choices until blood can be delivered.

Monitor the patient's hemodynamic status by making frequent blood pressure, pulse, CVP, and urine output determinations. Insert a Foley catheter, if indicated, to monitor fluid volume. Administer oxygen if the patient is hypotensive or anemic or has underlying cardiopulmonary disease. Keep the patient warm. A MAST suit can be used to provide increased resistance and raise BP.

2. Gastric lavage - Saline nasogastric lavage will initially control acute upper tract bleeding. Iced irrigation solution is not recommended. Continue to irrigate until returns become clear. To prevent aspiration, place the patient in mid-Fowler's position, if BP permits. Have suction readily available.

3. Bleeding esophageal varices can be treated with IV vasopressin, 0.4 units/min, administered via an infusion pump. Vasopressin causes a decrease in coronary artery blood flow and is contraindicated in patients with coronary artery disease. A Sengstaken-Blakemore tube, which is composed of a gastric and an esophageal balloon, may be inserted to compress varices if the patient is exsanguinating from varices. Label all ports, particularly the pharynx port, due to the danger of aspiration. Keep scissors available; the tube must be immediately deflated if the patient shows signs of respiratory distress. After ED stabilization, severe bleeding may be treated with endoscopic sclerotherapy. Intravariceal injections of a sclerosant solution (sodium morrhuate, sodium tetradecylsulfate) is a highly effective treatment for controlling acute and recurrent esophageal variceal hemorrhage.

ED Discharge Planning

It is the usual practice to admit any patient with a gross GI bleed (upper or lower) even if the patient is not severely ill, as the course may be unpredictable. Patients who bring up a few flecks of blood after repeatedly vomiting or who pass quaiac-positive stools without gross bleeding need not be admitted.

ED Discharge Instructions
1. Review the patient's and/or family's understanding of the patient's condition.
2. Give outpatient referrals for GI series, blood tests, etc.
3. Review medication dosage, action, and precautions.
4. Identify factors that can precipitate bleeding (alcohol, aspirin, stress).
5. Have the patient return to the ED if pain, bleeding, etc. recur.

PANCREATITIS

Acute inflammation of the pancreas is often associated with excess intake of alcohol, but it may also be caused by obstruction from gallstones, neoplasm, trauma (steering wheel injury), infection, and circulatory inadequacy.

Assessment

History

Pain is present in 90% of cases, ranging from mild to unbearable. It is often midepigastric but may be difficult to localize. It often radiates to the back and is described as constant or boring—usually not colicky. It typically begins acutely but may develop gradually. Some relief is gained by bending over or squatting on all fours, as gravity pulls the weight of the abdominal viscera forward and away from the inflamed retroperitoneal pancreas. Nausea and vomiting are common symptoms. Constipation may occur, but it is not common.

The history should concentrate on questions pertinent to the many possible etiologies of pancreatitis. Particularly important are history of gallstones, drug ingestion, endocrine disorders, or alcohol abuse that is often underestimated by the patient. Remember also that patients who present in alcohol withdrawal may have stopped drinking because of pancreatitis. Probably the most important historical point is a past similar episode diagnosed as pancreatitis.

Physical Findings

General - Look for signs of alcoholism; jaundice may be present in biliary pancreatitis as well. Tetany secondary to hypocalcemia and skin lesions secondary to fat necrosis are more unusual. Ecchymoses over flanks, if present, are associated with hemorrhagic pancreatitis.

Vital signs - Check for low-grade fever, tachycardia, orthostasis, and frank hypotension (massive fluid sequestration or hemorrhage).

Eyes - Look for scleral icterus.

Lungs - Listen for rales and percuss for pleural effusion (usually left-sided).

Abdomen - The abdomen may be flat or distended and tender, with decreased bowel sounds. Rebound may be present due to a severe chemical peritonitis from leakage of pancreatic enzymes into the peritoneal cavity. An abdominal mass (pancreatic pseudocyst) may be felt.

Diagnostic Tests

Amylase - The serum amylase is often elevated in pancreatitis. However, other causes of an elevated amylase include diseases that may present with predominantly intraabdominal symptoms such as penetrating ulcer, perforated gallbladder, infarcted bowel, ruptured ectopic pregnancy, or diabetic ketoacidosis and, in normal states, macroamylasemia. Amylase is partially cleared by the kidney, so patients with renal failure may also have elevated amylase. Most importantly, patients with pancreatitis may have normal amylase, either because of chronic calcific pancreatitis (the damaged pancreas cannot produce much amylase) or because of rapid clearance of amylase by the kidney. The level of amylase does not correlate with the severity of the attack of pancreatitis.

Lipase - Serum lipase determinations are available in many laboratores. The lipase level should be elevated in panreatitis and is more specific for the pancreas than is the amylase. It will help in establishing the diagnosis when the amylase is elevated due to conditions other than pancreatitis.

CBC - Note if the WBC is elevated or the Hct is abnormal.

SMA - Glucose is elevated in roughly one-half the patients with pancreatitis. Calcium may be decreased, and liver function tests may indicate hepatitis or the obstructive pattern suggestive of biliary disease.

ABGs - A blood gas should be drawn if the patient appears very ill, not only to assess for the possibility of acid-base imbalance but also because these patients may become hypoxic. There is an association between pancreatitis and respiratory distress syndrome.

X-rays - A chest film should be done to rule out the presence of a left pleural effusion or respiratory distress syndrome. A KUB should be done to look for gallstones, ascites, and pancreatic calcifications of chronic disease.

Patients with pancreatitis may be acutely ill, particularly with the hemorrhagic form of the disease. Complications include pancreatic pseudocyst, suppurative pancreatitis, fat necrosis, ascites, shock, acute tubular necrosis, DIC and respiratory distress syndrome (ARDS).

Ransom has developed criteria to predict severity in acute pancreatitis. They are as follows:

1. On admission: age > 55 years, WBC > 16,000, FBS > 200 mg%, LDH > 350, AST (SGOT) > 250, markedly elevated amylase.
2. Within 48 hours of admission, Hct falls by 10 points or more, BUN increases by 5 mg% or more, with a calcium < 8 mg%, pO_2 < 60 mm Hg, base deficit > 4 mEq/liter, and fluid sequestration > 6 liters.

Intervention

1. Hydration and electrolyte correction - Start IV line of Ringer's lactate; initial rate should be 200 ml/hr. Fluids will be regulated to maintain

hemodynamic and to compensate for peritoneal cavity "third spacing." Low serum albumin level will indicate the need for colloid administration.

2. Pain relief can be achieved with meperidine (Demerol), 75–100 mg IM every 4–6 hours, once other intraabdominal catastrophies have been ruled out.
3. Nasogastric intubation and lavage may be performed to check for upper tract bleeding. Whether the tube should be left in place with suction to rest the bowel remains somewhat controversial, but it should be utilized for the patient with persistent vomiting.

ED Discharge Planning

All patients with acute pancreatitis, regardless of severity, should be admitted. This will protect those who might become dehydrated or develop other serious complications.

VIRAL HEPATITIS

Etiology

Etiologies for hepatitis are:

1. Viral (common)
   a. Type A ("infectious hepatitis")
   b. Type B ("serum hepatitis")
   c. Non-A, non-B virus (-es)
   d. Epstein-Barr virus
   e. Cytomegalovirus
2. Bacterial (rare)
3. Toxic (alcohol, carbon tetrachloride)
4. Drug-induced (isoniazid, phenytoin, methyldopa, oral contraceptives)

Hepatitis A is usually transmitted by the fecal-oral route and has been associated with sewage-contaminated shellfish. The incubation period is short (roughly 15–50 days). Close to 50% of the North American population has undergone subclinical infection with hepatitis A, has hepatitis A antibodies, and is probably immune to reinfection.

Hepatitis B is usually transmitted by percutaneous, oral-fecal, oral-oral, and venereal routes. High-risk groups include IV drug abusers, homosexuals, medical personnel, and blood transfusion recipients. The incubation period is long (roughly 50–150 days). Antigen (hepatitis B surface antigen) and antibody (anti-hepatitis B core) appear early and may persist in carriers. Roughly 5-15% of the population have antibody to hepatitis surface antigen, indicating previous infection and immunity.

Non-A, non-B hepatitis is caused by an unknown agent or agents. The mode of transmission is percutaneous, and infection is currently the most common cause of posttransfusion hepatitis. The incubation period is roughly 25–75 days. There are no available serologic markers. Hepatitis due to Epstein-Barr virus or cytomegalovirus is usually mild and may be associated with the clinical syndrome of mononucleosis.

Assessment

History
Prodromal symptoms of viral hepatitis include general malaise, ano-rexia, nausea and vomiting, arthralgias, arthritis, urticaria, myalgias, low-grade fever, rash, dark urine, and clay-colored stools. Jaundiced pa-tients often have right-upper-quadrant pain. Important points to cover include:

1. Past history of hepatitis
2. Contact with others who have or have had hepatitis
3. Use of or exposure to alcohol or other hepatotoxins
4. Transfusions of blood products
5. IV drug abuse
6. Travel history
7. Prescribed medications
8. Sexual preference

Physical Findings
General - Patients may range from comfortable to toxic or shocky.
Vital signs - Always check the patient's rectal temperature. Do orthostatic pulse and pressure readings.
HEENT - Look for scleral icterus.
Abdomen - Palpate lightly for enlarged spleen and for liver tenderness, and check for ascites.
Rectal examination - Test stool for blood.
Extremities - Look for edema or track marks.
Skin - Note jaundice. Look for spider angiomata or palmar erythema (chronic alcohol abuse).
Neurologic signs - Note lethargy, confusion, stupor, or level of coma seen in hepatic encephalophy. Check for asterixis.

Diagnostic Tests
CBC - This will often show mild anemia and a normal or mildly elevated WBC with a relative lymphocytosis.
SMA - This will usually show a serum bilirubin in the range of 15–20,

with marked elevations of AST (SGOT), ALT (SGPT), and alkaline phosphatase.

PT - This may be mildly elevated (up to 15/12).

Antibodies - Hepatitis B surface antigen should be sent on all patients suspected of having hepatitis. Patients suspected of having hepatitis A should have IgM levels sent.

Intervention

1. Infection control measures - Place the patient on precautions; remember to use gloves when drawing bloods or handling body fluids. All specimens sent to the laboratory should be labelled for hepatitis precautions.
2. General measures - Rest and avoidance of hepatotoxic agents (drugs and alcohol) are standard. Patients with anorexia and vomiting will require IV hydration.

ED Discharge Planning

Admission criteria are:

1. Inability to keep fluids down with consequent dehydration
2. GI bleeding
3. Hypoglycemia
4. Altered mental status
5. Signs of fulminant hepatic failure (ascites, pedal edema, shock)
6. PT > 16/12 (prolonged by more than 4 seconds over control)
7. Concurrent complicating illnesses

Most patients who are able to eat and drink do not require admission. It should be explained to these patients that there is no specific therapy for hepatitis. They should be counselled to avoid alcohol and other toxins, as well as discontinue all potentially hepatotoxic drugs. Isolation is not necessary. Stool precautions and careful hygiene are reasonable. It may be appropriate for the patient to avoid contact with children and chronically ill or elderly adults until the diagnosis is clear. Patients should return weekly as outpatients for follow-up of blood tests until they show signs of recovery.

Prophylaxis

Prophylactic treatment to prevent hepatitis B infection after exposure to hepatitis B should be considered in needlestick or mucosal exposure to HBsAg-positive blood, and sexual exposure to a HBsAg-positive person.

Percutaneous exposure (needlestick, bite, etc.) in a recipient who has no Ag or Ab to hepatitis B should be treated with a single dose of hepatitis B immune globulin (HBIG), 5 ml IM within 24 hours, in addition to hepatitis B vaccine, 1 ml IM, at the same time but in a different site. The hepatitis B vaccine should be repeated at 1 and 6 months postexposure. Patients who refuse hepatitis B vaccine should receive HBIG, 5 ml IM within 24 hours, and again at 1 month postexposure. If HBIG is unavailable, standard immune globulin (gamma globulin) may be given in the same doses.

Sexual exposure should be treated with HBIG, 5 ml IM, within 14 days. In addition, a vaccination series as described above is recommended for homosexually active males and for regular sexual contacts of chronic hepatitis B carriers.

Prophylactic treatment to prevent hepatitis A or non-A, non-B hepatitis in needlestick or sexual exposures to known cases is standard immune globulin, 5 ml IM, as a single dose.

Nonsexual household contacts should be reassured that they are not at significantly increased risk of contracting hepatitis.

SUGGESTED READINGS

Acute Abdominal Pain

Burnett LS. Gynecologic causes of the acute abdomen. Surg Clin North Am 1988; 68:385–398.

Buschiazzo L. Careful assessment of abdominal pain. J Emerg Nurs 1986;12:72–75.

Munn NE. Diagnosis: acute abdomen. Nursing 1988;18:34-41.

Saclarides T, Hopkins W, Doolas A. Abdominal emergencies. Med Clin North Am 1986;70:1093–1110.

Sharp KW. Acute cholecystitis. Surg Clin North Am 1988;68:269–279.

Tollison AA. Danger signs, rebound tenderness. Nursing 1988;18:78–79.

Intestinal Obstruction

McConnell EA. Meeting the challenge of intestinal obstruction. Nursing 1987;17:34–41.

Richards WO, Williams LF. Obstruction of the large and small intestine. Surg Clin North Am 1988;68:355–376.

Sun EA, Snape WJ. Colon emergencies. In: Gitnick G, ed. Handbook of gastrointestinal emergencies. 2nd ed. New York: Medical Examination Publishing, 1987:121–175.

Gastrointestinal Bleeding

Buchman TG, Bulkley GB. Current management of patients with lower gastrointestinal bleeding. Surg Clin North Am 1987;67:651–664.

Lancaster JR. Upper gastrointestinal bleeding. Primary Care 1988;15:31–41.

Patras AZ, Paice JA, Lanigan K. Managing GI bleeding. Nursing 1988;18:68–74.

Ricci JA. Alcohol-induced upper GI hemorrhage: case studies and management. Crit Care Nurse 1987;7:56–63.

Schaffner J. Acute gastrointestinal bleeding. Med Clin North Am 1986;70:1055–1066.

Pancreatitis

Aitken DR, Ihde JK, Razzouk AJ. Acute pancreatitis. In: Inde JK, Jacobsen WK, Briggs BA, eds. Principles of critical care. Philadelphia: WB Saunders, 1987:272–282.

Blake R. Acute pancreatitis. Primary Care 1988;15:187–193.

Fain JA, Armato-Vealey E. Acute pancreatitis: a gastrointestinal emergency. Crit Care Nurse 1988;8:47–61.

Kannan CR. Acute pancreatitis. In: Gastroenterology, a problem oriented approach. New York: Medical Examination Publishing, 1986:411–419.

Potts JR. Acute pancreatitis. Surg Clin North Am 1988;68:281–299.

Viral Hepatitis

CDC. Update on hepatitis B prevention. MMWR 1987;36:354–360.

Kannan CR. Acute viral hepatitis. In: Gastroenterology, a problem oriented approach. New York: Medical Examination Publishing, 1986:446–450.

Swell RB. Acute and chronic viral hepatitis. In: Rakel RE, ed. Conn's current therapy. Philadelphia: WB Saunders, 1989:446–450.

Chapter 6

METABOLIC EMERGENCIES

DIABETIC EMERGENCIES

Metabolic problems in diabetes usually fall into one of these major categories:

1. Diabetic ketoacidosis (DKA)
2. Hyperosmolar nonketotic coma (HNKC)
3. Hyperglycemia
4. Hypoglycemia

DIABETIC KETOACIDOSIS (DKA)

Definition

Patients with DKA have a serum glucose over 300 with arterial pH* under 7.3. Young patients with a good glomerular filtration rate may have significant acidosis despite unimpressive glucose elevations. Roughly one-half of patients with DKA will also be hyperosmolar, reflecting a greater degree of volume depletion.

Pathophysiology

Hyperglycemia causes an osmotic diuresis that results in volume depletion with ensuing electrolyte depletion (K^+, Mg^{2+}, Ca^{2+}, phosphate). Shock occurs if volume depletion is profound. In response to the insulin deficiency and lack of available glucose the body breaks down fat (lipolysis) and some protein (proteolysis) for energy. The accumulation of ketone bodies in the blood results in metabolic acidosis.

---

*See "Appendix A" for definition of common abbreviations used in the text.

145

Assessment

History

Although DKA usually occurs in patients with known or newly diagnosed type I insulin-dependent diabetes mellitus (IDDM), it can also occur in the elderly. The patient's diabetic history should be elicited—years since diagnosis, level of control, previous hospitalizations, diabetic complications, and current insulin or drug regimen. Always look for the event precipitating the current episode of DKA. Most commonly, patients report a minor illness with poor oral intake and self-decreased or discontinued insulin. Other possible causes include myocardial infarction, stroke, pancreatitis, pregnancy, infection, or stress of any nature.

Patients may present with anorexia, abdominal pain, nausea, dehydration, and possibly altered mental status. Complications of DKA include hypothermia, hypotension, shock, gastric atony, gastrointestinal bleeding, pulmonary aspiration, possible respiratory distress syndrome, thrombosis, and hemorrhagic diathesis.

Physical Findings

Vital signs - Check the BP and pulse for orthostatic changes, and check the respiratory rate and pattern. Note deep, rapid (Kussmaul) breathing which is a compensatory mechanism to reduce acidity by blowing off carbon dioxide. Check the patient's breath for the fruity odor of acetone. Note the rectal temperature (hypothermia or mild elevations may be signs of infection).

Lungs - Listen for rales or wheezes.

Extremities - Look carefully for skin ulcers or abcesses.

Neurologic signs - Note level of consciousness. Examine for focal deficits. Use the Glasgow coma scale to assess consciousness and motor response.

Diagnostic Tests

Laboratory test - Do a Dextrostix for serum glucose stat. Draw blood for glucose and electrolytes, amylase, acetone, osmolarity, creatinine, phosphate, WBC, and RBC.

ABGs - Check an immediate ABG for pH and pO_2, and monitor the pH at regular intervals.

Urinalysis - Check a Chemstrip for ketones and leukocyte esterase.

X-rays - A chest x-ray is needed.

ECG - Check the rhythm strip for signs of hyperkalemia.

Nasogastric tube - A gastric aspirate is indicated to rule out gastrointestinal bleeding and to decompress the stomach to prevent subsequent aspiration.

Intervention

1. Fluid administration - The primary intervention in DKA is fluid replacement to correct hypovolemia, hemoconcentration, and dehydration. Vital signs, laboratory values, and fluid balance need to be carefully monitored. Start an intake and output flow sheet in the ED.
   a. Determine the patient's BP. If the patient is hypotensive, osmotic agents (e.g., beta starch or Plasmanate) are given to restore perfusion. Normal crystalloids (e.g., normal saline) can be given at the same time, but colloid is a more immediate volume expander.
   b. If the patient is not hypotensive, the osmolarity will determine fluid therapy. Normal plasma osmolality is 285 mOsm. Hyperglycemia will increase plasma osmolality and act to draw fluid from the cells into the intravascular space. In the resulting diuresis (polyuria) an extensive amount of fluid and electrolytes are lost. Normal saline (0.9%) or half-normal saline will be ordered according to the patient's osmolality. Administer half-normal saline to hyperosmolar patients with stable vital signs and administer normal saline to hypotensive patients. Osmolality can be estimated as follows:

$$mOsm = 2 (Na + K) + \frac{Glucose}{18} + \frac{BUN}{2.8}$$

   c. Administer volume - Volume is the single most important element in successful therapy. In fact, much of the metabolic derangement can be corrected by fluid alone. Fluids can be started at a rate of at least 1000 ml/hr. The acidotic hyperosmolar patient or the hypotensive patient will need even higher infusion rates. The nurse should monitor the patient's response to rapid hydration. Signs of fluid overload include neck vein distention, elevated CVP, pulmonary crackling or rales, and gallop rhythm.
2. Administer insulin - Appropriate therapy consists of regular insulin, which should be given IV in hypotensive patients and can be given either IV, IM, or SC after an IV loading dose in normotensive patients. We prefer the IV route, with a bolus followed by a constant infusion. The use of an infusion allows the serum glucose to be monitored at any time and offers more accurate control of insulin dose. An initial IV bolus of 0.2–0.4 units/Kg is followed by an IV infusion at 0.1 units/Kg/hr. The infusion is prepared by mixing 50 units in 250 ml normal saline (1 unit/5 ml). The tubing should first be flushed with albumin solution or primed with an insulin solution to prevent adsorption of insulin. Monitor serum glucose levels every hour. Be prepared to administer glucose in the event of hypoglycemia. To prevent overshoot hypoglycemia, D5W should be given when the serum glucose is under 250 mg/dl.

Insulin Preparations[a]

Insulin type	Route	Onset time (hours)	Peak time (hours)	Duration (hours)
Regular Actrapid, Humulin R, Velosulin, Iletin (short-acting)	SC, IV	½–1	2–3	6
Semilente (short-acting)	SC	½–1	5–7	12–16
NPH (Isophane insulin suspension) and Lente Humulin N (intermediate)	SC	1–1½	8–12	24
PZI (protamine zinc insulin suspension) (long-acting)	SC	4–8	14–20	36
Ultralente (long-acting)	SC	4–8	16–18	36

[a]Note: All insulin preparations should be refrigerated.

3. Electrolyte correction - Replacement of sodium and chloride is primarily accomplished by administration of normal or half-normal saline IV. Potassium levels require frequent monitoring in order to avoid hyperkalemia or hypokalemia. Patients should be placed on a cardiac monitor and the physician should be notified if the ECG shows signs of hypokalemia (prolonged QT interval, depressed T wave and U wave) or hyperkalemia (heart block, peaked T wave, wide QRS interval). Potassium will shift back into the intracellular space with the administration of insulin and fluids. Potassium acetate or potassium phosphate is preferred to potassium chloride in patients with DKA. Sodium bicarbonate should be used with caution because of the following effects:
   a. Bicarbonate will lower K and predispose to arrhythmias.
   b. Bicarbonate contributes to hyperosmolarity.
   c. The oxyhemoglobin dissociation curve will shift to the left, thus decreasing oxygen release to the tissues.
   d. Bicarbonate predisposes to subsequent alkalosis.
   e. Bicarbonate administration can cause a paradoxical worsening of coma as CO_2 diffuses through the blood-brain barrier and causes central nervous system acidosis.

However, bicarbonate is appropriate and should be given if hyperkalemia is known to be present or the ECG shows hyperacute T waves suggestive of life-threatening hyperkalemia. Note: Do not mix sodium bicarbonate and insulin.

HYPEROSMOLAR HYPERGLYCEMIC, NONKETOTIC COMA (HHNKC)

Definition

Patients with HHNKC have a serum glucose over 600 with serum osmolarity over 320. These patients are usually not acidotic, although mixed cases can occur. There is a "relative" insulin deficiency in HHNKC—insulin is present but not in adequate amounts to keep pace with rising glucose levels, which may reach 600–1000 mg/100 ml or higher.

Assessment

History
The patient's diabetic history should be elicited, as detailed earlier. HHNKC usually occurs in older, type II (NIDDM) diabetics who have mild renal dysfunction, but it may also occur in younger patients. Patients with HHNKC usually have a subacute presentation, and precipitating events are similar to those of DKA. Because glycosuria is present, similar complications occur, such as dehydration, electrolyte imbalance, and shock.

Patients with HHNKC are often lethargic and unable to take fluids; consequently, they present to the ED late and are often severely volume-depleted. Mental status changes are more common with HHNKC; coma, focal seizures, and even focal deficits have been described as a consequence of hyperosmolarity alone.

The assessment and diagnostic tests are essentially the same as for the patient with DKA.

Intervention

1. Fluid administration - The first priority is to correct existing hypotension with osmotic agents. Expect the patient with HHNKC to be extremely dehydrated. Start 2 large-bore (16-gauge) IV lines. Insertion of a CVP catheter will facilitate monitoring fluid balance. The appropriate fluid to give a normotensive patient is half-normal saline. Start an intake and output flow sheet, and if the patient is unconscious, insert a Foley catheter. The patient with HHNKC should receive 1 or

2 liters of fluids hourly for the first few hours of therapy. Although careful observation for signs of fluid overload or cerebral edema is required, the possibility of such complications should not prevent these patients from receiving adequate volume.
2. Insulin administration - These patients often require only low-dose insulin therapy, with frequent checking of the serum glucose to guide further administration. Initial dosage may be as small as 10–40 units.

HYPERGLYCEMIA

If a diabetic patient with an elevated serum glucose is well perfused, not acidotic, and not hyperosmolar, that patient is simply hyperglycemic.

History
It is important to determine why the patient's diabetes is uncontrolled; most likely reasons are infection and noncompliance with diet or medication.

Intervention

Hyperglycemic patients can be effectively managed by oral hydration and SC insulin. These patients do not need IV fluids or IV insulin; in fact, this aggressive approach is dangerous. If given SC insulin, these patients should be observed for a period of several hours in the ED, with a repeat Chemstrip or serum glucose performed prior to discharge.

Although all patients with DKA and HHNKC should be admitted, most patients with simple hyperglycemia can be treated in the ED and referred to outpatient follow-up. The only exceptions are hyperglycemic patients who are vomiting, are unable to take fluids or medications, or are becoming significantly dehydrated. If these patients are insulin dependent, they will need admission to prevent development of DKA.

HYPOGLYCEMIA

Hypoglycemia is defined as a plasma glucose below 55 mg/dl with symptoms. Common causes include:

1. Fasting hypoglycemia due to acquired liver disease (hepatitis, cirrhosis), drugs (ethanol, propranolol, diabetic medications, theophylline, dicumarol, salicylates), malnutrition, chronic renal failure or excess insulin production or administration, and sepsis
2. Postprandial hypoglycemia due to rapid gastric emptying (prior gastrectomy) or idiopathic postprandial hypoglycemia

Oral Hypoglycemic Agents

Generic name (trade name)	Duration (hours)	Common daily dosage (mg)
Tolbutamide (Orinase)	6–12	500–3000
Acetohexamide (Dymelor)	12–24	250–1500
Tolazamide (Tolinase)	12–24	100–750
Chlorpropamide (Diabinese)	12–24 (100 mg) 24–36 (250 mg)	100–500

Side effects and toxic effects include:

1. Allergic reactions
2. Gastrointestinal upset, weakness, headache, paresthesia, and intolerance to alcohol
3. Contraindicated in patients with hepatic disease

Assessment

History

If possible, the patient should give a clear history of the episode that prompted the ED visit, including symptoms, recent food intake or fasting, and time and amount of insulin administration or oral hypoglycemics. A history of diabetes, alcoholism, or major systemic disease should be sought. Occurrence of previous similar episodes and the symptoms should be elicited.

Symptoms of fasting hypoglycemia are considered central nervous system "neuroglycopenic" symptoms, have a fairly gradual onset, and include headache, fatigue, confusion, amnesia, seizures, loss of consciousness, irrational behavior, a glassy-eyed stare, diplopia, and dysarthria.

Patients with postprandial complaints describe a more sudden onset and adrenergic symptoms including anxiety, irritability, palpitations, sweating, tachycardia and tremors.

There can be a wide gamut of presenting complaints in hypoglycemia, including focal neurologic deficits, focal seizures, isolated aglossia, and acute violent behavior. Hypoglycemia should be suspected with any case of altered mental status, neurologic abnormality, or bizarre behavior. All patients with any alteration of consciousness, behavior, or neurologic function should have a Dextrostix determination and should receive thiamine (in a patient with a history of alcohol abuse) and naloxone.

Physical Findings
General - Note if the patient is obese (insulinoma, diabetes) or cachetic (malnutrition).
Skin - Note diaphoresis. Look for stigmata of alcohol abuse or liver disease.
Vital signs - Check for tachycardia. Note if the patient is febrile or slightly hypothermic (sepsis).
Neurologic signs - Note level of consciousness and mentation. Do a Glasgow coma scale, look for focal deficits, and check for tremors.

Diagnostic Tests
SMA - Do an immediate Dextrostix for an estimate of blood glucose. The diagnosis of hypoglycemia can be confirmed by a plasma glucose.

Intervention

Draw blood for a Dextrostix glucose and stat plasma glucose. The patient is then given 1 ampule of D50W, followed by an IV D10W drip until the patient is alert. It may be necessary to give more than 1 ampule of D50W if the patient responds incompletely. Check Dextrostix repeatedly. Do not give IV glucose solutions if the patient can eat. Hepatic glycogen stores cannot be repleted with IV glucose; thus oral intake of glucose is critical. In the absence of an IV line, a comatose patient may be treated with 1–2 mg of glucagon IM, provided he or she has adequate stores of liver glycogen.

ED Discharge Planning

The following patients should be admitted:

1. All patients with DKA and HHNKC
2. Hyperglycemic patients who are vomiting, are unable to take fluids or medication, or are significantly dehydrated
3. Patients with serious or life-threatening symptoms of hypoglycemia (e.g., seizures, coma)
4. Patients who have ingested long-acting sulfonylureas or self-administered insulin and have persistent hypoglycemia
5. Patients with hypoglycemia due to alcoholism or hepatic disease
6. Alcoholics who have taken insulin and become hypoglycemic

Diabetics with quickly relieved hypoglycemia or hyperglycemia who can supply a very cogent reason for the episode (e.g., took insulin but did not eat usual meals due to unusual circumstance) do not require admission. However, diabetics who took their usual dose of medications, who have a concomitant acute illness that prevented eating, or who cannot eat properly or administer medications properly without better social supports may need to be admitted for further observation and adjustment of medications.

ED Discharge Instructions
Discharge instructions should include:

1. Review of diet and medication prescription and instruction not to make changes without medical input
2. Referral to dietician if diet is poorly understood or a contributing factor in ED visit
3. Need for maintaining a consistent daily activity and exercise regimen
4. Instruction to carry a fast-acting carbohydrate for emergency use
5. Review of signs and symptoms of diabetic shock and hyperglycemia
6. Importance of wearing a diabetic identification tag (Medic-Alert bracelet) or carrying such a card in the wallet
7. Necessity of regular follow-up at an ambulatory care clinic or by the family physician

HEAT STROKE

Description

Classically, heat stroke has been defined as a triad of a temperature of $\geq 105°F$, altered mental status, and anhidrosis. Older patients and those on medications that interfere with the sweating mechanism will present with anhidrosis. However, younger patients and those exercising strenuously present with hyperthermia, central nervous system dysfunction, and diaphoresis. Younger patients with heat stroke are often athletes, military recruits, or psychiatric patients.

Heat cramps usually occur in the setting of intense physical activity and are caused by sodium depletion due to extensive sweating. Patients are afebrile with a normal mental status and painful muscle contractions. Heat exhaustion affects patients who are not physically conditioned or acclimatized to heat and who exercise in a hot or slightly elevated temperature. They may have nausea and vomiting, diarrhea, muscle cramps, and postural hypotension. There may be significant volume depletion due to the loss of salt and water.

Assessment

History

Exertional heat stroke is most commonly associated with high environmental temperature and humidity and physical exercise. Nonexertional heat stroke is seen in elderly, obese, or chonically ill patients. Risk factors for hyperthermia include:

1. Drugs (anticholinergics, alcohol, diuretics, neuroleptics, tranquilizers, and beta blockers, lithium, phencyclidine, or cocaine overdose)
2. Parkinson's disease
3. Chronic skin disorders
4. Hyperthyroidism
5. Spinal cord lesions
6. Previous stroke or thermal injury
7. Malnutrition

ED staff must be particularly alert and prepared for hyperthermia in hot, humid weather. Humid weather interferes with evaporative heat loss (sweating), which is the main mechanism of heat loss in hot weather. As the temperature humidity index (THI) rises above 65, the risk of heat stroke increases.

Note: Heat stroke is a medical emergency associated with a high mortality rate. Aggressive cooling measures should be started as soon as the condition is determined.

Physical Findings

Vital signs - An accurate temperature must be recorded with a thermocouple; the probe is left in place as examination and treatment proceed. Check for hypotension, tachycardia, and respiratory depression.

HEENT - Look for signs of trauma. Check pupil response.

Lungs - Auscultate for bilateral breath sounds, rales, rhonchi, or wheezes.

Extremities - Note if they are cold and clammy or cyanotic. Look for track marks.

Skin - Check for hot, dry skin (anhydrotic, particularly in elderly). A petechial rash may occur due to hemorrhage into sweat glands.

Neurologic signs - Note level of consciousness which can range from irritability to coma. Other central nervous system effects include headache, syncope, confusion, dizziness, focal deficits, and seizures.

Diagnostic Tests

Laboratory tests - CBC, BUN, glucose, SMA, PT, PTT, platelets (may see DIC).

ABGs - There is no need to correct the blood gases for temperature.

However, it should be remembered that hyperthermia elevates the pO_2 and that, despite a pO_2 in the "normal range," all hyperthermic patients should be given oxygen.

Urinalysis - Chemstrip and send for urinalysis. Hemoglobinuria and myoglobinuria may be detected.

ECG - Hyperthermia may cause ST or T wave changes, premature ventricular contractions, and arrhythmias.

Intervention

1. Support cardiac output and maintain airway - Start IV of normal saline and administer oxygen by cannula or mask. Place patient on cardiac monitor and initiate CPR as indicated.
2. Rapid cooling - Undress the patient, cover with a wet sheet, and place in a cool or air-conditioned room. Apply ice to the patient's neck, axilla, and inguinal areas. If the temperature does not begin to fall within 20 minutes, the patient can be placed in a tub filled with ice and water. In this situation, safety is a concern; hyperthermic patients are at risk for seizures, arrhythmias, and shock. Cooling must be terminated when the core temperature reaches 102°F to prevent overshoot and hypothermia.
3. Fluid administration - If the patient is not in shock or is sweating profusely, the fluid requirements are usually modest. An IV infusion of up to 1000 ml of normal saline may be given over the first 4 hours. Hypovolemic shock may be treated with Plasmanate or normal saline, as well as application of the MAST suit (see Chapter 1 for details on the treatment of hypovolemic shock). A CVP or Swan-Ganz catheter may be inserted to monitor fluid status. Potassium losses may be significant, and hypokalemia must be treated with potassium replacement. An intake and output flow record should be started in the ED. Urinary output needs to be closely monitored due to the possibility of acute tubular necrosis. Increased fluids, mannitol, and furosemide may be administered to improve renal perfusion.

ED Discharge Planning

All patients with heat stroke or heat exhaustion should be admitted. Milder forms of heat illness (heat cramps) may be treated and sent home. These patients should have adequate sodium replacement before discharge and should be told to refrain from exercise until they have fully recovered. Remember that the patient's temperature may have decreased spontaneously or in response to treatment en route to the hospital. Consequently, decisions regarding admission should be based not on temperature alone but on a total assessment of the patient.

1. Take preventive measures, i.e., decrease activity in hot weather, maintain an adequate intake of fluids and salt, take periodic rest periods, and stay cool in hot weather.
2. Gradually acclimatize to hot weather.
3. Seek medical care promptly if symptoms persist or return.

HYPOTHERMIA

Definition

Hypothermia is defined as a core temperature of <95°F. The diagnosis is often missed because standard thermometers do not register that low. Hypothermia must be identified by using special glass thermometers or thermocouple probes. Several mechanisms of heat loss may contribute to the development of hypothermia:

1. Conduction - loss by direct contact (lying on cold floor)
2. Convection - body to air loss (wind)
3. Radiation - loss to air (uncovered head)
4. Evaporation - sweating

In addition to exposure, other causes of impaired thermoregulation include hypothyroidism, DKA, hypoglycemia, liver disease, burns, drug and alcohol ingestion, sepsis, shock, and advanced age.

Assessment

History
Obtain a history of events leading to hypothermia, such as length of exposure, syncope or fall, or a cold apartment. Past medical history should focus on the presence of systemic disease, medications taken, and drug or alcohol abuse. Patient's social supports (e.g., lives in the streets, no heat in apartment) will be a major determinant in the patient's discharge plan.

Physical Findings
Vital signs - Check temperature with a thermocouple probe. There may be significant hypotension and hypoventilation if the patient's temperature is under 82°F. Bradycardia will result in a drop in cardiac output.
Lungs - Listen for rales and bilateral breath sounds.
Extremities - Note cyanosis or edema. Check distal pulses.
Neurologic signs - Do a Glasgow coma scale. Level of consciousness will range from dulled mentation to coma according to the degree of hypothermia.

Diagnostic Tests

Laboratory tests - Do a spun Hct and send a CBC with differential and platelets. (Platelets may be decreased if DIC is a complication.) Check SMA for electrolytes, liver function tests, muscle enzymes, glucose, and amylase. A Dextrostix for blood glucose will detect hyperglycemia that may result from decreased insulin and decreased glucose utilization.

PT - Look for prolongation, which may indicate impaired liver function as well as DIC.

ABGs - Check the pH and pO_2. In hypothermia, the oxyhemoglobin dissociation curve shifts to the left (decreased unloading). Blood gases show a metabolic acidosis.

ECGs - Hypothermia causes sinus bradycardia; flipped T waves; elevated PR, QRS, and ST segments; and J waves (see Fig. 6.1). There is increased myocardial irritability, and atrial fibrillation or ventricular fibrillation may occur.

Toxicologies - Appropriate drug levels should be determined. Hypothermia causes decreased liver function and slower clearance of intoxicants.

Intervention

1. Immediately evaluate vital signs. Place patient on cardiac monitor, and check frequently for arrhythmias. The risk of arrhythmias is highest in persons with severe hypothermia (<86°F). Accurate BP recording via arm cuffs may be difficult due to intense vasoconstriction. Bradycardia and hypotension usually respond to warming without the use of pressors.
2. Establish airway and circulation. Administer 100% oxygen via a heated nebulizer. Start a large-bore IV line for volume replacement with warm isotonic solution. (See Chapter 1 on treatment of hypovolemic shock.) Patients may require large amounts of fluids due to renal losses

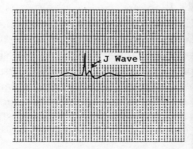

Figure 6.1. J wave. (From Pousada L, Osborn HH. Emergency medicine for the house officer. Baltimore: Williams & Wilkins, 1986:168).

and third spacing secondary to increased capillary permeability. A Foley catheter and CVP line will improve fluid balance monitoring. Perform CPR if needed—extended CPR may be necessary, as patients "come back from the dead" with rewarming. Hypothermia may block the physiologic response to resuscitation drugs. With rewarming, they may all act at once, and patients may show toxic reactions. In general, cardiotonics and pressors should not be used. Ventricular fibrillation is treated with aggressive rewarming (i.e., peritoneal lavage, femoral-femoral bypass), as its presence is related to hypothermia, not necessarily to heart disease. Bretylium has been reported to reverse ventricular fibrillation due to hypothermia. In any event, the combination of bradycardia and low cardiac output is highly compatible with low basal metabolic rate. As the temprature rises, fibrillation responds better and is more important to control. Remember that a patient cannot be declared dead until core temperature is 90°F.

3. Correct hypoglycemia. Check Dextrostix and give IV glucose (1 ampule of D50W) as prescribed. Thiamine, 100 mg IM or SC, is given to patients with a history of alcohol abuse.

4. If patient is hyperglycemic but not in diabetic ketoacidosis, hyperglycemia should be treated with fluids and not insulin initially. Rewarming will correct glucose metabolism, and muscle use will deplete glycogen stores, causing rebound hypoglycemia.

5. If overdose is suspected, naloxone (Narcan) at 2 mg IV is indicated. Repeated doses IV or IM may be given according to the patient's response.

6. Perform rewarming. All methods of rewarming are equally acceptable, as the prognosis is related to the underlying disease state, not to the degree or duration of hypothermia (with the exception of myxedema coma). Concentrate on core rewarming in moderate and severe hypothermia (<89.8°F). Patients have been successfully rewarmed from 61°F. The rate of rewarming should be 0.5–1.0°C/hr. Methods of rewarming include:
   a. Passive external - Blankets
   b. Active core - Electric or hot water blankets, warmed IV fluids, warm air ventilation, warm nasogastric lavage, warm peritoneal dialysis, and extracorporeal warming of blood via hemodialysis.
   All hypothermic patients should receive blankets and warm oxygen to breathe. Unstable patients (flat line, ventricular fibrillation) should receive continuous CPR (manual or mechanical oxygen-powered thumper) and aggressive rewarming with nasogastric or peritoneal lavage.

Frostbite should be treated by immersion in a warm water bath (104°F) or warm moist soaks for face or ears. See Chapter 15 for a further discussion of frostbite.

ED Discharge Planning

Most hypothermic patients will require admission for treatment of the underlying disease and further observation. Patients with mild hypothermia or frostbite may be discharged on the basis of the following considerations:

1. Patient's ability to provide safe self-care including housing and judgment
2. Social service and visiting nurse referrals, as indicated
3. Instruction of the patient and/or family on environmental hazards, proper clothing, etc.

ENDOCRINE EMERGENCIES

THYROID STORM

Definition

Thyroid storm is a severe and life-threatening extreme of thyrotoxicosis. It is manifested by exaggerated symptoms of thryotoxicosis, including fever and neurologic, cardiovascular, gastrointestinal, and hepatic dysfunction. Precipitating factors include:

1. Untreated or inadequately treated hyperthyroidism
2. Surgery (either thyroidectomy or unrelated surgery) in a poorly prepared hyperthyroid patient
3. Vigorous palpation of an enlarged, toxic thyroid gland
4. Trauma in a hyperthyroid patient
5. Medical disorders including intercurrent illness such as pneumonia, influenza, and DKA, in a hyperthyroid patient
6. Radioactive iodine therapy, exposure to inorganic iodine or exposure to organic iodine compounds during angiography, cardiac catheterization, and IV pyelography
7. Abrupt withdrawal of propranolol therapy in a thyrotoxic patient

Assessment

History
Common symptoms include weakness, weight loss, heat intolerance, diplopia, fever, palpitations, chest pains, anxiety, tremor, agitation, confusion, psychosis, diarrhea, nausea, and vomiting. Recent infections, trauma, or medical procedures should be noted. Past medical history

should include any chronic medical problems, previous thyroid disease, and all medications and dosages.

Physical Findings

General - Observe for restlessness, agitation, confusion, tremulousness, and jaundice.

Vital signs - Check for fever, tachycardia, widened pulse pressure, irregular heart beat, and tachypnea.

HEENT - Check for lid lag, extraocular muscle weakness, exophthalmos, and thyroid enlargement.

Cardiovascular system - Note heart sounds, and listen for murmur, rub, or S_3 (high output CHF).

Lung - Note presence of dyspnea, tachypnea, and rales.

Neurologic signs - Note alteration in mental status, e.g., confusion, agitation, and coma. Assess for peripheral muscle weakness and fine tremors.

Skin - This is usually warm, moist, and smooth. Look for pedal edema.

Diagnostic Tests

The physician will make a diagnosis based on clinical evaluation. Laboratory data will confirm the diagnosis, but therapy cannot wait for the results.

CBC - Check Hct and WBC with differential.

SMA - Note results of electrolytes, glucose, and liver function tests.

Thyroid function tests - Perform resin T_3 uptake and T_4 and T_3 radioimmunoassays. Draw serum cortisol (to rule out hypopituitarism).

Urinalysis - Look for infection.

X-rays - On chest film, note cardiomegaly or pulmonary infiltrate.

ECG - Note aberrant rhythms or tachycardia.

Thyroid scan and uptake - These are generally not available on an immediate basis.

Intervention

1. Correction of fluid and electrolyte imbalance. Start an IV of D10W with B vitamins to meet metabolic needs. Monitor fluid intake and output; fluid overload will tax an already decompensated cardiac system. Check vital signs, neck veins, and lung sounds for signs of CHF.
2. Reduce patient's temperature - Place the patient on a cooling blanket or sponge with ice water. Give nonaspirin antipyretic (aspirin may displace thyroid hormone from binding sites).
3. Medications to block thyroid hormones (T_3 and T_4)

   a. Propylthiouracil (PTU), 200–250 mg every 4 hours PO, or methimazole, 20–25 mg every 4 hours PO, inhibits thyroid hormone synthesis.

   b. Sodium iodide, 1–2 gm/day by slow IV infusion, or Lugol's iodide, 5 drops every 4 hours PO, acts to inhibit thyroid hormone release.

   c. Propranolol, 1–5 mg every 4 hours IV or 20–40 mg every 4 hours PO, or reserpine, 0.25–2.5 mg every 4–6 hours IM, block overstimulating the sympathetic nervous system.

   d. PTU (dose above), or propranolol (dose above), or dexamethasone, 2 mg every 6 hours IV or IM, will inhibit the conversion of T_4 to T_3.

   e. Hydrocortisone, 200 mg IV, if panhypopituitarism is a possibility.

4. Supportive measures - Due to the high metabolic rate, all patients should be given oxygen by mask. Other measures to reduce complications include:

   a. Reduce environmental stressors, e.g., cool darkened room, limit visitors.

   b. Limit activity, and place patient in mid-Fowler's position.

ED Discharge Planning

All patients in thyroid storm should be admitted to the hospital, preferably to an ICU for close monitoring. Nursing priorities for an admitted patient include:

1. Promote rest and energy conservation.
2. Maintain normal body temperature.
3. Monitor for hypertension and CHF.
4. Reduce anxiety
5. Provide for intake of high-calorie, high-vitamin fluids and diet.
6. Prevent complications, e.g., eye injury.

OTHER ENDOCRINE EMERGENCIES

Other endocrine emergencies are listed in Table 6.1, along with their signs and symptoms, causes and interventions.

Table 6.1.
Other Endocrine Emergencies

Signs and symptoms	Causes	Intervention
Adrenal crisis (Addisonian crisis)		
Weakness, anorexia, nausea, vomiting, and weight loss. Increased pigmentation of elbows, knees, and lips. Personality changes from irritability to psychosis. Course hair, dry skin, and alopecia.	Hemorrhage or tumor invasion of adrenal glands. Acute stress or infection in patient with known adrenal insufficiency.	IV D5/NS for dehydration and possible hypotension. IV steroid replacement with hydrocortisone or dexamethasone. NG tube, Foley catheter, and oxygen. Treat hypotension aggressively. Treat underlying cause, e.g., infection.
Hypercalcemia		
Lethargy, stupor, thirst, fatigue, weakness, and anorexia. Depressed mentation and altered level of consciousness. Abdominal pain, pancreatitis, renal stones, and peptic ulcer are relevant.	Increased calcium uptake (milk-alkali syndrome, adrenal insufficiency), increased movement from bone and decreased calcium output (thiazide diuretics), dehydration.	IV NS 250–500 ml/hr. Monitor intake and output, CVP, and electrolytes. Furosemide to enhance calcium diuresis. Hydrocortisone or oral phosphate may be prescribed.
Hypocalcemia (tetany)		
Neuromuscular irritability, muscle cramps, paresthesias, carpopedal spasms, seizures, bronchospasm, laryngospasm, and prolonged QT interval.	Inadequate dietary intake, multiple blood transfusions, trauma to parathyroid gland, intestinal malabsorption, hepatic and biliary disorders, hypoparathyroidism postoperatively, and idiopathic trauma.	IV calcium chloride or gluconate. Check magnesium level. Hypomagnesemia may also be present. Monitor IV calcium chloride for infiltration. Monitor ECG and QT interval.

ELECTROLYTE IMBALANCES

Some degree of electrolyte imbalance accompanies any critical or chronic illness. Electrolytes affect all body systems—serum osmolality, nerve conduction, muscular contraction, and cardiac conduction as well as acid-base balance. The ED nurse needs to be alert for signs of electrolyte imbalance, the situations in which the imbalance is most likely to occur and preventive measures.

Assessment

History
The patient should be questioned as to systemic disease, such as cirrhosis, renal disease, CHF, and diabetes. A medication history should include drugs known to affect fluid and electrolyte balance such as diuretics and those known to cause the syndrome of inappropriate antidiuretic hormone (SIADH), such as chlorpropamide (Diabinese), chlorpromazine (Thorazine), carbamazepine (Tegretol). A recent history of nausea and vomiting, diarrhea, polyuria or oliguria, hyperventilation, or major change in fluid intake will be contributory to fluid and electrolyte imbalance.

Physical Findings
Vital signs - Check for orthostatic changes. Always take a temperature.
Lungs - Listen for rales (CHF, pneumonia).
Heart - Note the presence of gallops or rubs and regularity of rhythm.
Skin and extremities - Note peripheral edema or sign of dehydration, e.g., poor skin turgor, wrinkling, and sunken eyes.
Neuromuscular signs - Assess for fatigue, weakness, abdominal cramps, and muscle spasms.

Diagnostic Tests
SMA - Check all electrolytes, BUN, and creatinine. Remember that osmotically active substances, such as glucose, mannitol, lipids, and proteins, will effect the movement of water and electrolytes between the intravascular and extravascular spaces.
Osmolarity - Check both urine and serum osmolarity.
ECG - Abnormalities in cardiac conduction are particularly seen in disorders of potassium balance.

HYPONATREMIA

Hyponatremia is defined as a serum sodium under 135 mEq/liter, and it implies deficit of body sodium in relation to body water. The signs and symptoms associated with hyponatremia include hypotension, anorexia, nausea, vomiting, confusion, seizures, and coma. Symptoms increase in severity with lower sodium levels. With levels below 110 mEq/liter, particularly on an acute basis, seizures and coma may occur.

Intervention

Specific treatment will depend on the specific etiology of hyponatremia, but all of the following will need to be done:

1. Correct fluid imbalance. For dehydrated patients, administer isotonic saline as prescribed. On occasion, patients with severe hyponatremia and seizures or coma will be treated with hypertonic saline (3%). Patients with water intoxication and SIADH will be placed on fluid restriction.
2. Monitor intake and output every hour.
3. Place the patient on seizure precautions, and assess CNS function and vital signs every hour.

HYPERNATREMIA

Hypernatremia is defined as a serum sodium over 145 mEq/liter. It results from either an excessive intake of sodium or a loss of water without a corresponding loss in sodium. Signs and symptoms associated with hypernatremia include thirst, lethargy, fatigue, somnolence, and irritability. Causes of hypernatremia include excessive water loss due to diabetes insipidus, osmotic diuretics, excessive sodium intake, and decreased water intake seen in debilitated patients unable to drink freely.

Intervention

1. Fluid replacement. If patient's condition permits, encourage oral fluid intake. If the hypernatremia is severe or the patient is unable to take fluids PO, administer D5W or hypotonic saline (0.45% NaCl) as ordered.
2. Monitor vital signs and intake and output every hour.

HYPOKALEMIA

Hypokalemia is defined as a serum potassium under 3.5 mEq/liter, although the serum potassium is only a rough reflection of total body potassium. Manifestations of hypokalemia include weakness, hyporeflexia, paresthesias, cardiac abnormalities, ileus, and mental status changes. ECG changes include flat or inverted T waves, prominent U waves, and depressed ST segments. Causes of hypokalemia include gastrointestinal losses, diuretics, inadequate intake, and alkalosis.

Intervention

1. Potassium replacement. Whenever possible, oral potassium replacement will be prescribed in doses of 40–80 mEq of KCl elixir, Slow-K,

or K-Lor. IV potassium is necessary if the potassium level is below 2.5 mEq/liter. Potassium may be given as 40–60 mEq/liter KCl diluted in NS or D5W. In an emergency, 10–20 mEq KCl in 100 ml of D5W or NS may be given in 30–60 minutes. Potassium is never given by SC, IM, or IV bolus.

2. Monitor vital signs, and monitor the heart for T wave changes and arrhythmias, particularly PVCs. Consult a physician before administering digitalis.

HYPERKALEMIA

Hyperkalemia is defined as a serum potassium over 5.5 mEq/liter. A rapidly rising potassium level is especially dangerous and may be life-threatening.

Manifestations of hyperkalemia include weakness, paresthesias, areflexia, and muscular or respiratory paralysis. Cardiovascular effects are frequent with levels at or above 8.0 mEq/liter and include bradycardia, hypotension, ventricular fibrillation, and cardiac standstill. The ECG shows tall peaked T waves, depressed ST segments, decreased amplitude of R waves, prolonged PR interval, decreased or absent P waves with a widening of the QRS complex, and prolonged QT interval. Causes of hyperkalemia include acute and chronic renal failure, excessive use of potassium supplements, cell breakdown (e.g., burns, crush injuries, surgery, hemolysis), administration of high doses of penicillin and acidosis from any cause.

Intervention

Immediate intervention in a case of hyperkalemia may be lifesaving and consists of the following:

1. Restore membrane potential. In cases of life-threatening hyperkalemia the physician may order calcium gluconate 10% solution, 5–10 ml by slow IV push. Calcium is a potassium antagonist, and it acts to restore membrane potential and cardiac conduction. It is the quickest form of therapy, but its effects dissipate quickly.
2. Shift potassium into the cells.
   a. Sodium bicarbonate, 1 ampule (44 mEq) given by slow IV push, will shift potassium into the cells. Sodium bicarbonate takes about 15 minutes to take effect and lasts 1–2 hours.
   b. Administration of IV glucose and insulin will force potassium into the cells. The dose is 50 ml of D50W (25 gm dextrose) and 5–10 units regular insulin. Effects are seen within 30 minutes and last for several hours.
3. Take measures to eliminate potassium.

a. Administration of sodium polystyrene sulfonate (Kayexalate) via nasogastric tube or retention enema—Kayexalate removes potassium on an ion-exchange basis with sodium. It may be given PO in a dose of 20–50 gm dissolved in 100–200 ml sorbitol 20% solution to avoid constipation. Doses may be repeated every 2–3 hours. Because of the sodium load, Kayexalate should be used with caution in patients with CHF.

b. Hemodialysis - A renal consultant should be called in all cases of severe hyperkalemia. Hemodialysis is very useful in correcting acidosis and hyperkalemia and may be indicated.

4. Monitor vital signs every hour and observe cardiac monitor for bradycardia, peaked T waves, wide QRS complexes, and depressed ST segments.
5. Monitor and record intake and output.
6. Observe for signs of hyperkalemia and hypokalemia and send blood for repeat SMA according to protocol.

ED Discharge Planning

Patients treated in the ED for severe electrolyte imbalance will be admitted for stabilization of fluid and electrolyte balance and for treatment of any underlying condition. Patients with mild electrolyte imbalance may be discharged with the following considerations:

1. Patient needs to follow diet or take medication as prescribed, or the family should be instructed as necessary.
2. Consider visiting nurse and dietician referrals for follow-up instruction and monitoring.
3. Stress the importance of continued medical care.
4. Instruct the patient to return to the ED for recurrence of symptoms.

ACID-BASE IMBALANCE

The balance between bodily acids and base is maintained by the use of dynamic regulatory systems. The body's acid-base balance is expressed in terms of hydrogen ion concentration and is written as pH. The normal body pH is 7.35–7.45. pH is a negative logarithm of the hydrogen ion (H^+) concentration; therefore, a fall in pH denotes a rise in the H^+ concentration. The three acid-base regulatory mechanisms are the buffer systems, the respiratory system, and the renal system. The major attributes of these three complementary systems are described below:

1. Buffer system - Composed of weak acids and bases, the buffers react

chemically to neutralize acid-base imbalance. The system responds immediately. The most important of the body's buffers is the carbonic acid-bicarbonate system in which a strong acid is combined with bicarbonate to form carbonic acid (H_2CO_3) which is a weak acid. Carbonic acid further breaks down to form water and carbon dioxide (CO_2). The CO_2 and, in effect, acid are then excreted by the lungs.

$$H^+Cl^- + Na^+HCO_3^- \rightarrow Na^+Cl^- + H_2CO_3$$
$$H_2CO_3 \leftrightarrow H_2O + CO_2$$

2. Respiratory system - The lungs affect the acid-base balance by regulating the amount of CO_2 expired. There is a direct correlation between respiratory rate, carbonic acid, and H^+ concentration. An increase in the rate and depth of respirations will reduce or "blow off" CO_2, causing less H_2CO_3 to be produced and thereby lowering the pH. The opposite is also true. Slow, shallow respirations cause CO_2 to be retained and increase the acid level in the blood. Respiratory regulation of acid- base balance can be initiated within minutes.

3. Renal system - The kidneys regulate pH by affecting the amount of bicarbonate (HCO_3^-) and H^+ excreted. An elevated blood pH (alkaline) will precipitate the excretion of bicarbonate and the retention of H^+. The renal system is the slowest regulatory mechanism, taking 1–2 days to respond fully.

Acid-base imbalance - A significant alteration in the ratio between carbonic acid and bicarbonate (20 parts base:1 part acid) will produce an acid-base imbalance. If the regulatory mechanisms are unable to compensate and maintain a pH within normal limits, then a condition of acidosis or alkalosis exists. Acid-base imbalances are categorized as respiratory or metabolic.

Normal values	
pH	7.35–7.45
pCO_2	35–45 mm Hg (torr)
pO_2	80–100 mm Hg (torr)
HCO_3^-	22–26 mEq/liter
O_2 saturation	96–100%

Respiratory acidosis - Hypoventilation causes a retention of CO_2 and, subsequently, carbonic acid. Respiratory acidosis will occur in any condition that impedes gas exchange, including COPD, barbiturate overdose, pneumonia, flail chest, and aspiration. When the pulmonary condition has been present for over 24 hours, the renal system will attempt to normalize (compensate) the pH by retaining HCO_3^- and increasing the H^+ secreted. ABG levels will indicate the primary disorder and the compensatory mechanism. Note that regardless of the effectiveness of the compensation the pH will not be completely normalized. The direction (acid or alkaline) of the pH indicates the primary problem, as is indicated in the following examples of acute and compensated acidosis:

Acute acidosis	Chronic acidosis (>24 hours)
pH 7.21 mm Hg (torr)	pH 7.32
pCO$_2$ 66	pCO$_2$ 66
HCO$_3^-$24 (normal)	HCO$_3$ 34
(uncompensated)	(compensated)

Respiratory alkalosis - Hyperventilation causes the "blow off" (expiration) of CO_2, which decreases carbonic acid and results in an imbalance in the ratio of acids to base. Respiratory alkalosis may be caused by anxiety, central nervous system disease, fever, and mechanical overventilation. Respiratory alkalosis is most often an acute short-term condition, but when it is prolonged, the kidneys will compensate by excretion of HCO_3^-, as is indicated in the following examples of respiratory alkalosis:

Acute alkalosis	Chronic alkalosis
pH 7.6	pH 7.46
pCO$_2$ 26	pCO$_2$ 26
HCO$_3^-$26 (normal)	HCO$_3^-$16
(uncompensated)	(compensated)

Note: A change in pCO$_2$ of 10 mm Hg (torr) in either direction (up or down) is accompanied by a change in pH of 0.08 units. The change in pH is reciprocal to the change in pCO$_2$, e.g., in hypoventilation:

In this example the pCO$_2$ = 60 mm Hg
Normal CO$_2$ = 40 mm Hg
pCO$_2$ difference = +20
20 mm Hg ÷ 10 mm Hg = 2
2 × 0.08 = 0.16
pH = 7.40 (normal pH) − 0.16 = 7.24

pH should be 7.24, if acute. A pH > or < 7.24 implies compensation or some other primary acid-base disorder, e.g., in hyperventilation:

In this example the pCO_2 = 20 mm Hg
Normal pCO_2 = 40 mm Hg
pCO_2 difference = −20
20 mm Hg ÷ 10 mm Hg = 2
2 × 0.08 = 0.16
pH = 7.40 (normal pH) + 0.16 = 7.56

pH should be 7.56, if acute. Within 24–36 hours the pH should decrease, indicating renal (metabolic) compensation. As indicated previously, a pH > or < 7.56 implies compensation or another primary acid-base disorder (see Fig. 6.2 on pp. 170 and 171).

Metabolic acidosis - An excess of acid (other than carbonic acid) or a loss of bicarbonate results in metabolic acidosis. DKA, uremia, and lactic acidosis (shock) cause a relative bicarbonate deficit. Direct loss of bicarbonate will result from severe diarrhea and renal disease. The lungs react by increasing the respiratory rate and depth, thereby "blowing off" CO_2. Kussmaul's breathing is a mechanism by which the lungs' compensate, as indicated by the following example:

	Metabolic acidosis	
pH	7.32	
pCO_2	32	(compensated)
HCO_3	16	

Metabolic alkalosis - A loss of acid or an increase in bicarbonate intake results in metabolic alkalosis. Prolonged vomiting and nasogastric suction causes a loss of gastric HCl and diuretic therapy without adequate potassium supplement and can result in metabolic alkalosis. To compensate for the overbalance of base, the lungs slow the respiratory rate in order to retain CO_2, and the kidneys excrete bicarbonate, as is indicated in the following example of compensated metabolic alkalosis:

	Metabolic alkalosis	
pH	7.48	
pCO_2	48	(compensated)
HCO_3	34	

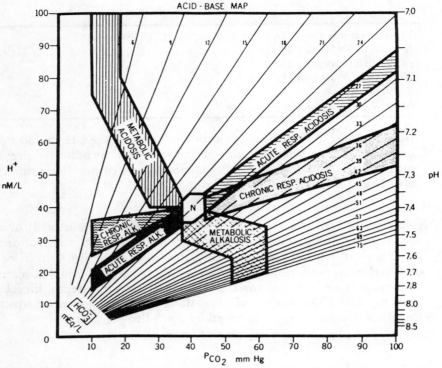

Figure 6.2. Acid-base map. *N*, area of normal values. Map actually extends further up than shown (to a pH of 6.6.) and further to the right than shown (to a pCO_2 of 180 mm Hg). *Numbered lines* represent isopleths for bicarbonate (in milliequivalents per liter).

1. Locate the point where the pH and pCO_2 values (from an ABG determination) intersect on the acid-base map.
2. If the point is within a labelled band (e.g., "metabolic acidosis," "acute respiratory acidosis," etc.), the patient may have a "single" or "simple" acid-base disturbance *with* its appropriate, physiologic compensation.
   Example: A patient with DKA and *no other medical (respiratory) problem* has a pH of 7.20 and a pCO_2 of 20 mm Hg. The pH/pCO_2 values intersect *within* the "metabolic acidosis" band, meaning that the patient has a metabolic acidosis with the appropriate *compensatory* respiratory alkalosis.
3. If the point is outside any of the labelled bands, the patient has at least two primary acid-base disturbances (within a 95% probability used to construct the in vivo confidence bands).
   Example: A patient who is thought to have DKA alone has a pH of 7.30 and a pCO_2 of 20 mm Hg. The pH/pCO_2 values intersect *below* the "metabolic acidosis" band, i.e., *between* the "metabolic acidosis" band and the two (acute and chronic) "respiratory alkalosis" bands, meaning that the patient has a *mixed* acid-base disturbance consisting of a "metabolic acidosis" and a (primary) "respiratory alkalosis"—*not a compensatory* respiratory alkalosis. Such an acid-base picture may characterize an acute adult salicylate overdose, in which case the

respiratory alkalosis is an *acute* respiratory alkalosis (i.e., mentally erase the *chronic* respiratory alkalosis band from the map).

4. If the point is within a labelled band, the *patient's clinical situation* will help determine whether or not he or she is suffering from a simple of mixed acid-base disturbance.

   Example: Case 1: 70-year-old man with barrel chest, wheezing, rhonchi, rales, very mild respiratory distress, flattened diaphragm on chest x-ray, arterial pH of 7.35, and pCO_2 of 60 mm Hg.

   Case 2: 18-year-old previously healthy man with history of vomiting for days, then aspiration and acute respiratory distress. Arterial pH of 7.35 and pCO_2 of 60 mm Hg.

   Case 1 probably represents a chronic respiratory acidosis (with its appropriate compensatory metabolic alkalosis), whereas case 2 probably represents a mixed acid-base disturbance characterized by a metabolic alkalosis due to protracted vomiting and an acute respiratory acidosis due to aspiration pneumonia. (Again, mentally erase the chronic respiratory acidosis band for case 2.)

5. The intersection of the pH and pCO_2 values on the acid-base map may also be used to *predict* a serum bicarbonate value. The bicarbonate lines run from the lower left to the top and right side of the map. The bicarbonate values are listed on the top and right side and are calculated from the Henderson-Hasselbalch equation.

(From Goldberg M, Green SB, Moss ML, Marbach CB, Garfinkel D. Computed based instruction and diagnosis of acid base disorders. JAMA 1973;223:270, ©1973, American Medical Association.)

Clinical Manifestations of Acidosis and Alkalosis

Acidosis	Alkalosis
Respiratory — ↑ CO_2	Respiratory — ↓ CO_2
Drowsy	Lethargic
Coma	Confusion
Disoriented	Tetany
↓ BP, ↑ HR	Hyperventilation
Asterixis	Hyperreflexia
Tachypnea	
Metabolic — ↓ HCO_3^-	Metabolic — ↑ HCO_3^-
Coma	Stupor
Dehydration	Coma
Disorientation	Confusion
Abdominal pain	Anorexia
Nausea, vomiting	Nausea, vomiting
Diarrhea	Tremors
Asterixis	Tetany
Hyperventilation	Muscle cramps
	Hypoventilation

ABG Examples

Example 1	
pH	7.3
pCO_2	35
H_2CO_3	17
pO_2	88
O_2 saturation	95%

1. pH is <7.35; therefore, it is acidotic. A fall in pH reflects a rise in H^+ concentration.
2. Check pCO_2. 35 torr is within normal limits. This normal pCO_2 shows that the acidosis (pH 7.3) is not of respiratory origin.
3. The HCO_3 (CO_2 content) is below normal. There is a deficit of base, and the ratio of 20 parts bicarbonate to 1 part carbonic acid is upset. Since the HCO_3^- and the pH are both shifted to acidosis, this is a metabolic acidosis.
4. The pO_2 is within normal limits (80–100 torr). For further information on the relationship between pO_2, O_2 saturation, and O_2 availability to tissues refer to Chapter 2 and the oxyhemoglobin dissociation curve.
5. Compensatory efforts. Within a short period of time the lungs will attempt to increase the amount of CO_2 excreted. Kussmaul's breathing will lower the body's carbonic acid level and normalize the pH.

Example 2	
pH	7.28
pCO_2	60
HCO_3	26
pO_2	60
O_2 saturation	80%

1. The pH shows an overall acidosis.
2. The pCO_2 is markedly elevated. Since both the pH and the pCO2 are shifted toward acidosis, this is a respiratory acidosis.
3. If the condition continues with no correction of the primary respiratory problem, the kidneys will start to retain HCO_3 in an attempt to normalize the pH. As the pH rises toward 7.35, the condition would be termed compensated respiratory acidosis.
4. This pO_2 indicates hypoxemia. This and the elevated pCO_2 indicate hypoventilation.

Nursing Implications

Acid-base imbalances must either be corrected or compensated to avoid further patient injury. Nursing diagnoses that apply to patients in acid-base imbalance include:

1. Ineffective breathing pattern
2. Ineffective airway clearance
3. Impaired gas exchange
4. Anxiety

SUGGESTED READINGS

Diabetic Emergencies

Bacchus H. Metabolic and endocrine emergencies. 2nd ed. Baltimore: University Park Press, 1984.

Butts DE. Fluid and electrolyte disorders associated with diabetic ketoacidosis and hyperglycemic hyperosmolar nonketotic coma. Nurs Clin North Am 1987;22:827–836.

Christman C, Bennett J. Diabetes, new names, new test, new diet. Nursing 1987;17:34–41.

Haire-Joshu DH, Flavin K, Clutter W. Contrasting type I and type II diabetes. Am J Nurs 1986;86:1240–1243.

Kent RA. Triage decisions—an adult diabetic man with a depressed sensorium. J Emerg Nurs 1987;13:186–187.

McAdams RC, Birmingham D. When diabetes races out of control. RN 1986:46–53.

Sabo CE, Michael SR. Diabetic ketoacidosis: pathophysiology, nursing diagnoses and nursing interventions. Focus Crit Care 1989;16:21–28.

Heat Stroke

Callaham ML. Hyperthermia. In: Kravis TC, Warner CG, eds. Emergency medicine. Rockville, Maryland: Aspen Publishers, 1987:629–637.

Goldfrank LR, Osborn H, Weisman RS. Heatstroke. In: Goldfrank LR, Flomenbaum NE, Lewin NA, Weisman RS, Howland MA, Kulberg AG, eds. Goldfrank's toxicologic emergencies. 3rd ed. Norwalk, Connecticut: Appleton-Century-Crofts, 1986:789–799.

Knochel JP. Hyperthermia. In: Parrillo JE, ed. Current therapy in critical care medicine. Toronto: BC Decker, 1987:326–330.

Posey VM, Caruso CC. Life-threatening heat-related emergencies. Dimens Crit Care Nurs 1986;5:216–225.

Hypothermia

Heller K, Salata S. Cardiopulmonary arrest after cold water immersion and hypothermia. J Emerg Nurs 1988;14:5–8.

Kolb RH. Why is this patient unconscious? RN 1986:49–50.

Rich J. Hypothermia. J Emerg Nurs 1983;9:8–10.

Steinman AM. Cardiopulmonary resuscitation and hypothermia. Circulation 1986;74(Suppl IV):29–31.

Zell SC, Kurtz KJ. Severe exposure hypothermia: a resuscitation protocol. Ann Emerg Med 1985;14:335–338.

Endocrine Emergencies

Bybee DE. Saving lives in parathyroid crises. Emerg Med 1987:62–78.

Howton JC. Thyroid storm presenting as coma. Ann Emerg Med 1988:17;343–345.

Ihde JK. Endocrine emergencies. In: Ihde JK, Jacobsen WK, Briggs BA, eds. Principles of criticl care. Philadelphia: WB Saunders, 1987:133–151.

Mathewson MK. Thyroid disorder. Crit Care Nurse 1987;7:74–85.

Ragland G. Thyroid storm. In: Tintinalli J, Rothstein RJ, Krome RL, eds. Emergency medicine, a comprehensive study guide. New York: McGraw-Hill, 1986:640–644.

Electrolyte Imbalances

Barta MA. Correcting electrolyte imbalances. RN 1987:30–33.

Janson CL. Fluid and electrolyte balance. In: Rosen P, Baker FJ, Barkin RM, Braen GR, Dailey RH, Levy RC, eds. Emergency medicine. 2nd ed. St Louis: CV Mosby 1988:1969–2019.

Schwartz MW. Potassium imbalances. Am J Nurs 1987;87:1292–1299.

Stroot VR, Lee CA, Barrett CA. Fluids and electrolytes. 3rd ed. Philadelphia: FA Davis, 1984.

Toto KH. When the patient has hyperkalemia. RN 1987:34–37.

Acid-Base Imbalance

Chenevey B. Overview of fluids and electrolytes. Nurs Clin North Am 1987;22:749–759.

Fell WL, McLeish KR, Stremel RW. Clinical arterial blood gas analysis. St Louis: CV Mosby, 1987:162–197.

Mennen M, Slovis CM. Severe metabolic alkalosis in the emergency department. Ann Emerg Med 1988;17:354–357.

Neff JA, Tidwell SL. Acid-base balance: a tool for rapid evaluation. J Emerg Nurs 1984; 10:322–324.

Poyss AS. Assessment and nursing diagnosis in fluid and electrolyte disorders. Nurs Clin North Am 1987;22:773–783.

Romanski SO. Interpreting ABGs in four easy steps. Nursing 1986;16:58–63.

Shapiro B. Arterial blood gases. In: Parrillo JE, ed. Current therapy in critical care medicine. Toronto: BC Decker, 1987:14–19.

West JB. Pulmonary pathophysiology—the essentials. 3rd ed. Baltimore: Williams & Wilkins, 1987:19–41.

Chapter 7

TOXICOLOGIC EMERGENCIES

DRUG OVERDOSE: A GENERAL APPROACH

Drug and alcohol abuse may be seen in every facet of emergency care. The signs of drug abuse may be obscure or, as in the case of a drug overdose, blatant; it may present as a single entity or in conjunction with another problem or injury such as trauma from a motor vehicle accident; and it may involve abuse of illicit drugs or very commonly prescribed or over-the-counter drugs. No form of drug abuse, accidental or intentional, can be taken lightly; drugs from aspirin to alcohol to heroin can complicate ED* care and cause death.

Assessment

History
If the patient is unable or unwilling to give a history, a member of the medical team should interview family, friends, or ambulance personnel or police. If possible, the bottle or containers of ingested substances should be obtained. Important historical points include:

1. Name and quantity of substances ingested (if a substance is unknown, ask about medications and other drugs belonging to other household members)
2. Time of ingestion
3. Behavior changes or symptoms since ingestion (e.g., level of consciousness, seizures)
4. Previous drug overdoses

---

*See "Appendix A" for definition of common abbreviations used in the text.

5. Alcoholism or illicit drug use
6. Chronic illnesses, especially mental illness
7. Chronic medications and doses
8. History of recent trauma

Physical Findings

General - Note agitation, stupor, or incoherency.

Vital signs - Always check a rectal temperature, as well as respirations, pulse, and blood pressure.

Skin - Note if the patient is flushed, pale, cyanotic, sweating or dry. Look for track marks.

Neck - Check for stiffness or thyromegaly.

Lungs - Listen for rales or consolidation (aspiration).

Cardiovascular system - Check for murmurs and arrhythmias.

HEENT - Make sure the airway is patent, and test for the gag reflex. Note the eye movements and presence of nystagmus.

Neurologic signs - Note the level of consciousness, motor activity, and pupil reactivity as indicated by the Glascow coma scale. Assess the cranial nerves. Check for signs of head trauma.

Classification of Coma

0 Asleep but can be aroused and can answer questions
1 Comatose; withdraws from painful stimuli; reflexes are intact
2 Comatose; does not withdraw from painful stimuli; most reflexes are intact; no respiratory or circulatory depression
3 Comatose; most or all reflexes are absent; no respiratory or circulatory depression
4 Comatose; reflexes are absent; respiratory depression with cyanosis, circulatory failure, or shock

Classification of Hyperactivity

1+Restlessness, irritability, insomnia, tremor, hyperreflexia, sweating, mydriasis, flushing
2+Confusion, hyperactivity, hypertension, tachypnea, tachycardia, extrasystoles, sweating, mydriasis, flushing, mild hyperpyrexia
3+Delirium, mania, self-injury, marked hypertension, tachycardia, arrhythmias, hyperpyrexia
4+Above, plus convulsions, coma, circulatory collapse

Specific Toxicologic Signs

Pupils
    Pinpoint (meiosis) - Opiates, cholinergics, antihypertensives, beta blockers, phenothiazines, barbiturates, chloral hydrate

Dilated (mydriasis) - Anticholinergics, sympathomimetics, phencyclidine, cocaine, cyanide, carbon monoxide

Note: Pupil size may be unpredictable in mixed overdose

Breath odor

Garlic - Arsenic, organophosphates

Almond - Cyanide

Plastic - Placidyl

Pear - Chloral hydrate

Violets - Turpentine

Sweet - Chloroform

Shoe polish - Nitrobenzene

Fermented - Ethanol

Fruity - Ketosis (alcoholic ketoacidosis, DKA, etc.)

Skin

Flushed - Anticholinergics, phenothiazines, sympathomimetics, ethanol, hypoglycemia

Hyperventilation

Primary (aspirin)

Secondary

Anoxia (carbon monoxide, cyanide)

Acidosis

Extrapyramidal signs

Phenothiazines

Butyrophenones

Sympathomimetics (tachycardia, tachypnea, pyrexia, tremors, sweating)

Amphetamines

Cocaine

Phencyclidine

LSD

Alcohol, sedative and/or hypnotic withdrawal

Anticholinergics (tachycardia, agitation, flushed, dry skin, urinary retention)

Polycyclic antidepressants

Antihistamines

Belladonna alkaloids

A mnemonic useful in determining anticholinergics is:

Mad as a hatter

Red as a beet

Dry as a bone

Hot as a hare

Blind as a bat

Cholinergics (bradycardia, hypersecretions, urinary and fecal incontinence; may see tachycardia, mydriasis, or hypertension if sympathetic ganglia are involved)

Organophosphates

Carbamates

Overtreated myasthenics

A mnemonic useful in determining cholinergic overdose is:
S Salivation
L Lacrimation
U Urinary incontinenace
D Defecation

Diagnostic Tests

Laboratory tests - CBC, spin a Hct. Check a Dextrostix for blood glucose. Note electrolytes.

Urinalysis - Check for glucose or ketones.

Blood gas - Must be done if any possibility of respiratory alteration or acid-base disturbance is considered.

X-rays - A chest film may show signs of aspiration. Other films may be taken as clinically indicated.

Toxicologies - Drug levels will be ordered selectively, based on the physician's clinical assessment of the individual patient. Availability of specific drug levels varies from one institution to the next. In general, "routine" drug screens are of academic interest but add little to the clinical management of the patient.

Intervention

1. Provide for a patent airway - Administer oxygen and prepare for the intubation of obtunded patients.
2. Fluid administration - Start an IV of normal saline or Ringer's lactate and administer at a volume to keep the vein open. An increased rate of IV fluid and/or vasopressors is indicated for hypotensive patients.
3. Treatment of acutely reversible syndromes
   a. Naloxone (Narcan), 2 mg IV, is given with an additional 2 mg IM in patients who show a response. Patients with codeine or propoxyphene ingestions may require much larger amounts. Duration of narcotic may exceed that of naloxone; therefore, be prepared to repeat naloxone. If the patient responds, start a continuous IV infusion, giving two-thirds of the reversal dose every hour.
   b. Unconscious patients are given standard measures: glucose, 50 ml D50W IV, and thiamine, 100 mg IM or IV. Glucose is given to treat potential hypoglycemia and to compensate for increased glucose utilization. Thiamine should accompany glucose to prevent Wernicke's encephalopathy, a particular possibility in alcoholics. If glucose is elevated on Dextrostix, give only the thiamine. Give oxygen in the face of pulmonary congestion or suspected carbon monoxide overdose.
4. Prevent absorption

a. Dilution with water or milk can be used for caustic ingestions.
b. Emesis may be induced with syrup of ipecac, 30 ml PO with 300–500 ml of water. In the majority of patients, ipecac will induce vomiting in 15–30 minutes. Remember that patient must have an intact gag reflex to receive ipecac. Contraindications to emesis include seizures, ingestion of a drug that can cause seizures, petroleum product ingestion, caustic ingestion, ingestion of a sharp object, hemorrhagic diathesis, or need for urgent removal of ingested substance. In practice, ipecac has little use in the clinical situation any longer. It may lead to aspiration and prevents the administration of charcoal (the mainstay of therapy) and oral antidotes such as *N*-acetylcysteine.
c. Gastric lavage, when indicated, should be performed by using a 36–40 French Lavacutor hose or Ewald tube. Pill fragments will not pass through smaller tubes. The patient must have an intact gag reflex or be intubated with a cuffed endotracheal tube before lavage. Lavage is contraindicated in caustic ingestions.
   Indications for lavage include:
   i. Ingestion of 2 hours duration or less
   ii. Unconscious or ill patient
   iii. Ingestion of a seriously toxic substance
   iv. Salicylate ingestion
   v. Overdose with substance that decreases intestinal motility (e.g., opiates, anticholinergics)
   Rules of lavage are:
   i. Always protect the airway.
   ii. Place the patient in the left-lateral decubitus position with the head tilted down.
   iii. Always confirm tube placement. Listen in three positions (over both lungs and stomach).
   iv. Use the barrel of a 50-ml catheter tipped syringe as a funnel.
   v. Lavage with aliquots of 200 ml. Remember that the large-bore tubes have 25–50 ml of dead space. Use of a volume over 200 ml might distend the stomach and cause material to pass through the pylorus.
   vi. Use normal saline as the lavage fluid. Use $NaHCO_3$ with iron ingestions.
d. Activated charcoal adsorbs toxic substances. It is given after vomiting or lavage and should not be given with ipecac—wait until ipecac has produced vomiting. Give 60 gm PO or through a lavage tube 1–2 hours as a slurry of 1:4 parts water. Charcoal is useful for most intoxications. Repeated doses of charcoal PO may draw toxins out of the blood into the gut lumen (GI dialysis). Give repeated doses of 60 gm PO every 1–2 hours until the patient is awake.

5. Increase elimination
   a. Cathartics can be given with charcoal. Oil-based cathartics should never be given. Give 30 gm of magnesium sulfate ($MgSO_4$) or sodium sulfate (Na_2SO_4) or 30 ml of FLEET Phospho-soda diluted 1:4. Contraindications include adynamic ileus, severe diarrhea, abdominal trauma, intestinal obstruction, renal failure ($MgSO_4$), and CHF (Na_2SO_4).
   b. Diuresis - Forced diuresis (urine output of 200 ml/hr or more) is usually ineffective and can also be quite dangerous if not monitored closely. It is contraindicated in patients with renal, respiratory, or cardiac failure.
   c. Ion trapping - Urine is alkalized or acidified to facilitate elimination of specific substances. Alkalinization with sodium bicarbonate ($NaHCO_3$) IV will speed the elimination of phenobarbital, salicylates, and isoniazid among others. Vitamin C IV is given to acidify urine and may promote removal of amphetamines, strychnine, phencyclidine, and quinidine. pH and acid-base balance must be determined before any attempt is made to manipulate the pH.
   d. Peritoneal dialysis and hemoperfusion may be utilized for the removal of specific substances according to their permeability, molecular weight, etc. Hemoperfusion is perfusion of blood over activated charcoal or polystyrene resin.
   e. Whole bowel irrigation (WBI) has been introduced recently to assist in toxin removal when patients present late or have taken drugs that are slowly adsorbed or not adsorbed by charcoal. Lavage is performed with an isosmotic solution containing glycol polyethylene and electrolytes (GoLYTELY) which is also used as a surgical bowel preparation. The fluid is delivered via a nasogastric tube at a rate of 2 liters/hr until the returns are clear.
   Indications for WBI include:
      i. Late presentation (>4 hours) of an ingestion of a possible toxin
      ii. Ingestion of a slow release medication or an enteric-coated medication
      iii. Ingestion of substances not adsorbed by charcoal (iron, lithium, etc.)
      iv. Ingestion of a large amount of toxin
   Contraindications for WBI include:
      i. Intestinal ileus and/or obstruction
      ii. Intestinal perforation
      iii. GI bleeding
      iv. Protracted vomiting
   f. Use of antidotes for agents identified by toxicology screening or by history - All EDs should have an antidote kit or poison cart with necessary equipment and medication to treat toxic ingestion. An

antidote kit should include: naloxone (Narcan), atropine, Mucomyst, physostigmine (Antilirium), diphenhydramine hydrochloride (Benadryl), ephrinephrine, methylene blue, Lilly cyanide kit, activated charcoal, ipecac, magnesium citrate, and sodium sulfate.

6. Potential for self-injury - The agitated or combative patient presents a serious management problem to the ED staff. Patients may respond to a calm approach. They need to be closely observed. The patient's behavior cannot be allowed to prevent rapid assessment and emergency treatment. The physician can order a mental health hold and restraints if the patient attempts to leave the ED or is a danger to himself or herself.

7. All patients who take an overdose or who overdose on illicit drugs should see a psychiatrist before they are discharged from the ED.

ED Discharge Planning

All patients who do not respond to therapy or who have ingestions with possible late-onset effects should be admitted for observation and further therapy. Very sick patients should be admitted immediately to an ICU. Suicidal patients who are medically stable should be admitted to a psychiatric unit.

ED Discharge Instructions

1. Review arrangements for psychiatric follow-up if indicated.
2. Discuss medication and toxic substance safety.
3. Consider the need for social service or visiting nurse evaluation.
4. Notify the patient and/or family that the patient's stools will be black if he or she has been treated with charcoal.

NARCOTIC OVERDOSE

Chronic narcotic abusers run very high risks of numerous acute and chronic complications resulting from unsterile injection techniques and adulterated drug samples, as well as from the pharmacologic effects of narcotics. The terms "narcotics" and "opioids" refer to any drugs with actions similar to those of morphine. The pharmacologic effects of the narcotics are all similar, with differences being mainly quantitative. Compounds that are chemical modifications of morphine include:

Diacetylmorphine (heroin)   Hydromorphone (Dilaudid)
Methoxymorphine (codeine)   Oxycodone (Percodan)

Purely synthetic opioid analgesics include:

Meperidine (Demerol)   Methadone (Dolophine)
Levorphanol (levo-Dromoran)   Propoxyphen (Darvon)
Diphenoxylate (main ingredient in Lomotil)

Mild narcotic intoxication results in marked euphoria, accompanied by anorexia, nausea and vomiting, constipation, and decreased libido.

Addicts develop "track" marks from repeated venipunctures and the resulting scar formation. Tracks are most often found on the forearms, hands, and feet. Addicts may present with a variety of physical complaints in an attempt to obtain ED treatment with narcotics.

Narcotic overdose will result in decreased mentation and depression of consciousness with eventual coma and respiratory depression. Hypotension and bradycardia can lead to circulatory collapse and cardiopulmonary arrest.

A widely known hallmark of narcotic overdose, specifically morphine and related drugs, is pinpoint fixed, equal pupils (meiosis). However, meperidine (Demerol) may dilate the pupils, and severe hypoxia may result in bilaterally dilated and fixed pupils.

Intervention

1. Provide life support - Place the patient on a cardiac monitor, start an IV, and be prepared to intubate and ventilate with a bag/mask device. (See "Acute Respiratory Failure" in Chapter 2 and "Shock" in Chapter 1.)
2. Narcotic antagonist naloxone (Narcan), 2 mg, is considered the safest drug to use when the cause of respiratory depression is induced by narcotics or when the cause is uncertain. Given as a 2-mg IV bolus, it may also be given IM, SC, or via an endotracheal tube. IV naloxone should result in increased respiratory rate and improved mental status within 1–2 minutes. If no change occurs, the same dose should be repeated immediately and every 5 minutes to a total of 10–20 mg. If IV access cannot be obtained rapidly, patients with stable vital signs and an adequate airway may receive the same dose IM; a response should be seen within 3–5 minutes. If IV access cannot be obtained and the vital signs are unstable, the patient should be intubated, and the same dose can be given down the endotracheal tube; a response should be evident within 2 minutes. An IV naloxone drip is useful for patients who respond clinically to the administration of a bolus, because the effects dissipate within 45 minutes and respiratory depression may recur. Place 10 mg naloxone in 500 ml D5W and run at 100 ml/hr. As a rough guide, every hour a patient should receive about two-thirds of the dose it took to revive him or her. A naloxone infusion can be maintained as long as clinically indicated, and it is particularly useful

in cases of overdose from long-acting narcotics such as methadone. The only proven side effect of naloxone is induction of narcotic withdrawal and consequent agitation. Be prepared for the possibility of an extreme reaction; i.e., have the side rails up; have help available; and consider applying restraints.
3. Continued observation is necessary. All patients who show a clinical response to naloxone should be observed for at least 4 hours following a bolus or IV infusion and for 6 hours following IM injection. If a patient refuses to remain in the ED for appropriate observation, naloxone (2 mg) IM may be given to help prevent immediate recurrence of coma.
4. Further treatment via the general approach to drug ingestion outlined earlier in this chapter under "Drug Overdose: A General Approach" should be given to those patients who do not respond or respond incompletely to naloxone therapy. Patients who remain comatose should be evaluated as detailed under "Coma—The Unconscious Patient" in Chapter 3.

ED Discharge Planning

Ideally, all patients who present with coma or respiratory depression should be admitted. Unfortunately, many of these patients will refuse admission upon awakening. Clearly, all patients with continued coma or unstable vital signs will require admission. See "ED Discharge Planning" in "Drug Overdose: A General Approach" for further discussion.

BARBITURATE OVERDOSE

Description

Barbiturate use in the United States is associated with a high incidence of addiction, suicide, and accidental death. Barbiturates are sedative-hypnotics that can be divided into short-, intermediate-, and long-acting preparations. Over 50 barbiturate preparations are commercially available, but the most frequently encountered include:

Short-acting preparations
   Thiopental (Pentothal)
   Pentobarbital (Nembutal)
   Secobarbital (Seconal)
   Thiamylal sodium (Surital)
Intermediate-acting preparations
   Amobarbital (Amytal)

Butalbital (found in Fiorinal)
Long-acting preparations
    Phenobarbital (Luminal; found in Donnatal)
    Barbital (Veronal)
    Primidone (Mysoline)

Barbiturates are frequently taken in conjunction with other drugs, particularly alcohol, whose depressant effects may be additive. Symptoms of mild intoxication include drowsiness or light sleep from which the patient can be easily aroused. History should include what was taken, the amount, and the time elapse since ingestion. Expect that the barbiturate abuser will underestimate drug intake. Mentation is slow, and the patient may exhibit mild disorientation, impaired judgment, slurred speech, nystagmus, and ataxia. These patients often appear drunk.

Severe intoxication is seen with ingestion of 15–20 times the oral hynotic dose. The patient cannot be aroused, and corneal and gag reflexes may be impaired or absent. The pupillary light reflex is ordinarily unaffected and is lost only if the patient is significantly hypoxic. Respiration is typically slow and shallow or irregular; vital signs may reveal hypothermia, hypotension, and tachycardia. Hypotension is due to cardiac depression and vasodilatation.

Intervention

1. Provide any necessary life support (see "Acute Respiratory Failure" in Chapter 2 and "Shock" in Chapter 1).
2. Follow the general approach to drug ingestion as outlined in "Drug Overdose: A General Approach" in this chapter, namely, lavage followed by charcoal and a cathartic.
3. Alkalinization of the urine will enhance excretion of most long-acting barbiturates. Alkalinization is ineffective in overdose with short- or intermediate-acting preparations or with primidone (Mysoline). Sodium bicarbonate ($NaHCO_3$), 2 mEq/Kg in 500 ml IV solution is tritrated to a urine pH of 8. Blood gases are checked frequently to monitor serum pH. Adequate potassium must be given if the serum potassium is low or the urine will not remain alkaline.
4. Forced diuresis enhances excretion of all barbiturates. Sufficient fluid should be given IV to maintain a urine output of at least 200 ml/hr. If necessary, furosemide, 20 mg, may be given IV to maintain urine flow. Hypotensive patients should not be diuresed aggressively, although administration of parenteral fluids is generally part of the treatment of shock. Forced diuresis is not without hazards (fluid overload, pulmonary edema, and electrolyte disturbance) and should be undertaken with great caution.

5. Monitor electrolytes and fluid balance closely, watching particularly for hypokalemia as a result of alkalinization and forced diuresis.

The mainstay of treatment is supportive. Patients will do well if their airways are protected and if they are well oxygenated and receive adequate hemodynamic support.

ANTICHOLINERGIC AND POLYCYCLIC OVERDOSE

Description

Anticholinergics are available in a variety of prescription and over-the-counter medications. Polycyclic antidepressants, which have serious cardiac toxicity in addition to anticholinergic activity, are also frequently prescribed and widely available. Preparations with anticholinergic properties include:

Polycyclic antidepressants	Amitriptyline (Elavil)
	Imipramine (Tofranil)
	Doxepin (Sinequan)
	Desipramine (Norpramin)
	Amoxapine (Asendin)
	Trazodone (Desyrel)
Antiemetics	Prochlorperazine (Compazine)
Antihistamines	Diphenhydramine (Benadryl)
Cholinergic blockers	Benztropine mesylate (Cogentin)
	Trihexyphenidyl (Artane)
Antipsychotics	Haloperidol (Haldol)
	Chlorpromazine (Thorazine)
	Thioridazine (Mellaril-S)
	Trifluoperazine (Stelazine)
	Thiothixene (Navane)
Antispasmodics	Dicyclomine (Bentyl)
	Propantheline (Pro-Banthine)
Ophthalmoplegics	Tropicamide (Mydracyl)
	Scopolamine
Over-the-counter drugs	Chlorpheniramine maleate (Allerest)
	Pyrilamine maleate (Sominex)
Plants	Jimson weed, Henbane, nightshade

Pharmacology

Anticholinergic drugs block acetylcholine and other muscarinic agents by competitive inhibition at peripheral and central receptor sites.

Peripheral effects of anticholinergics include dry skin and mucous membranes. Suppression of sweating and increased activity result in hyperthermia. Smooth muscle blockade leads to urinary retention and intestinal ileus with decreased bowel sounds. The pupils are dilated, and vision is blurred. Hypertension occurs due to increased heart rate (anticholinergic effect) and blockade of reuptake of norepinephrine and epinephrine. Increasing intoxication may cause shock and hypotension. Dilatation of cutaneous vessels occurs via an unknown mechanism and results in flushing of the skin.

Cardiac effects of all anticholinergics include sinus and supraventricular tachycardia. The polycyclic antidepressants block the reuptake of norepinephrine and epinephrine and have a direct quinidine-like effect on the heart, in addition to their anticholinergic properties. They may commonly cause ventricular arrhythmias, including PVCs, ventricular tachycardia, torsades de pointes, and ventricular fibrillation. Conduction abnormalities may occur particularly with the polycyclics, including bundle branch block widening of the QRS and atrioventricular dissociation. With polycyclic antidepressants, prolongation of the QRS to longer than 0.10 second is closely correlated with significant toxicity. Conduction defects may persist up to 1 week after ingestion, although associated fatal arrhythmias usually occur in the early phase of poisoning.

Central effects of anticholinergic intoxication include agitation and disorientation. Patients may be dysphasic or hyperreflexic, and seizures can occur.

Assessment

History
The quantity and kind of drug(s) ingested should be ascertained, if possible, along with the time elapsed since ingestion. A history of depression or suicidal ideation should be elicited if present. Note any reported symptoms consistent with significant toxicity. Past medical history should reveal any underlying cardiac or neurologic disease.

Physical Findings
General - Note the patient's mental status and level of consciousness.
Vital signs - Look for hyperthermia, tachycardia, and hypertension. Hypotension is a later finding and may lead to shock.
HEENT - Pupils will be dilated, and the face will be dry and flushed. Vision is blurred, and the mouth is dry.

Abdomen - Listen carefully for bowel sounds, and palpate and percuss the bladder to check for distention.

Neurologic signs - Look for hyperreflexia and myoclonus. Note any focal findings.

Skin - Examine the axilla and trunk for evidence of sweating.

An anticholenergic overdose must be distinguished from other illnesses, such as infections (e.g., meningitis), that can present in a similar manner. The sympathomimetic toxidrome due to overdose of substances such as cocaine and amphetamines and withdrawal from sedatives and/or hypnotic agents such as alcohol, benzodiazepines, and barbiturates can be confused with the anticholinergic toxidrome. Essential features that separate the anticholinergic syndrome from all the rest are the absence of sweating and the presence of bowel atony and urinary retention; remember the mnemonic:

Mad as a hatter, red as a beet, dry as a bone, hot as a hare, blind as a bat.

Intervention

1. Provide basic life support (see "Acute Respiratory Failure" in Chapter 2 and "Cardiopulmonary Arrest" in Chapter 1). Monitor cardiac rate and rhythm, and an ECG must be done to look for conduction abnormalities.
2. Follow the general approach to drug ingestion as outlined in this chapter under "Drug Overdose: A General Approach."
3. Physostigmine (a reversible cholinesterase inhibitor that crosses the blood-brain barrier) is given for severe toxicity. The dose is 2 mg as a slow IV push; this dose may be repeated every 20 minutes according to the patient's response. Physostigmine can precipitate seizures, bradycardia, or asystole. Therefore, physostigmine should not be used routinely. Use should be restricted to the following situations: supraventricular tachycardia with hypotension, choreoathetosis, seizures, and arrhythmias refractory to conventional agents.
4. Sodium bicarbonate is the drug of choice for the treatment of conduction abnormalities, ventricular arrhythmias, and hypotension. It may be given as a continuous IV infusion of 2 ampules of $NaHCO_3$ in 100 ml of D5W with the rate titrated to a serum pH of 7.50. When $NaHCO_3$ therapy is given, serial blood gases are needed to monitor the serum pH. Sodium bicarbonate should be administered prophylatically to all patients with a QRS of 0.10 second or longer.
5. IV phenytoin may be prescribed for conduction abnormalities and ventricular arrhythmias refractory to $NaHCO_3$ therapy. The usual

dose is 30 mg/min via an IV pump, with the total dose not to exceed 18 mg/Kg. Lidocaine may be given for ventricular arrhythmias but may be ineffective.

ED Discharge Planning

Patients with signs of central nervous system toxicity and/or cardiac toxicity (conduction abnormalities, arrhythmias) must be admitted to a monitored bed. It is prudent to observe asymptomatic patients on a cardiac monitor in the ED for at least 6 hours prior to discharge. For a further discussion of ED discharge planning, see "Drug Overdose: A General Approach" earlier in this chapter.

COCAINE

Cocaine, which is one of the oldest local anesthetics, is derived from the South American *Erythroxylon coca* plant. Used locally, cocaine produces surface anesthesia, which lasts about 1 hour. It also causes local vasoconstriction. Due to its toxic effects, cocaine is not used medically for other than local anesthesia. Systemically, cocaine potentiates the effects of catecholamines and increased sympathetic stimulation.

Direct CNS stimulation gives rise to a garrulous, excited state, a feeling of euphoria, increased motor activity, and resistance to fatigue. There is a rise in pulse and respiratory rate, and blood pressure elevation and vomiting may occur.

Toxic effects include depression of the central and autonomic nervous systems and stimulation of lower motor centers. Signs of toxicity include seizures, tachycardia, hypertension, and hyperthermia.

The onset of action depends on the dose and route of administration. Peak levels are seen in 3–5 minutes with IV use and via smoking; in 20–60 minutes with intranasal use: and in 60–90 minutes following oral ingestion.

Cocaine powder can be inhaled nasally ("snorted") or dissolved and taken IV. "Crack" is a form of free-base cocaine crystals made by combining cocaine HCl with a basic substance such as bicarbonate of soda, which can be placed in a pipe or cigarette and smoked; as it is smoked, it makes a cracking or popping sound. Crack gives an intense high, lasting only 15 minutes or so and is followed by a period of depression that encourages repeated use of the drug. Due to the high purity of crack compared with other street cocaine, overdose and toxicity are more likely.

"Speedballing" is the IV administration of a combination of heroin and cocaine. The pharmacologic effects depend on the relative quantities used in the mixture. Complications of this method include the many complications of unsterile injection techniques and adulterated drug samples in addition to the effects of the drugs themselves.

The toxicity of cocaine is not necessarily dose related. The mean lethal dose by oral administration is said to be 500 mg, but death has been reported with as little as 20 mg intranasally. Some chronic users can tolerate 650 mg daily without serious consequence. Although tolerance of this sort can develop, cocaine was not thought to be physically addicting; however, psychologic dependence clearly may occur, and withdrawal dysphoria has been noted.

Assessment

History

The patient who uses cocaine will initially experience a euphoric feeling with decreased fatigue, increased alertness and mental ability, and talkativeness. With continued use, negative effects emerge, such as paranoia and restlessness. These symptoms wear off rapidly and depression may develop, causing the patient to use the drug again and continue the cycle.

Acutely intoxicated patients may present to the ED with complaints of palpitations and a feeling that their heart is running away with them. They may be agitated and frightened or even frankly psychotic. Hallucinations can occur, as can a crawling sensation under the skin (formications). Vomiting may be prominent. Serious presentations include seizures or status epilepticus, acute cerebrovascular accident, myocardial infarction, and even cardiopulmonary arrest.

Patients must be questioned as to the kind and quantities of drugs taken, as well as time and route of administration. Patients who inject IV should be questioned as to other complications of IV drug abuse.

Physical Findings

Vital signs - Check for hyperthermia, hypertension, tachycardia, or irregular pulse.

HEENT - Pupils should be dilated.

Lungs - Listen for rales (aspiration).

Cardiovascular system - Check for irregular pulse and heart murmurs.

Neurologic signs - Do a neurologic assessment and note any deficits.

Diagnostic Tests

Toxicology - A serum and a urine sample for cocaine assay may be requested if the diagnosis is in doubt.

ECG - Check for ST and T wave changes indicative of myocardial ischemia infarction.

CAT scan - A CAT scan is indicated to rule out CVA in patients with neurologic findings or those in coma.

Intervention

1. Provide any necessary life support (see "Cardiopulmonary Arrest" in Chapter 1).
2. Provide reassurance if the patient is agitated or psychotic and the vital signs are stable. Try to maintain verbal contact and keep the patient oriented as to time and place. Decrease environmental stimulation.
3. Avoid use of physical or chemical restraints, if possible. If the patient is at risk of harming himself or herself or of harming others, physical restraints may be employed. If the patient remains very agitated, small doses of IV diazepam may be given.
4. Administer naloxone for mixed drug overdose (see "Narcotic Overdose" earlier in this chapter).
5. Monitor the patient closely for cardiac arrhythmias, such as sinus tachycardia, supraventricular and ventricular tachycardias, and fibrillation. See "Supraventricular Tachycardia" and "Cardiopulmonary Arrest" in Chapter 1 for detailed discussions of these arrhythmias and their therapy. For cocaine-induced ventricular irritability, lidocaine can be given IV; propranolol can be given subsequently if no response is achieved. Supraventricular arrhythmias will generally respond to propranolol.
6. Monitor blood pressure closely to prevent and treat cocaine-induced hypertensive crisis early. IV propranolol is generally the drug of choice. See "Hypertension" in Chapter 1 for details of management.
7. Hyperthermic crisis is treated with external cooling, such as hypothermia blankets, ice baths, and fans; monitor temperature continuously with a rectal thermocouple, and follow vital signs closely. See "Heat Stroke" in Chapter 6 for further details.
8. Implement seizure precautions. Seizures or status epilepticus is treated with IV diazepam as discussed under "Seizures" in Chapter 3.
9. Sedation should be provided with the use of benzodiazepines (Valium, 5–10 mg IV, or midazolam, 2–5 mg IM.)

ED Discharge Planning

Patients with mild intoxication can be treated in the ED. All patients with serious complications should be admitted, including those with the following:

1. Cardiac arrhythmias
2. Myocardial ischemia or infarction
3. Status epilepticus
4. Hyperthermia
5. Hypertensive crisis

6. CVA
7. Severe psychotic problems

ED Discharge Instructions
1. Provide the patient with drug rehabilitation information.
2. Encourage the patient to contact self-help groups such as Cocaine Anonymous or to call 1-800-COCAINE.
3. Instruct the patient to return to the ED for chest pain, palpitations, and other signs of toxicity.

PHENCYCLIDINE

Description

Abuse of phencyclidine (PCP, "angel dust") is a frequent drug problem encountered among young adults. PCP is a dissociative anesthetic that is easily synthesized and highly potent. It is used for its hallucinogenic effects, and one of its most dangerous aspects is the risk of self-inflicted damage due to behavioral changes.

PCP can be taken orally, intravenously, or intranasally but is most frequently smoked with marijuana. When PCP is taken by mouth, the effects are felt within 30–60 minutes, and when smoked, within 2–5 minutes. The effects usually last approximately 6 hours but may last intermittently for days or weeks.

Low-dose intoxication (ingestion of up to 5 mg) will result in sensations of body distortion, such as the limbs enlarging or the head detaching. Patients sometimes experience auditory or visual hallucinations, but more commonly they experience delusions. Patients intoxicated with PCP exhibit a wide spectrum of behavioral changes. They are typically disoriented with amnesia; they may be anxious, fearful and withdrawn, euphoric, or agitated and violent.

Neurologic effects of low-dose PCP intoxication include ataxia, slurred speech, decreased perception of pain, numbness, increased muscle tone and rigidity, hyperreflexia, facial grimacing, grinding teeth, athetosis, and myoclonic jerking. Excessive involuntary isometric motor activity may lead to skeletal muscle injury and necrosis (rhabdomyolysis) and the excretion of a muscle protein through the kidneys (myoglobinuria).

The patient may have a blank stare with pupils that are midsize or small but that remain reactive. Vertical or horizontal nystagmus is characteristic. Sinus tachycardia and hypertension are common findings. Patients may have an increased rate and depth of respiration. Fever may occur as a result of autonomic hyperactivity.

Intoxication with moderate to high doses (5–10 mg) will result in heightened motor activity, and hypertension can progress to hypertensive crisis and encephalopathy. Seizures and coma may occur. Unlike the coma associated with sedative-hypnotics, the coma caused by PCP may be accompanied by brisk reflexes and elevated blood pressure. Probably the most common causes of injury and death associated with PCP are self-inflicted. Apart from bodily injury, respiratory arrest is the most common cause of death from PCP intoxication.

Assessment

History
Patients are frequently brought to the ED by concerned friends and family or by the restraining police officers. If the patient is acutely psychotic, it may be impossible to obtain a medical history. In addition, the patient may have unknowingly taken PCP, either by addition of the drug by others to food or marijuana or by misrepresentation of it as another drug (e.g., cocaine). It is important to attempt identification of any other drugs taken simultaneously with the PCP.

Diagnostic Tests
Urine PCP level - Stat testing for PCP is extremely helpful in making the diagnosis. Urine assay gives a higher yield than does serum.
Urinalysis - Check the urine for color (brownish red with myoglobinuria) and look for blood on the Chemstrip (positive with myoglobinuria).

Intervention

1. Follow the general approach to drug overdose as outlined earlier in this chapter under "Drug Overdose: A General Approach". If the patient took PCP orally, use emesis, charcoal, and a cathartic. Unless necessary, use of a nasogastric tube should be avoided, as PCP predisposes to laryngospasm. Prevent patient self-injury. Attempt to calm the patient by using quiet verbal contact and reduction of environmental stimulation (e.g., dim lights, quiet room). Limit the number of staff in contact with the patient. Physical restraints should be avoided, if possible, but if they must be used, be certain the patient is restrained in a side-lying position to avoid aspiration. Diazepam (Valium) in doses of 5–10 mg IV or haloperidol (Haldol) in doses of 5–10 mg IM may be used if the patient is very agitated or psychotic, but when they are used, the patient must be closely monitored for seizures and hypotension.
2. Monitor the patient for hypertension. Propranolol (Inderal) or diazoxide may be given (see "Hypertension" in Chapter 1 for details of hypertensive emergencies).
3. Increase excretion of PCP by acidifying the urine. Because PCP is a

weak base, excretion can be enhanced by acidifying the urine to a pH of <5.5. Ascorbic acid, 1 gm in 500 ml of D5W, is given IV at a rate of approximately 150 ml/hr, titrating the rate to the urine pH. Prior to acidification the patient's CPK and urinalysis should be reviewed for indications of muscle damage. Urine can be checked for myoglobin by using a Chemstrip. Acidification of urine should not be performed in the face of rhabdomyolysis, as acidification may increase the incidence of renal failure or systemic acidosis.

ED Discharge Planning

All patients with cardiovascular abnormalities, myoglobinuria, or severe, prolonged psychosis should be admitted. All other patients should be observed for several hours in the ED and should have a psychiatric consultation prior to discharge.

ED Discharge Instructions
1. Patient should return to the ED if he or she experiences a return of symptoms.
2. Recommend or refer the patient for drug or mental health counselling.
3. Convey that PCP is an unpredictable drug with dangerous physical and mental effects.

SALICYLATE POISONING

Etiology

The ready availability of over-the-counter aspirin, both in pure form and hidden in combination drugs, makes salicylate poisoning one of the most commonly encountered lethal drug overdoses. Intoxication may occur unwittingly, by overuse of analgesic tablets or cold remedies containing aspirin or by incorrect oral ingestion of oil of wintergreen (methyl salicylate) found in skin liniments. Intentional overdose in suicide attempts is also commonly seen.

In general, the ingestion of 50 regular-strength or 35 extra-strength tablets of aspirin in an adult represents a 200–300 mg/Kg dose and is associated with significant toxicity. One teaspoon of oil of wintergreen contains the equivalent of 21 regular-strength aspirin tablets.

Pathophysiology

Toxic doses of salicylates will initially stimulate the respiratory center, causing hyperventiltion with consequent decrease in pCO_2 and respiratory alkalosis. Subsequent renal excretion of bicarbonate, sodium, and potassium will cause the pH to return to normal, producing a compensated respiratory alkalosis but significantly decreasing the buffering capacity of the extracellular fluid. This renal compensation is protective, as alkalinization of urine leads to increased excretion of salicylate.

After the initial respiratory alkalosis, patients with serious salicylate intoxication may develop a combined respiratory and metabolic acidosis due to several factors. First, increasingly high concentrations of salicylate will ultimately depress the respiratory center, causing an increase in pCO_2 and subsequent respiratory acidosis. In addition, patients with combined drug ingestions may have taken additional respiratory depressants. Second, dehydration and hypotension will result in impaired renal function with accumulation of inorganic metabolic acids. Third, salicylates impair carbohydrate metabolism, resulting in accumulation of lactic acid and ketones. Fourth, salicyclic acid derivatives can lower blood bicarbonate. The combination of these factors will result in a significant acidosis.

Other metabolic effects of salicylate poisoning may include hyperglycemia and glycosuria or even profound hypoglycemia. Bleeding disorders may occur, usually as a result of reversible hypoprothrombinemia and platelet dysfunction. Renal tubular defects with proteinuria have been described that may progress to renal failure. Noncardiogenic pulmonary edema may occur, apparently as a result of increased pulmonary vascular permeability. Hypokalemia is seen secondary to acidosis and urinary loss.

Assessment

History
Patients must be questioned as to the quantity and type of salicylate taken, as well as the time elapsed since ingestion. Ask about underlying medical conditions and if aspirin or over-the-counter drug containing aspirin is regularly used.

Symptoms of early salicylate toxicity include vertigo, tinnitus, and hearing impairment. Increasing toxicity results in diaphoresis, nausea and vomiting, fever, confusion or drowsiness, headache, blurred or decreased vision, and slurred speech. The patient may become agitated, restless, and talkative and in cases of very severe toxicity may progress to seizures, to hallucinations, and ultimately to coma.

Diagnostic Tests
Laboratory tests - CBC (spin a Hct), SMA (monitor glucose and potassium), and PT.
Urinalysis - Check for protein, pH, ketones, RBC, and WBC.
ABGs - Monitor pH, pCO_2, and pO_2 at regular intervals.
Serum salicylate level - Send 5 ml of venous blood in a tube with anticoag-

ulant (green-stoppered tube). Send at time of presentation in patients who appear symptomatic and in those with an unknown time of ingestion. For all others, blood levels will be taken at 6 hours postingestion (Fig.7.1).

Treatment

1. Provide life support for patients who present with tachypnea and deep labored respirations, seizures, coma, or cardiovascular collapse. Have airway equipment readily available; place the patient on a cardiac monitor and start an IV line with D5/0.45 NaCl.
2. Follow the general approach to drug ingestion as outlined earlier in this chapter under "Drug Overdose: A General Approach" namely, emesis or lavage followed by charcoal and a cathartic. Because

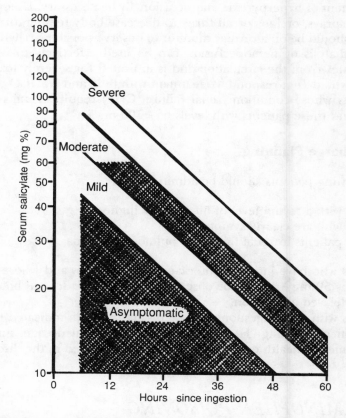

Figure 7.1. This nomogram relates serum salicylate concentrations and expected severity of intoxication at varying intervals following the ingestion of a *single* dose of salicylate. (From Pousada L, Osborn HH. Emergency medicine for the house officer. Baltimore: Williams & Wilkins, 1986:206.)

salicylates slow gastric emptying, be aggressive in utilizing them to empty the stomach irregardless of the time of ingestion.

3. Fluid and electrolyte therapy - Most patients require initial correction of dehydration. Sodium bicarbonate may be added to the IV solution to correct metabolic acidosis. High doses of sodium bicarbonate (2 mEq/Kg in 500 ml D5W) may be given over a 2-hour period to alkalize the urine and enhance renal excretion; aim for a urinary pH of 8–9. Supplemental potassium may be required to maintain serum level above 4.0. Alkalosis due to either hyperventilation or treatment with $NaHCO_3$ can result in severe hypokalemia. Fluid and electrolyte balance must be carefully monitored with hourly intake and output. A Foley catheter should be inserted in acute patients to facilitate monitoring urine output and urine pH levels. Signs of fluid retention, i.e., decreased urine output, pulmonary rales, should be immediately reported to the physician.

4. Treatment of hyperpyrexia may occasionally be necessary. Use sponge baths, sprays, or fans or all three to decrease body temperature. Patients should be on a cardiac monitor to observe possible arrhythmias.

5. Hemodialysis or hemoperfusion can be used effectively to remove salicylates from the circulation and is indicated for severely toxic patients who do not respond to treatment with fluid and $NaHCO_3$, those patients whose condition (renal failure, CHF) requires fluid restriction, and those patients with levels of ≥100 mg%.

ED Discharge Planning

The following patients should be admitted:

1. Those with a serum level of 50 mg% or higher
2. Those who are clearly symptomatic
3. Those patients in renal failure or pulmonary edema

Patients who have ingested enteric-coated salicylates and whose initial levels are <50 mg% should be observed in the ED for several hours because of delayed absorption.

Patients with mild ingestions may be discharged with indicated poison prevention counselling. Home aspirin storage, usual dosage, and the need for mental health evaluation should be considered in the discharge plan.

ACETAMINOPHEN POISONING

In recent years, as the popularity of acetaminophen for minor analgesia has increased, it has also become one of the most common overdoses seen in the ED. Despite its safety in therapeutic doses, acetaminophen in large doses may result in severe hepatotoxicity.

Therapeutic doses of acetaminophen are metabolized by sulfonation and gluconation. When these metabolic pathways are saturated, a hepatotoxic intermediate is formed. This intermediate can be metabolized in the liver because there are adequate stores of hepatic glutathione to bind the toxic by-products of metabolism. When massive doses are consumed, the liver's detoxification properties are overwhelmed, and hepatotoxicity and necrosis result. Acetaminophen is rapidly absorbed from the GI tract. Peak plasma levels are reached generally in 30–120 minutes following ingestion. Although the amount of hepatic necrosis correlates poorly with the dose ingested, damage to the liver can be seen in adults with 10–15-gm ingestion, and a dose of 25 gm or more is potentially fatal.

Assessment

History
It is extremely important to question the patient and/or family as to the quantity of acetaminophen ingested, the strength of the acetaminophen (regular, "extra," or "maximum"), and the time elapsed since ingestion. There are a large number of combination drugs available over the counter that contain acetaminophen. Ask if the patient vomited and, if so, how long after ingestion. Any history of underlying hepatic disease or concurrent ingestion of other hepatotoxic medications should be elicited.

Most patients will have no specific complaints at the time of presentation; this should not be misconstrued as a sign of minor ingestion. The clinical course of acetaminophen overdose can be divided into three phases:

1. First 24 hours - Gradual onset of nausea, vomiting, cramping, abdominal pain, pallor, and diaphoresis.
2. Latent phase (roughly 24–48 hours) - May be asymptomatic, with elevation of liver ensymes, bilirubin, and PT. Right-upper quadrant pain may occur secondary to hepatic swelling.
3. Three to five days - Generalized malaise, jaundice, coagulation defects, hypoglycemia, renal failure, cardiomyopathy, hepatic encephalopathy, and fulminant hepatic failure.

Diagnostic Tests
Serum acetaminophen levels (see Fig. 7.2) - Obtain a level no sooner than 4 hours after ingestion and another 4 hours after the first. Results may be plotted on a nomogram to determine the risk of hepatotoxicity.

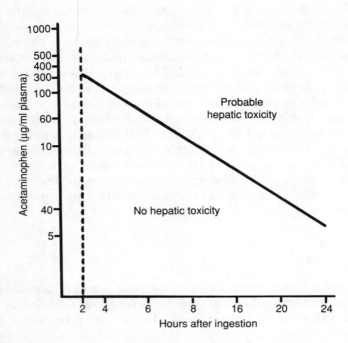

Figure 7.2. Serum level of acetaminophen. (From Pousada L, Osborn HH. Emergency medicine for the house officer. Baltimore: Williams & Wilkins, 1986:209.)

Intervention

1. See "Drug Overdose: A General Approach" outlined earlier in this chapter. Prevention of GI absorption of acetaminophen should be attempted up to 24 hours after ingestion. Charcoal should be administered with *N*-acetylcysteine, as the charcoal will not interfere greatly with the antidote's absorption. To be safer, an additional 40% of the first dose (i.e., 200 mg/Kg instead of 140 mg/Kg) can be administered. With mixed overdoses, charcoal may be given and continued every 3 hours while Mucomyst is administered every 4 hours.
2. Treatment with *N*-acetylcysteine (Mucomyst) - *N*-Acetylcysteine is a specific antidote for acetaminophen poisoning that acts as a glutathione substitute and directly inactivates hepatotoxic metabolites. Indications for use of the antidote include a potentially toxic overdose on the nomogram or an ingestion 8 or more hours prior to presentation. The loading dose is 140 mg/Kg PO, diluted with soda or juice. The maintenance dose is 70 mg/Kg PO every 4 hours for a total of 17 doses. Completion of the full 17 doses is necessary if the first level exceeds the potentially hepatotoxic dose. If not, the therapy may be stopped.

Patients who present relatively late should always be started on therapy until the level is available. If the patient vomits the loading dose within 1 hour, the dose should be repeated. Diluting the terrible-tasting N-acetylcysteine to a 5% solution helps to reduce the incidence of vomiting. It may be given via nasogastric tube if the patient refuses to drink the solution. For persistent vomiting, antiemetics or metoclopramid may be given, or a Miller-Abbott or Cantor tube can be inserted, and the antidote can be instilled directly into the duodenum. IV N-acetylcysteine is not yet available for general use in the United States.

ED Discharge Planning

All patients requiring N-acetylcysteine therapy should be admitted. Patients will require monitoring for fluid and electrolyte balance and hypoglycemia. Suicide precautions must be employed if the ingestion was intentional.

CARBON MONOXIDE POISONING

Etiology

Carbon monoxide poisoning results from inhalation of smoke from fires; fumes from home heating devices using fossil fuels; motor exhaust fumes; and, occasionally, from paint remover. It is also seen in inhalation of fumes during occupational exposure; groups at risk include toll and turnstile workers, miners, foundry workers, and, most commonly, firefighters. Natural gas (i.e., gas used for cooking), unlike coal gas, has neglible amounts of carbon monoxide. Carbon monoxide competes with oxygen for binding sites on the hemoglobin molecule. The affinity of carbon monoxide for hemoglobin is 240 times that of oxygen. Carbon monoxide inhalation results in a decrease in the blood's oxygen-carrying capacity and a decrease in oxygen dissociation from hemoglobin at the tissue level (i.e., the oxygen/hemoglobin dissociation curve shifts to the left).

Assessment

History
The symptoms of carbon monoxide poisoning depend on the patient's level of carboxyhemoglobin (COHb) and length of exposure. Patients with a long exposure time may have excessive body loads of carbon monoxide and may be symptomatic despite paradoxically low COHb levels.

Symptoms include headache, nausea, dizziness, dyspnea, fatigue, chest pain, or confusion. Determine the type and duration of carbon monoxide exposure as well as possible inhalation of other toxic fumes. Ask if oxygen was used following exposure, since O_2 therapy will lower COHb levels. Question the patient about occupational exposure or suicidal intent. A past smoking history is pertinent, as smokers may chronically have a COHb level of up to 20%. Underlying anemia or cardiac, pulmonary, or neurologic disease places a patient at greater risk. ECG changes and anginal symptoms have been observed with COHb levels below 5%.

Physical Findings
General - Cyanosis may be masked by the cherry-red color of COHb. Assess the level of consciousness.
Vital signs - Increased respiratory and pulse rates are generally present.
Skin - The lips and nail beds may or may not be cherry-red.
HEENT - Note soot around the nose, lips, and mouth if the patient has suffered smoke inhalation. Look for signs of pharyngeal edema or thermal damage to the airway.
Neck - Listen for stridor (laryngeal edema due to thermal injury).
Lungs - Listen for rales or wheezes (smoke inhalation induced ARDS).

COHb level[a]	Findings
10%	Tightness across forehead, flushing, mild dyspnea on exertion
20%	Throbbing headache, dyspnea on moderate exertion
30%	Severe headache, dizziness, fatigue, irritability, disturbed judgment, dyspnea on mild exertion
40–50%	Severe headache, confusion, syncope on exertion
60–70%	Coma, convulsions, respiratory failure

[a]Note: Patients with prolonged exposure to carbon monoxide may be severely affected (e.g., coma, cardiac arrest) from relatively low levels. The correlation of symptoms with COHb levels does not apply in all situations.

Diagnostic Tests
COHb level - This must be obtained in all patients with any history of smoke inhalation or fumes exposure. Draw 3–5 ml of arterial or venous blood with heparin as for an ABG analysis.
Blood gas abnormalities - Carbon monoxide competes with oxygen for hemoglobin binding. Therefore, it affects oxygen saturation but not oxygen tension (partial pressure of oxygen). Look for signs of metabolic acidosis (tissue hypoxia). Note: The pO_2 can be normal or high if the patient is receiving oxygen. Moreover, the oxygen saturation may be falsely reported as normal because it is calculated from the pO_2 on a

routine ABG analysis. Ask for a direct oxygen saturation determination. It should be low.

CBC - Anemia will result in a greater degree of tissue hypoxia at a given COHb level.

X-rays - A chest x-ray should be obtained on all patients to rule out pulmonary edema and aspiration.

ECG - All patients with smoke inhalation or fumes exposure should have a cardiogram to rule out ischemia. Tachycardia over 120/min, PVCs, and ST wave changes should be brought to the physician's attention.

Intervention

1. Oxygen therapy - All patients should be placed on 100% oxygen by nonrebreathing mask or via endotracheal tube, if necessary, in order to reverse tissue hypoxia and eliminate carbon monoxide from the blood. Oxygen not only improves tissue oxygenation but also aids in carbon monoxide elimination. Air breathing alone will eliminate 50% of carbon monoxide in 4–5 hours; breathing 100% oxygen will eliminate 50% in 1 hour; and breathing 100% oxygen in a hyperbaric chamber at 3 atm pressure reduces the half-life to 20 minutes. Extrapolate back, using these values, to estimate what the maximum COHb level was at the site of exposure. Patients should receive oxygen until the CoHb level is below 10%.

2. Monitor for altered breathing pattern and respiratory failure; observe rate, depth, and degree of respiratory effort every 15-30 minutes. Use of accessory muscles, increased tachycardia, and acidosis are signs of respiratory failure. The patient may require intubation and ventilation with 100% oxygen. Indirect laryngoscopy should be performed by an ENT specialist if thermal or toxic injury to the airway is suspected.

3. Hyperbaric oxygen therapy - Patients should receive hyperbaric oxygen for the following conditions: cardiac arrest, hypotension, seizures, coma, neurologic signs, angina, ischemia, and maximum levels > 25%.

ED Discharge Planning

All patients with signs or symptoms should be admitted to the hospital. Asymptomatic patients with low COHb levels may be discharged. Report the case to the local health department, and in the case of faulty burners, gas leaks, etc., call in the Environmental Protection Agency (EPA).

ED Discharge Instructions
1. Discuss methods of prevention, safe use of home heaters, and proper ventilation when petroleum or chlorine products are used.

2. Have the patient return to the ED if symptoms, respiratory difficulty, hoarseness, or loss of voice recur.

ALCOHOL ABUSE AND WITHDRAWAL

Alcohol abuse and alcohol-related injuries are common to every ED. It is important to stress that the effects of severe alcohol intoxication and withdrawal may be life-threatening. Alcohol may mask and delay diagnosis of head injury, drug overdose, and diabetic emergencies.

Assessment

History
It may be necessary to obtain the history from relatives if the patient is not able or willing to discuss his or her condition. History should include what, how much, and when the patient last drank. Ask about other drugs or medication taken, and obtain a history of any medical or surgical problems. Look for an Antabuse card. A history of pancreatitis, GI bleeding, liver disease, seizures, or delirium tremens is significant.

Physical Findings
General - Look for diaphoresis, tremors, and tachycardia. Note the stigmata of chronic alcoholism, including icterus, spider angiomata, gynecomastia, and ascites.
Vital signs - Check for orthostasis, and take blood pressure with the patient both lying and standing, if possible. Take a rectal temperature (fever may be due to withdrawal).
Lungs - Listen for signs of pneumonia.
Abdomen - Evaluate for guarding and tenderness caused by gastritis, pancreatitis, or ulcer.
Neurologic signs - Note level of consciousness, lethargy, stupor, paresthesia, delirium, and focal or grand mal seizures. If seizures occur, there are usually no more than two or three seizures, which are invariably grand mal in type and occur within 6 hours after cessation of drinking, peak at 24 hours, and are usually gone within 2–3 days. Focal seizures must be explained by an alternate diagnosis, such as subdural or epidural hematoma from occult head trauma. All patients with new-onset focal seizures should have a CAT scan. Alcohol intoxication and withdrawal can cause hallucinations.

Diagnostic Tests
Laboratory tests - CBC, SMA including liver function tests and amylase, and PT. Check blood glucose by Dextrostix immediately.

Urinalysis - Do a Chemstrip for glucose and ketones.
ABGs - Check pH. Compensatory respiratory alkalosis (Kussmaul respirations) and metabolic alkalosis from vomiting may normalize the pH
in a patient with alcohol acidosis.

Intervention

1. Provide for the patient's safety. Keep the patient in an area where he
   or she can be continuously observed. Take seizure precautions. Avoid
   use of restraints, if possible. Application of restraints may precipitate
   agitation, struggling, and elevated blood pressure and heart rate. On
   the other hand, patients often attempt to climb over the side rails and
   must be protected from harming themselves. Chlordiazepoxide (Lib-
   rium) or diazepam (Valium) may be ordered for patients in alcohol
   withdrawal for their sedating and anticonvulsant effects. The dose of
   chlordiazepoxide is 50–100 mg PO or IV, titrated to sedation level. Diazepam, 5 mg IV, may be given every 10–15 minutes until the patient
   is calm but awake. Pentobarbital or phenobarbital may also be used to
   treat alcohol withdrawal.
2. Airway management - The most serious risk to airway and oxygenation
   is aspiration. Place the patient in side-lying or mid-Fowler's position
   and suction, if needed. Oxygen administration is indicated by abnormal blood gas results, hypotension, ECG changes, and cardiac arrhythmias.
3. Thiamine administration - Always give thiamine, 100 mg IM or IV,
   prior to administration of glucose in an alcoholic. Without adequate
   thiamine, giving glucose may precipitate Wernicke's encephalopathy.
4. Glucose administration - A Dextrostix for glucose should be performed routinely. Glucose, 50 ml D50W (25 gm), should be given IV
   if the Dextrostix is low or normal. Patients who respond to an IV bolus
   of glucose should receive a constant infusion of D10W.
5. Fluid balance deficit - Patients may have fluid deficits of 3–5 liters or
   more due to fever, hyperactivity, sepsis, third-space losses, or vomiting. Start a well-placed IV line for administration of normal saline,
   with the consideration that the agitated patient may cause IV dislodge-
   ment and infiltration. Keep an accurate intake and output record.
6. Magnesium sulfate - Alcoholics are frequently magnesium deficient,
   and this deficiency may exacerbate alcohol withdrawal. The usual dose
   of $MgSO_4$ (50%) is 4 ml (2 gm) IM.
7. Blood alcohol level - If the test for a blood alcohol level is ordered,
   draw a 10-ml sample and label with the patient's name, the date, and
   time. Use a solution that does not contain alcohol for the skin preparation. Refer to the hospital's policy on obtaining the patient's informed
   consent and on the labelling and handling of the specimen.

204 Emergency Nursing—A Practice Guide

Acute alcohol intoxication must be distinguished from drug overdose, hypoglycemia, head injury, stroke syndromes, CNS infections, sepsis, etc. The alcohol level may be very helpful in this regard. A low or negative alcohol level in a patient with altered mental status should prompt an immediate search for other causes. It is helpful to know that alcohol is metabolized at a fixed rate (10–15 mg% per hour in normal subjects and up to 25–30 mg% per hour in chronic alcoholics). An inebriated patient who shows no sign of recovery despite a falling alcohol level should be evaluated for additional pathology. Guard against the tendency to let a once-noisy alcoholic patient sleep for a prolonged period without reevaluation. Acute alcohol withdrawal must be differentiated from drug withdrawal, seizure disorders either primary or secondary to another illness, hypoglycemia, CNS infections, or acute psychosis. The evaluation must be meticulous and thorough in order to exclude the various possibilities. An alcohol level is not helpful in this regard, since alcoholics can develop withdrawal at levels from negligible to high, depending upon their daily consumption.

ED Discharge Planning

Patients with the following conditions should be admitted for continued therapy and observations:

1. Alcoholic ketoacidosis
2. Hallucinations, severe agitation, marked tachycardia or fever
3. Global confusion or delirium
4. Concurrent medical or surgical conditions
5. Seizures (all alcoholics with seizures deserve admission, and focal seizures or status epilepticus necessitate a stat CAT scan)
6. Associated illnesses such as pneumonia, and pancreatitis
7. Withdrawal from a combination of drugs
8. Head injury with loss of consciousness
9. Hypoglycemia (in the setting of alcohol abuse, correction of hypoglycemia may take a long time)
10. Compelling social factors and inability to provide safe self-care

Prior to discharge, assess the patient for:

1. Orientation to person, place, and time
2. Ability to ambulate
3. Stable vital signs

Consider the need for social service intervention for patients being discharged.

Patients may need assistance in obtaining adequate clothing and transportation prior to leaving the ED. Refer the patient and/or family to the hospital's alcohol treatment program or an inpatient detoxification unit.

Encourage contact with Alcoholics Anonymous (AA) for the patient and with Al-Anon for the patient's family.

SUGGESTED READINGS

Drug Overdose: A General Approach

Auerbach PS, Osterloh J, Braun, et al. Efficacy of gastric emptying: gastric lavage versus emesis induced with ipecac. Ann Emerg Med 1986;15:692–698.

Guzzardi L, Bayer MJ. Emergency management of the poisoned patient. In: Bayer MJ, Rumack BH, Wanke LA, eds. Toxicologic emergencies. Bowie, Maryland: Robert J Brady, 1984:1–17.

Joubert DW. Use of emetic, absorbent, and cathartic agents in acute drug overdose. J Emerg Nurs 1987;13:49–51.

Kulig K, Bar-Or D, Cantrill SV, Rosen P, Rumack BH. Management of acute poisoned patients without gastric emptying. Ann Emerg Med 1985;14:562–567.

Newton M, Bartek JK, Fitzgerald A, Cawthorn-Sippel M, Schnell C. Drug update, descriptive outline of major poisoning treatment modes. J Emerg Nurs 1987;13:102–106.

Sullivan JB, Rumack BH, Peterson RG. Management of the poisoned patient in the emergency department. In: Bayer MJ, Rumack BH, eds. Poisoning & overdose. Rockville, Maryland: Aspen Publications, 1983:1–12.

Narcotic Overdose

Freitas PM. Narcotic withdrawal in the emergency department. Am J Emerg Med 1985; 3:456–460.

Goldfrank L. Narcotics. In: Bayer MJ, Rumack BH, Wanke LA, eds. Toxicologic emergencies. Bowie, Maryland: Robert J Brady, 1984:119–125.

Goldfrank L, Weisman RS, Errick JK, Lo M, et al. A dosing nomogram for continuous infusion intravenous naloxone. Ann Emerg Med 1986;15:566–570.

Platt JJ. Heroin addiction theory, research and treatment. Melbourne, Florida: Robert E Krieger Publishing, 1986:80–102.

Barbituate Overdose

Bryson PD. Comprehensive review in toxicology. Rockville, Maryland: Aspen Publications, 1986:199–217.

Dreisbach RH, Robertson WO. Handbook of poisoning: prevention, diagnosis and treatment. 12th ed. Norwalk, Connecticut: Appleton & Lange, 1987:318–344.

Anticholinergic and Polycyclic Overdose

Dreisbach RH, Robertson WO. Handbook of poisoning: prevention, diagnosis and treatment. 12th ed. Norwalk, Connecticut: Appleton & Lange, 1987:459.

Rosen MJ. Tricyclic antidepressant overdose: clinical features & management. Heart Lung 1983;12:222–225.

Cocaine

Acee AM, Smith D. Crack. Am J Nurs 1987;87:614–617.

Allen T. Narcotics. In: Rosen P, Baker FJ, Barkin RM, Braen GR, Dailey RH, Levy RC, eds. Emergency medicine. 2nd ed. St. Louis: CV Mosby, 1988:2125–2181.

Loveys BJ. Physiologic effects of cocaine with particular reference to the cardiovascular system. Heart Lung 1987;16:175–182.

Nuckols CC, Greeson J. Cocaine addiction: assessment and intervention. Nurs Clin North Am 1989;24:33–43.

Phencyclidine

Bayer MJ, Norton RL. Solving the clinical problems of phencyclidine intoxication. ER Rep 1983;4:7–12.

Goldfrank L, Lewin N, Osborn H. Dusted (PCP). Hosp Phys 1982;5:61–73.

Pearlson GD. Psychiatric and medical syndromes associated with phencyclidine abuse. John Hopkins Med J 1981;148:25–33.

Salicylate Poisoning

Bryson PD. Comprehensive review in toxicology. Rockville, Maryland: Aspen Publications, 1986:91–109.

Goldfrank L, Weisman R. The minor analgesic overdose: salicylates and acetaminophen. Heart Lung 1983;12:215–221.

Rosenberg PJ, Livingstone DJ, McLellan BA. Effect of whole- bowel irrigation on the antidotal efficacy of oral activated charcoal. Ann Emerg Med 1988;17:681–683.

Temple AR. Aspirin poisoning. In: Bayer M, Rumack BH, Wanke LA, eds. Toxicologic emergencies. Bowie, Maryland: Robert J Brady, 1984:109–117.

Acetaminophen Poisoning

Goldfrank LR, Howland MA, Weisman RS, Kirstein RH. Acetaminophen. In: Goldfrank LR, Flomenbaum NE, Lewin NA, Weisman RS, Howland MA, Kulberg AG, eds. Goldfrank's toxicologic emergencies. Norwalk: Appleton-Century-Crofts, 1986:222–232.

Rumack BH. Acetaminophen overdose: a high index of suspicion. In: Bayer MJ, Rumack BH, eds. Poisoning and overdose. Rockville, Maryland: Aspen Publications, 1983: 43–49.

Rumack BH, Kulig K. Acetaminophen overdose. In: Bayer MJ, Rumack BH, Wanke LA, eds. Toxicologic emergencies. Bowie, Maryland: Robert J Brady, 1984:99–108.

Thurkauf GE. Acetaminophen overdose. Crit Care Nurse 1987; 7:20–28.

Wall C. The real risk of acetaminophen overdose. RN 1985: 35–37.

Carbon Monoxide Poisoning

Brands A. Asphyxiant gases. In: Haley TJ, Berndt WO, eds. Handbook of toxicology. Washington, DC: Hemisphere Publishing, 1987:472–503.

Turnbull TL, Hart RG, Strange GR, et al. Emergency department screening for unsuspected carbon monoxide exposure. Ann Emerg Med 1988;17:478–483.

Alcohol Abuse and Withdrawal

Becker CE. The alcoholic patient as a toxic emergency. Emerg Med Clin North Am 1984;2:47–61.

Fisk NB. Alcoholism: ineffective family coping. Am J Nurs 1986;86:586–587.

Gilmore GM. Behavioral management of the acutely intoxicated patient in the emergency department. J Emerg Nurs 1986;12:13–17.

Kelly FM. Caring for the patient in acute alcohol withdrawal. Crit Care Q 1986;8:11–19.

Morris JC, Victor M. Alcohol withdrawal seizures. Emerg Med Clin North Am 1987; 5:827–839.

Powell AH, Minick MP. Alcohol withdrawal syndrome. Am J Nurs 1988;88:312–315.

Tweed SH. Identifying the alcoholic client. Nurs Clin North Am 1989;24:13–32.

Chapter 8

ALLERGIC REACTION

ANAPHYLAXIS AND URTICARIA

Description

Anaphylaxis is any or all of an acute symptom complex that includes generalized erythema, pruritus, urticaria, angioedema (swelling of areas of skin, mucous membrane, or viscera), nausea, vomiting, abdominal cramps, diarrhea, bronchial constriction, laryngeal edema, and cardiac arrhythmias, with or without cardiovascular collapse. Anaphylactic reactions may be graded as follows:

Grade I - Large local skin reaction, >15 cm in diameter
Grade II - Generalized pruritus and urticaria, with or without mild dyspnea
Grade III - Any of the above plus at least two of the following: generalized angioedema, mild wheezing, nausea and vomiting, dizziness
Grade IV - Any of the above plus at least one of the following: severe dyspnea or asthma, dysphagia with tongue swelling, hoarseness with laryngeal edema, hypotension, syncope

Etiology

There are innumerable substances that may cause anaphylaxis. The most common include:

Antibiotics - Penicillin, penicillin analogs, cephalosporins
Drugs - Aspirin, iodides
Anesthetics - Procaine, cocaine, benzocaine
Dyes - Iodinated contrast media
Stinging insects - Wasps, yellow jackets, hornets
Foods - Eggs, milk, nuts, seafood, citrus fruits, legumes

Assessment

History

Patients should be questioned closely as to personal and family history of allergies such as hay fever, asthma, eczema, drug reactions, or anaphylaxis, because the incidence of serious drug reactions is much higher in patients with a positive history. If possible, have the patient identify the causative agent and determine the time interval between exposure and onset of symptoms—the longer the time, the less the likelihood of a severe reaction. Most acute anaphylactic reactions occur within 1 hour of exposure, although a secondary anaphylactic reaction occurring 4–6 hours after an initial reaction has recently been described.

Physical Findings

Vital signs - Check for tachycardia, arrhythmia, hypotension, or tachypnea.

HEENT* - Look for angioedema, drooling, and inability to handle secretions, and listen for hoarseness.

Neck - Listen for stridor.

Lungs - Auscultate the patient for wheezing or decreased breath sounds. Loss of voice should be noted.

Extremities - Note if extremities are cold and clammy or cyanotic.

Skin - Examine carefully for erythema (diffuse redness) or urticaria (raised wheals with severe itching).

Intervention

The triage nurse should immediately bring a patient suspected of having a severe allergic reaction to the physician's attention.

Appropriate therapy should be instituted immediately at the first sign of a severe anaphylactic reaction. In severe (grade III or IV) reactions, every second counts. In fatal cases, the reaction may occur within seconds to minutes after exposure, and death may occur in under 15 minutes. Therapy consists of:

1. Airway maintenance - Administer oxygen at 2–6 liters/min. Be prepared for the use of intubation or emergency cricothyrotomy. An oropharyngeal airway will often relieve obstruction caused by the tongue or soft tissues of the pharynx. Position the patient in Fowler's position, if blood pressure permits.

---

*See "Appendix A" for definition of common abbreviations used in the text.

2. Fluid administration - Start a large-bore IV line with normal saline. IV access is required for drug therapy and for volume administration in case of shock.
3. Drug therapy
   a. Epinephrine is essential for immediate therapy in all grades of reaction. It causes peripheral vasoconstriction and bronchodilation. Give epinephrine (1:1000 solution), 0.3–0.5 ml SC as ordered. In life-threatening reactions, epinephrine may be given IV in 2 ml boluses (1:100,000 solution). Epinephrine for IV use may be prepared by diluting 1 ml of the 1:10,000 solution with 9 ml of normal saline. For continuing hypotension or bronchospasm, an epinephrine infusion can be given IV as 1–2 ml of 1:1000 solution in 500 ml normal saline. For markedly hypotensive patients with poor venous access, 0.3–0.5 ml of 1:1000 can be given into the posterior ventral tongue, where vascularity ensures rapid absorption.
   b. Antihistamines are indicated following epinephrine. Antihistamines act to reduce urticaria and angioedema. Grade I reactions usually respond to epinephrine plus diphenhydramine (Benadryl), 25–50 mg PO or IM, along with cold compresses locally. Grade II reactions should be advised to continue Benadryl, 25–50 mg PO, every 6 hours for 24–43 hours. In grade III or IV reactions, Benadryl, 25–50 mg, may be given as an IV push, and the dose may be repeated every 6 hours prn.
   c. Aminophylline by IV drip is indicated when bronchospasm persists despite administration of epinephrine. Patients receiving aminophylline or epinephrine IV should be on a cardiac monitor to check for arrhythmias. Aminophylline should be administered according to guidelines approved for the treatment of asthma (see Chapter 2). For those not on xanthines already, a loading dose of 6 mg/Kg IV should be given by an infusion (0.3–0.9 mg/Kg/hr).
   d. Pressors may be necessary in hypotensive patients who fail to respond to fluids. Have a MAST suit available. The vital signs should be monitored continuously, and dopamine, 2–10 μg/Kg/min, may be administered IV via an infusion pump for sustained vasopressor action.
   e. Local tourniquet placement proximal to the site of an insect bite or drug injection may be useful if done immediately. Epinephrine, 0.3 ml of 1:1000, should be injected directly into the site for grades III and IV.
   f. Steroids should be given for anaphylaxis. The dose of hydrocortisone (Solu-Cortef) is 100–200 mg IV every 4–6 hours.
4. Reassurance and comfort - Provide reassurance and comfort to the pa-

tient, who can be expected to be apprehensive and, possibly, agitated. Stay with the patient, and keep the family informed.

ED Discharge Planning

Patients with any serious anaphylactic reactions should be admitted for continued observation and therapy. This includes all those with grade III or IV reaction and specifically those with angioedema of the face and pharynx or any respiratory or cardiovascular manifestation.

Most patients with grade I or II reaction will respond to a single dose of epinephrine SC, followed by antihistamines PO. They should be counselled to avoid further exposure to the allergen. An identification tag (Medic-Alert bracelet) may be useful in the case of drug allergies. Instruct the patient to return to the ED immediately if a reaction recurs.

SUGGESTED READING

Lew DB, Herrod HG. Anaphylaxis, anaphylactoid reactions, and serum sickness. In: Rakel RE, ed. Conn's current therapy. Philadelphia: WB Saunders, 1989:661–663.

Chapter 9

INFECTIOUS DISEASE

MENINGITIS

Meningitis is an inflammation of the meninges of the brain and spinal cord. Meningeal infection is most commonly seen in patients with systemic bacteremia or upper respiratory or adjacent local infection or in patients who have suffered invasive head trauma or have undergone surgery.

Acute meningitis is most often the result of bacterial or viral infection. *Streptococcus pneumoniae, Neisseria meningitidis,* or staphlococci are most commonly the causative organisms.

Meningococcal meningitis is the only bacterial meningitis that occurs in outbreaks. It usually occurs among groups living in close quarters (in camps, institutions, etc.)

Pneumococcal meningitis is the most common cause of bacterial meningitis in adults; the infection is often secondary to acute otitis media and mastoiditis (30%), pneumonia (10–25%), nonpenetrating head injury (5–10%), CSF* fluid rhinorrhea or otorrhea (5%), or acute sinusitis (less common). Immunocompromised patients account for 10–25% of cases; these include people with sickle cell anemia, alcoholism, and asplenia (absence of spleen).

Viral (aseptic) meningitis in adults is most often caused by enteroviruses, which include coxsackieviruses A and B and echoviruses. Although the responsible virus is not identified in the majority of cases, other viruses encountered include mumps, varicella-zoster, herpes simplex, and lymphocytic choriomeningitis virus. Viral meningitides often occur during the spring or summer in epidemics; they usually carry a much better prognosis than bacterial meningitis.

---

*See "Appendix A" for definition of common abbreviations used in the text.

211

Tuberculous meningitis is currently a disease of the elderly. It is typically less abrupt in onset than bacterial or viral meningitis—patients have only general manifestations of infection for 2–3 weeks before meningeal irritation develops. Tuberulosis and fungal meningitis (e.g., crytococcus, coccidioidomycosis) are seen in immunocompromised hosts (e.g., AIDS patients) and may develop as a result of disseminated infection weeks to months after an initial infection.

Assessment

History

Meningitis commonly presents as fever and headache or a change in mental status. Time elapsed since onset of symptoms is a vital part of the history, as is information about any recent infection (e.g., upper respiratory tract infection, otitis) or cranial trauma. An important associated complaint is the presence of a rash. Past medical history should focus on underlying disease states resulting in immunocompromise.

Patients with bacterial meningitis will often give a history of a recent upper respiratory tract infection, pneumonia, or otitis. The onset is usually sudden (over 24–36 hours), but sometimes symptoms may evolve over 3–5 days. Early symptoms include fever, headache, stiff neck, vomiting, and myalgias. Later, the patient may progress to confusion and, ultimately, coma. Additional neurologic manifestations may include cranial nerve palsies, focal or generalized seizures, hemiparesis, dysphasia, and hemianopsia (blindness in half the visual field). Cerebral edema may develop, with hypertension, bradycardia, and coma. Meningitis caused by *N. meningitidis* is typically associated with a maculopetechial or purpuric rash that reaches the face and neck after extensively covering the rest of the body (centripetal).

Patients with viral meningitis generally have symptoms of sudden onset, with high fever, stiff neck, myalgias, and arthralgias. Echovirus may produce a maculopetechial rash that covers the face and neck before extending to the trunk and extremities (centrifugal). Patients with mumps meningitis will have a concomitant parotitis; those with herpes simplex type II meningitis will give a history of sexual contact and often have identifiable genital lesions. Because viral meningitis is generally self-limited and resolves in 3–5 days, more severe or lasting neurologic sequelae are uncommon.

Tuberculous meningitis may present as several weeks of symptoms that include headache, fever, and stiff neck. Patients can develop cranial nerve palsies as well as other focal deficits, confusion or delirium, focal or generalized seizures, cerebral edema, and coma. Fever is minimal, and signs of meningeal irritation are often missing.

Physical Findings

Vital signs - Check for fever, hyperpnea (increased respiratory rate or depth), hypotension, and bradycardia (seen with cerebral edema).

HEENT - Examine for evidence of head trauma.

Neck - Look for stiffness on anterior flexion. Abrupt neck flexion may cause involuntary hip flexion (Brudzinski's sign).

Lungs - Listen for rhonchi or rales.

Extremities - Extension of the knee while the hip is flexed may be met by strong passive resistance and involuntary neck flexion (Kernig's sign).

Neurologic signs - Note the level of conscious and mental status. Perform a Glasgow coma scale. Check the patient for pupil response, and note any focal deficits.

Skin - Check the skin carefully for lesions, purpura, or petechiae.

Diagnostic Tests

Lumbar puncture - This should be performed immediately in patients strongly suspected of having acute meningitis. In suspected meningitis, lumbar puncture is important to the diagnosis and should not be delayed. However, in patients with liver disease, with clotting disorders, or on anticoagulant therapy, a platelet count and PT should be obtained first, if at all possible. In the face of focal neurologic signs, suspected brain edema or brain abscess, and signs of head trauma, lumbar puncture should be deferred until a CAT scan of the head is obtained. The initiation of treatment for suspected meningitis should not be deferred, however. After three sets of blood cultures, the patient may be started on empiric broad-spectrum antibiotics. After the CAT scan the lumbar puncture may be performed in the absence of increased intracranial pressure.

CSF - Fluid should be immediately evaluated for cell count, glucose and protein, and Gram stain. The fluid should be sent for bacterial culture and sensitivity, including cultures for fungus and acid-fast bacilli.

Blood cultures - Blood cultures are indicated prior to initiation of antibiotic therapy.

CBC - Send for WBC, differential, and platelet count.

SMA - Note electrolyte imbalances, BUN/creatinine ratio, and glucose.

CIE - Counterimmunoelectrophoresis or CIE is generally not of value. It is only diagnostic when there are bacteria in the CSF that are identifiable by Gram stain.

X-rays - A chest x-ray may reveal an infiltrate. Sinus, mastoid, or skull films may be ordered.

CAT scan - An emergency CAT scan should be performed prior to lumbar puncture in patients with signs of increased intracranial pressure (e.g., papilledema) or focal neurologic deficits suggestive of intracranial abscess.

Intervention

1. Provide necessary life support - See "Cardiopulmonary Arrest" in Chapter 1 and "Acute Respiratory Failure" in Chapter 2. Monitor the patient for signs of shock and seizure activity. Start an IV of 0.45% NaCl. Consult a physician for IV fluid orders; avoid overhydration. Monitor the patient's intake and output. Keep an oral airway and intubation equipment on standby. Oxygen therapy may be prescribed.
2. Provide comfort measures - Assist the patient to a comfortable position, usually side-lying or mid-Fowler's with the head slightly extended. Codeine may be prescribed for head and neck pain. Patients may be confused or experiencing hallucinations; take measures to prevent self-injury.
3. Reduce fever - An elevated temperature increases the patient's metabolic rate, cerebral edema, and seizures. Aspirin, a hypothermia blanket, and sponge baths can be used to lower the temperature.
4. Antibiotic therapy - Antibiotics are indicated for proven or suspected bacterial meningitis. Check the patient's record for drug allergies. In many cases, infection is due to either pneumococcal or meningococcal meningitis, and treatment with aqueous penicillin G, 24 million units daily given as 2 million units IV every 2 hours for 10–14 days, will be effective. Meningitis caused by *Haemophilus influenzae* may be treated with chloramphenicol, 500–1000 mg IV every 6 hours or ampicillin, 12–14 gm daily, divided into IV doses every 2 hours. Staphylococcal meningitis can be treated with nafcillin, 20 gm/day, or oxacillin, 16 gm/day, in divided IV doses every 4–6 hours. Gram-negative meningitis requires treatment with chloramphenicol, 4 gm IV daily, and gentamicin, 5 mg/Kg IM or IV daily.
5. Infection control measures - Patients with meningococcal meningitis or with meningitis of uncertain origin require respiratory isolation. Staff in contact with the patient must wear gloves, gown, and mask. Consult the infectious disease department concerning treatment of patient contacts (staff, family, coworkers).

ED Discharge Planning

All patients with proven or suspected meningitis will require admission for treatment or continuing observation. Although patients with viral meningitis often follow a benign and self-limited course, admission is warranted on the grounds of observation for development of uncommon sequelae and for results of spinal fluid cultures and studies. Arrange for an isolation room, if indicated, and notify all staff of required precautions.

ENDOCARDITIS

Endocarditis, an inflammation of the inner lining of the heart, is usually limited to the heart valves. The picture of endocarditis has been changing in recent decades. This change is attributed in part to improved laboratory and diagnostic techniques and in part to the increasing number of cases seen in IV drug abusers and patients with nosocomial infections related to prosthetic valves and invasive procedures.

The causative organism is most commonly a streptococcal species, including viridans and beta-hemolytic streptococci, or enterococci. Staphlococci, Gram-negative bacilli, and *Candida albicans* may cause endocarditis.

Previously damaged heart valves and an abnormal hemodynamic state often underlie the development of endocarditis. In most patients the left side of the heart is predominantly involved, with the mitral valve affected more often than the aortic. However, in IV drug abusers, involvement of the right side of the heart is a common finding.

Assessment

History
A patient with subacute endocarditis will have slow and subtle onset of symptoms, which may persist for months before the patient seeks treatment. Low-grade fever, weakness, muscle and joint pain, fatigue, and anorexia are common. Probing into the history will result in description of recent dental procedure, cystoscopy, bowel instrumentation, or oropharyngeal surgery in many of the cases. Patients will often give a history of congenital heart problems, rheumatic fever, or cardiac surgery.

The patient with acute endocarditis often describes an abrupt onset with high fever and shaking chills. Questioning may reveal recent bacterial infection (e.g., pneumonia, furunculosis, abscess) or may provide a likely predisposition (IV drug abuse, recent instrumentation, etc.). The infection is rapidly progressive, and the patient is usually acutely ill and toxic.

Physical Findings
General - Note the level of consciousness if the patient is acutely toxic or chronically ill in appearance.
Vital signs - Look for tachycardia, tachypnea, and hypotension. Check the patient's rectal temperature.

Neck - Note if the patient's neck is supple. Jugular venous distention may indicate tricuspid insufficiency.

Lungs - Listen for rales, rhonchi, or rubs.

Heart - Note rate and rhythm. Listen for murmurs, gallops, and rubs. Diastolic murmurs not previously heard are significant.

Abdomen - Note bowel sounds or local areas of tenderness.

Extremities - Note cyanosis or edema. Check for track marks.

Skin - Examine the skin carefully for petechiae, pustules, or purpura.

Diagnostic Tests

Laboratory tests - Obtain a CBC with WBC and differential. Send for SMA, PT, and ESR (almost always elevated). An elevated BUN and creatinine can be seen in renal failure.

Urinalysis - Check for hematuria or red cell casts.

Blood cultures - Should be obtained prior to antibiotic therapy. Three separate sets should be obtained. If the patient appears very ill, the sets can be obtained within minutes of each other.

ECG - An ECG may show conduction abnormalities due to myocardial abscesses.

X-rays - Chest films may reveal pulmonary involvement (septic pulmonary emboli), effusions, or pneumonia.

Intervention

1. Provide basic life support, if needed. (See "Cardiopulmonary Arrest" in Chapter 1 and "Acute Respiratory Failure" in Chapter 2). Assess critically ill patients for signs of decreased cardiac output. Patients with severe congestive heart failure due to valvular insufficiency may require surgery for valve replacement.
2. Provide antibiotic therapy. All diagnostic specimens should be obtained before antibiotic therapy is started. The antibiotic regimen should include a combination effective against the common causal organisms. One such regimen is ampicillin, nafcillin, and gentamicin. Vancomycin and gentamicin may be prescribed for penicillin-allergic patients.

ED Discharge Planning and Instructions

All patients with known or suspected endocarditis must be admitted for further observation and to await culture results. The nurse should provide all patients at risk for endocarditis with information on prevention. In particular, patients with cardiac murmurs and valvular disease should consult their physicians concerning prophylactic antibiotic therapy prior to having any dental or other invasive procedure.

PERICARDITIS

Pericarditis is an inflammation of the pericardium, the two layered sac that contains the heart. The causes of acute pericarditis can be categorized as follows:

1. Infectious—viral, bacterial, and fungal
2. Noninfectious—acute myocardial infarction, postinfarction (Dressler's syndrome), uremia, trauma, drug induced (e.g., hydralazine, procainamide), and collagen vascular

Assessment

History
The most common manifestation is anterior chest pain that is worsened by deep breathing and lying prone. The pain is often described as pleuritic and may be aggravated by swallowing if the posterior aspect of the heart is involved.

If the diaphragmatic surface of the pericardium is involved, pain will be referred to the left shoulder. There may be a decrease in severity when the patient sits up and leans forward. Occasionally, the pain may mimic angina, appearing as a dull and steady retrosternal pain with radiation to one or both arms, shoulders, and/or the epigastrium.

Many patients report an antecedent viral syndrome, usually an upper respiratory tract infection, about 10–12 days prior to onset of precordial pain. Fever may be noted.

Physical Findings
General - Weakness, malaise.
Vital signs - Fever may be as high as 104° or 105°F. Note any tachycardia or tachypnea. Monitor blood pressure for hypotension and pulsus paradoxus. The presence of a pulsus paradoxus (respiratory variation in auscultated pressure spanning more than 10 mm Hg) is indicative of cardiac tamponade.
Neck - Examine the patient for neck vein distension (seen with tamponade).
Lungs - Listen for rales or a pleural rub.
Heart - The pericardial friction rub is the cardinal sign of pericarditis. It is a scratchy sound that is best heard on forced inspiration with the patient sitting and leaning forward with hands on knees. Classically, it has three phases—atrial systole, ventricle systole, and diastole. Because the rub is inconstant and transitory, its absence does not rule out the diagnosis.
Extremities - Note pedal edema or cyanosis.

Diagnostic Tests

Laboratory tests - Obtain a CBC, WBC, and SMA. ESR is almost always significantly elevated.

X-rays - A chest film is helpful in ruling out pulmonary causes of chest pain and in checking for signs of congestive heart failure and the cardiomegaly of large pericardial infusion.

ECG - Elevation on the ECG of ST segments in two or three limb leads and V_2–V_6 occurs, with reciprocal depressions in aVR and V_1. There is no change in the QRS. After several days the ST segments return to baseline. PR segment depression may also be noted in leads II, aVF, and V_4–V_6, and may be the earliest ECG abnormality noted. There may be T-wave inversion in leads formerly showing ST-segment elevations.

Echocardiogram - An echocardiogram is indicated in patients with pericarditis to evaluate the presence of a pericardial effusion.

Pericardiocentesis - Aspiration of fluid with laboratory analysis and culture is helpful in evaluation of patients with significant pericardial effusions. It may be used therapeutically as an emergency procedure in patients with acute complications such as cardiac tamponade.

Intervention

1. Promote cardiac function - Place the patient on a cardiac monitor. Both atrial and ventricular arrhythmias may occur, and frequent ECG monitoring is therefore imperative. (See "Selected Cardiac Arrhythmias" for a discussion of supraventricular tachycardia and heart block, and see "Cardiopulmonary Arrest" for details of therapy (all in Chapter 1).) It is notable that procainamide should be avoided due to its known ability to produce a lupus-like syndrome that may cause pericarditis. Tachycardia, hypotension, distended neck vein, edema, and fatigue warn of interference with cardiac output. Pericardial effusion, cardiac tamponade, and pericardial constriction affect cardiac output and may require emergency intervention. Patients should be placed on bed rest. Start oxygen at 3–6 liters/min by nasal cannula in patients who are symptomatic.

2. Provide drug therapy - In the majority of cases, aspirin or, if aspirin is ineffective, indomethacin (Indocin) will be given to reduce inflammation, chest pain, and fever. Acute viral or idiopathic pericarditis is generally self-limited and resolves in several days to weeks, but it may recur. If bacterial or fungal pericarditis is suspected, a pericardiocentesis with Gram and fungal stains and cultures of the aspirate should be performed. Antibiotic therapy should be started parenterally in aggressive dosages to prevent complications of tamponade and constriction. When pericarditis is due to a systemic ill-

ness (malignancy, uremia, hypothyroidism), treatment should center around control or reversal of the underlying disease process.

3. Promote patient comfort - In addition to administration of aspirin or indomethacin, placing the patient in a high-Fowler's position, i.e., leaning forward on a bedside stand, will reduce chest pain. Once a diagnosis is made, the nurse can help allay the patient's fears concerning the origin of the chest pain and usual course of the disease.

ED Discharge Planning

All patients with newly diagnosed pericarditis should be admitted to the hospital for further diagnostic tests and monitoring. Pericardial effusions may occur in all forms of pericarditis, even viral, with serious consequences.

EAR, NOSE, AND THROAT DISORDERS

The incidence of ENT infections is affected by seasonal changes. During the winter months, adults and children spend more time indoors in close proximity with each other. Influenza outbreaks during the winter are of particular concern for patients with chronic diseases, as well as for the elderly.

Assessment

History
Important points to cover include: (1) time course of infection, (2) presence of fever, chills, or rigors, (3) associated symptoms, such as headache or joint pains, (4) possible contacts with known causes, and (5) presence of underlying disease associated with immunosuppression.

Physical Findings
Check for fever, and note any difficulty breathing or swallowing. Drooling may indicate an airway obstruction. Signs of a peritonsillar abscess include trismus (tonic contraction of the muscles of mastication), inability to swallow, and excessive salivation. Assess the patient for pain or tenderness and for nose or ear drainage. Note voice hoarseness and any gross hearing deficit.

Diagnostic Tests
Throat cultures and streptococcal slide test - All patients with suspected streptococcal pharyngitis should have a quick test for streptococcal organisms or a throat culture done on blood agar with neomycin. Patients

with a high likelihood of streptococcal infection or with a positive quick test may be treated without a culture. Patients in whom gonococcal infection is suspected should also have a culture on Thayer-Martin agar.

CBC - May show a moderate increase in WBC.

X-rays and other noninvasive tests - X-rays, indicated by signs of acute sinusitis, will show sinus air-fluid levels, opacification, and structural lesions. CAT scan, sinoscopy, and ultrasound will also provide diagnostic information.

Sinus aspiration - Provides relief of pressure through drainage, as well as specimens for culture and Gram stain. Aspiration is usually reserved for the seriously ill, the immunosuppressed, and the patient who is not responding to therapy.

PHARYNGITIS

Intervention

In the majority of cases of pharyngitis the patient should be sent home with palliative measures to await the result of throat cultures. If the throat culture is positive, the patient should be recalled to the ED to receive appropriate therapy. It is important to explain to these patients that most sore throats are due to viruses, which penicillin cannot treat, and that the purpose of treatment with penicillin is primarily to prevent acute rheumatic fever.

In patients with the following conditions, treatment should be started immediately without waiting for culture results:

1. Previous positive culture with noncompliance
2. Fever higher than 37.7°C, tender anterior cervical nodes, exudative tonsils, and the absence of a cough
3. Past history of rheumatic fever, especially with carditis
4. Scarlatiniform rash
5. Underlying immunosuppression (e.g., in diabetics)
6. Known epidemic of a nephritogenic streptococcus
7. Contact with young children
8. Adverse social situation

Appropriate therapy for streptococcal pharyngitis consists of oral penicillin VK, 250 mg qid for 10 days (with a risk of noncompliance), or benzathine penicillin, 1.2 million units IM in a single dose (assuring compliance). Therapy should be started within 9 days of onset to avoid risk of acute rheumatic fever. Penicillin-allergic patients should receive erythromycin, 250 mg PO qid for 10 days.

If the patient looks toxic, oral penicillin can be given for 2–3 days along with IM benzathine penicillin (the suspension is easier to swallow). Palliative measures include bed rest, fluids, saline gargles, and lozenges.

If the patient has trismus, excessive salivation, and a fluctuant tonsillar inability to swallow, peritonsillar abscess should be suspected, and an ENT consult should be obtained.

SINUSITIS

Sinusitis is an inflammation of one or more of the four pairs of paranasal sinuses (ethmoid, frontal, maxillary, sphenoid). It occurs when the passages between each sinus and the nasal cavity become obstructed due to congestion and tenacious mucus production, leading to decreased drainage of fluid and impaired air exchange. In some cases, incubation of bacteria results in subsequent pain and inflammation.

Sinusitis may also be due to noninfectious causes including allergies and asthma, vasomotor rhinitis, tumors and polyps, foreign bodies, and trauma, and cigarette smoking.

Frontal sinusitis produces pain and tenderness over the lower forehead, whereas maxillary sinusitis causes pain over the cheeks or referred pain to the teeth. Pain may be worse upon arising or leaning forward. Other less common and less specific symptoms include malaise, lethargy, and dizziness.

A purulent nasal discharge may or may not be seen. Pain may be elicited by percussing the affected sinus. Possible complications include osteomyelitis (from frontal sinus), orbital cellulitis, cavernous sinus thrombophlebitis, brain abscess, or meningitis.

Intervention

1. Promote sinus drainage - Decongestants and/or antihistamines may be given via nasal spray or PO. A rebound effect may occur if topical spray is used for more than 3–5 days.
2. Provide symptomatic relief - Aspirin, acetaminophen, and codeine can be given. The use of a heated humidifier and the application of heated wet packs can be of help.
3. Give antibiotics - Antibiotics given PO are acceptable for uncomplicated sinusitis of the frontal or maxillary sinus. Multiple sinus sinusitis, ethnoid or sphenoid sinusitis, and sinusitis with spread require admission of the patient for IV administration of antibiotics.

Treatment response is usually noticeable within 48 hours, with complete resolution of symptoms occurring in 5–10 days. Follow-up sinus films may be recommended. Referral to an ENT specialist is advised in all cases of facial pain, headache, and fever that do not respond to conventional therapy after 10 days.

OTITIS

Otitis externa (often called "swimmer's ear") is a common, usually benign inflammation of the ear canal caused by moisture, trauma, or dermatitis. It is seen in all age groups.

Otitis externa is treated as follows:

1. Bacterial - Apply topical ear drops with an antibiotic and steroid to decrease swelling.
2. Fungal - Avoid steroids. Use Burrow's or acetic acid solution drops. (It may be necessary to gently cleanse the external canal if there is so much discharge and debris that the drops will not penetrate. Irrigation should be avoided because it will cause more maceration of the canal and may penetrate the middle ear if there is a drum perforation.)
3. Systemic antibiotics should be prescribed if there is regional cervical adenopathy or a spreading cellulitis or if the patient is a diabetic. Appropriate regimens include penicillin, ampicillin, or amoxicillin for 7–10 days. Analgesics (aspirin, acetaminophen, codeine, etc.) may be needed.

Acute otitis media (suppurative or purulent otitis media) is an infection of the normally sterile middle ear, which is usually caused by extension of a nasopharyngeal infection. It may be seen in adults but is most commonly seen in children.

Treatment includes:

1. Decongestant/antihistamine nasal sprays and oral agents.
2. Systemic antibiotics - These should be prescribed for all cases of acute otitis media.
3. Analgesics - Aspirin, acetaminophen, codeine, etc. can be given prn.
4. Myringotomy - This procedure is indicated for patients with intractable pain, progressive hearing loss, early mastoiditis, or poor response to medical therapy. These patients should be referred to an ENT specialist. Ear drum perforations should be treated with systemic antibiotics and kept dry, as they usually close spontaneously.

If neglected or recurrent, acute otitis media may result in a chronic condition with mild ear pain, hearing loss, and discharge. Rare and serious complications of acute otitis media include mastoiditis, meningitis, brain abscess, facial paralysis.

Serous otitis media, a noninfectious effusion of the middle ear space, is usually caused by a blocked Eustachian tube. It also may be seen in adults but is most commonly seen in children. Serous otitis media is the second most common cause of deafness in the general population, pointing up the importance of careful follow-up.

Intervention

1. Topical sprays, decongestants (antibiotics are of no value).
2. Antihistamines - These are controversial because they thicken secretions and slow ciliary action.
3. Humidification with cool mist - Humidification may be helpful.
4. Myringotomy - This procedure may be necessary for aspiration of the fluid and for insertion of a tympanostomy tube, which allows ventilation of the middle ear and ameliorates the Eustachian tube obstruction.

ED Discharge Planning

Patients who appear toxic, are unable to swallow, require IV antibiotics, have ethmoid or sphenoid sinusitis, are diabetics, are immunocompromised patients, and have infection extending to the mastoids, labyrinths, or intracranial regions should be admitted.

ED Discharge Instructions
Topical nasal sprays (sympathomimetics) such as phenylephrine HCl (Neo-Synephrine) and oxymetazoline HCl (Afrin) should be used for only 3–5 days and not more than 3–4 times/day. Note that these agents are contraindicated in patients with hypertension or thyroid disease and are to be used with caution in patients taking monoamine oxidase inhibitors and tricyclic antidepressants.

Patients taking antihistamines should be cautioned against using heavy machinery or driving, because of the sedative effect of these medications.

Instruct the patient as indicated, on the use of warm saline gargles, increased fluid intake, warm soaks, and rest.

Patients should feel better in 2–3 days; if the patient's condition is unimproved, he or she should return in 1 week for further evaluation. Patients with acute otitis media and serous otitis media should have follow-up evaluation and hearing test.

Advise all patients that the normal ear does not need to be cleaned. Tell them to keep fingers, instruments, and cotton swabs out of their ears. After water exposure the swimmer can dry out the ear with a drop of 70% alcohol.

TETANUS

Tetanus is a clinical syndrome caused by the release of a potent neurotoxin produced by *Clostridium tetani*. The principal manifestation of tetanus is neuromuscular dysfunction. The spores of *C. tetani* have been cultured from soil, dust, water, and animal and human feces. According to the United States Public Health Service CDC annual statistics report, 64 cases of tetanus were reported in the United States for 1986. Most people are exposed to tetanus infection in wounds that are soil contaminated. Because the organism is an obligate anaerobe, puncture wounds or wounds involving deep necrotic tissue provide the best media.

Assessment

History
Important points to include are type of injury, conditions under which injury occurred, time elapsed since injury, and previous history of tetanus immunization. So-called "tetanus-prone" injuries include compound fractures, gunshot wounds, burns, crush injuries, wounds with retained foreign bodies, deep punctures, soil- or feces-contaminated wounds, wounds untended for more than 24 hours, wounds infected with other organisms, necrotic wounds, and induced abortions. IV drug abusers are prone to tetanus infections because of unhygienic practices and possible depressed immunity.

Once tetanus sets in, the patient may initially complain of difficulty swallowing and excessive yawning. Stiffness of the jaw (lockjaw or trismus) and neck or back pain will develop, followed by tonic muscle spasms that can be either local or generalized. Severe cases include paroxysmal muscle spasms, board-like rigidity, opisthotonus (extreme arching of the back and retraction of the head), and respiratory compromise. Environmental stimuli (noise, lights, motion) may trigger convulsions. Because extrapyramidal reactions may mimic tetanus, obtain a history of psychotropic medication ingestion.

Mild cases have an incubation period of 10 days or more; patients initially have a low-grade fever, irritability, and local rigidity near the wound site, followed by mild stiffness of the neck and jaw lasting about 1 week. Moderate cases have a slightly shorter incubation; patients present with severe trismus (tonic contractions of the muscles of mastication), dysphagia, and generalized paroxysmal muscle spasms triggered by such stimuli as noise, motion, or temperature change. Severe cases have an incubation of less than 1 week; these patients have frequent violent and prolonged paroxysms. Complications include pneumonia, fracture of thoracic vertebrae, and death due to respiratory arrest.

Diagnostic Tests

Laboratory tests - Send for a CBC, and check the WBC and differential for a rise indicative of infection. Obtain a SMA for electrolytes and calcium. Do a Dextrostix for blood glucose.

ABGs - Check pH and pO_2.

Intervention

Generalized Tetanus

1. Maintain airway and adequate breathing pattern - Oxygen administration and endotracheal intubation are often required to prevent hypoxia. Position the patient to facilitate drainage of oral secretions; suction the patient's mouth via a Yankower suction tip.
2. Prevent and treat convulsions (see "Seizures" in Chapter 3). Protect the patient from injury. Keep the patient's room as quiet and dark as possible to avoid triggering spasms.
3. Provide immunization for tetanus - Administer tetanus immune globulin (TIG) (3000 units IM given as three 1000-unit doses at separate sites) and diptheria-tetanus (dT) toxoid booster early to neutralize any circulating toxins and to begin tetanus immunization (tetanus toxin is so toxic it does not confer immunity). When administering dT and TIG concurrently, use separate syringes and injection sites.
4. Provide tetanus prophylaxis - Patients who have been immunized and have superficial minor wounds should have their wounds cleaned and should receive a dT toxoid booster injection if they have not received a booster in the past 10 years. dT toxoid should always be used, as there have been recent reports of diphtheria infections in patients without adequate vaccinations. Previously immunized patients with dirty wounds should have meticulous debridement, as well as a dT toxoid booster, if they have not received a booster in the past 5 years.

Nonimmunized adults with clean wounds should receive 3 doses of dT toxoid 1 month apart, followed by a booster dose after 1 year. Nonimmunized adults with dirty wounds should receive careful surgical debridement, dT toxoid, and 250 units TIG. Antibiotics are of questionable efficacy against *C. tetani*; although the organism is sensitive to penicillin. Very high doses are needed to penetrate the necrotic or devascularized tissue in which *C. tetani* thrives.

IV drug users are especially prone to tetanus infections despite previous immunization and, when treated for wounds, should receive dT boosters regardless of immunization status (see Table 9.1).

ED Discharge Planning and Instructions

All patients with generalized tetanus should be admitted to an ICU.
  Nursing diagnosis for a patient with tetanus includes:

1. Breathing pattern, ineffective - Related to laryngeal and respiratory spasms and dysphagia.
2. Potential for injury - Related to tonic convulsions and muscle rigidity. Vertebral fractures may result.
3. Nutrition, less than body requirements - Nasogastric feedings or parenteral nutrition will be required.
4. Fear and knowledge deficit - Except when sedated or hypoxic, the patient remains alert throughout.

Preventive health instruction is an important component of the ED nurse's role. All patients should be encouraged to complete their immunization schedule and seek prompt attention for high-risk puncture or infected wounds.

Table 9.1.
Indications for Immunization[a]

	Clean wound		Dirty wound	
Previous immunization	dT toxoid	TIG	dT toxoid	TIG
No previous immunization or uncertain	Yes*	No	Yes*	Yes
One previous injection of dT or dPT	Yes*	No	Yes*	Yes
Two previous injections of dT or dPT	Yes*	No	Yes*	Yes
Three or more previous injections of dT or dPT	No[†]	No	No[‡]	No

[a]Abbreviations and symbols: dT, indicates diptheria-tetanus toxoid; TIG, tetanus immune globulin; dPT, diptheria, pertussis, tetanus toxoid; *, the series should be completed; [†], unless more than10 years have elapsed since the last booster; and [‡], unless more than 5 years have elapsed since the last booster.

ACQUIRED IMMUNODEFICIENCY SYNDROME

Human immunodeficiency virus (HIV) has been identified as the agent responsible for acquired immunodeficiency syndrome (AIDS). HIV interferes with the body's immune response and leaves the victim defenseless to infection. The clinical manifestations of AIDS are variable, particularly in the early stages.

The patient may or may not tell the triage nurse he or she has AIDS while describing the reason for the ED visit. Those considered at high risk for contracting the HIV infection are homosexual men, IV drug abusers, recipients of contaminated blood products, infants born of mothers with HIV infections, and sexual partners of persons with HIV infections. Although HIV has been found in a number of body fluids, only semen and blood have been shown to be a source of transmission.

Assessment

History

In addition to the chief complaint, include associated symptoms and time frame. Ascertain whether the symptoms have been progressive and whether the patient has been previously treated for these symptoms. Barring severe infection, patients often complain of prolonged feelings of weakness and malaise, weight loss, and night sweats. The most common opportunistic infections include:

1. *Pneumocystis carinii* pneumonia - The patient has dyspnea, nonproductive cough, and chest pain. Symptoms can range from those of mild respiratory dysfunction to overt respiratory failure. There has also been a significant increase in the incidence of tuberculosis among AIDS patients in New York City as reported by the CDC.
2. Central nervous system dysfunction is often due to the HIV virus itself, bacterial agents, other viral infections, or malignancy. Neurologic complications include encephalitis, aseptic meningitis, dementia, toxoplasmosis, behavior and personality changes, ataxia, and seizures.
3. GI complications - Oral candidiasis (thrush) and severe diarrhea can rapidly debilitate a patient, and due to fluid and electrolyte imbalance, hospitalization may be required.
4. Lymphadenopathy - Enlarged lymph nodes may or may not be painful.
5. Karposi's sarcoma - A previously rare skin cancer. An aggressive form of Karposi's sarcoma is seen in patients with AIDS. The lesions are flat or slightly raised with a pink to dark purple appearance. Visceral lesions of the lung, lymph nodes, and GI tract carry a poorer prognosis.

Intervention

1. Provide appropriate, considerate care. Patients with suspected or diagnosed AIDS must be treated in the same manner as other patients seeking treatment. Patients' rights to treatment and confidentiality are protected by a number of state and federal laws. The ED nurse needs to be knowledgeable of hospital policy and legal regulations concerning:
   a. Confidentiality
   b. Patient consent for human T-lymphotrophic virus type III (HTLV-III) testing
   c. Reporting of AIDS as a communicable disease
2. Precaution: Since ED staff are called upon to act rapidly, often with minimal patient history, precautions to prevent transmission of HIV should be employed universally without regard for diagnosis. Prudent precautions include:
   a. Safe disposal of needles and sharp instruments - Large puncture-resistant containers should be kept in all treatment areas, utility room, laboratory, and medication room. Do *not* recap needles after use.
   b. Use of gloves - When in contact with blood or body fluids, gloves should be worn on both hands. Remove gloves and wash the hands if gloves become soiled, as well as between patients.
   c. Use of mask, goggles, and gowns - When at risk of blood splattering during resuscitation of trauma patients, emergency deliveries, etc., full precautions should be employed.
   d. Contaminated stretchers, work areas, etc. should be washed with a 1:10 dilution of sodium hypochlorite (bleach) (see Appendix F).

ED Discharge Planning

Admission should be provided to all patients with AIDS or suspected AIDS (e.g., IV drug abusers) with serious infections, fever without an obvious source, and altered mental status. Patients with oral candidiasis who are otherwise stable, and those with self-limited conditions (e.g., skin abscess) may be discharged on treatment.

Consider the patient's need for further medical or social service referrals; i.e.,

1. Review outpatient follow-up.
2. Refer the patient to the hospital's HIV counsellor.

The following organizations can be contacted concerning AIDS information, educational materials, and support groups:

AIDS hot line - 1-800-551-2728

Gay Men's Health Crisis
Box 274
132 West 24th Street
New York, N.Y. 10011
212-807-6655

National AIDS Hotline
1-800-342-2437
Spanish - 1-800-344-7432

Project Inform
1-800-822-7422

AIDS Blue Cross-Blue Shield Insurance information
1-800-831-3141

Centers for Disease Control
404-639-2891

People with AIDS Coalition
212-532-0568

AIDS Resource Center
212-481-1270

Association for Drug Abuse Prevention and Treatment
718-834-9585

Women and AIDS Resource Network (WARN)
718-596-6007

Body Positive - HIV Positive information
212-633-1782

SEXUALLY TRANSMITTED DISEASES

There are over 20 infectious diseases that are spread primarily by inti-
mate sexual contact. Syphilis and gonorrhea are the most common sexually transmitted diseases. In 1986 the United States Public Health Service
CDC reported 27,883 and 900,868 civilian cases of syphilus and gonorrhea, respectively. Although the number of reported cases has leveled off

or declined in the past 5 years, the statistics for the first 3 months of 1987 show a 23% increase in the number of reported cases of syphilis, and there has also been a dramatic increase in resistant strains of gonorrhea since 1980. All cases of gonorrhea and syphilis in the United States are to be reported to the state or local health department.

Assessment

History
Obtain a history of recent sexual activity and previous history of un-treated or incompletely treated infections. Women should be questioned as to the possibility of pregnancy and the presence of an interuterine de-vice (IUD). Symptoms of vaginal, urethral, and anal itching, burning, drainage, or lesion (chancre) should be noted. A low-grade fever and in-termittent maculopapular rash are common in cases of syphilis.

Diagnostic Tests
Gram stain and cultures - Specimens from the urethra, rectum, cervix, and pharynx should be obtained. In males the presence of Gram-negative diplococci is diagnostic. In females, the presence of these or-ganisms in white blood cells is diagnostic. A Thayer-Martin culture medium is used, and all cultures should be checked for penicillin resistance.
Blood cultures - In disseminated disease, blood cultures are intermittently positive.
VDRL - All patients should have VDRL performed to determine the pres-ence of syphilis.
Viral titers - Herpes virus cultures or viral titers can be obtained in the case of primary infection.
Darkfield examination - diagnosis of syphilis can be made when motile spirochetes are observed under a darkfield lens on a specially prepared slide.

GONORRHEA

Clinical Syndromes

Gonorrhea is a local or systemic infection caused by *Neisseria gonorrhoeae* and is transmitted by sexual contact of any sort. The incubation period is 48 hours to 1 week. There are a variety of clinical syndromes that may occur, including asymptomatic carrier state, acute state, acute urethritis, acute cervicitis, acute salpingitis, acute proctitis, acute pharyngitis, and disseminated gonococcemia (arthritis-dermatitis syndrome).

Intervention

For asymptomatic patients or those with urethritis, simple cervicitis, proctitis, or pharyngitis, the treatment of choice is now ceftriaxone, 250 mg IM. Patients who are allergic to penicillin should receive spectinomycin, 2 gm IM. Doxycycline, 100 mg PO bid for 10 days, should be prescribed for all patients to treat concomitant *Chlamydia* infections. Pregnant women should be treated with erythromycin, 500 mg qid for 5 days.

The above methods produce symptomatic relief within 24 hours and render the patient noninfectious in 72 hours. Patients should be advised to either refrain from intercourse or use condoms for the next 72 hours after treatment. Patients with acute pelvic inflammatory disease (PID) and an IUD in place may need to have the IUD removed, although this is a controversial issue. All patients should be referred to clinic to have the VDRL checked and should be told to have their sexual partners treated.

HERPES PROGENITALIS

Herpes progenitalis is a venereal infection caused by the herpes simplex virus (HSV). Classically, type 1 (HSV 1) causes gingivostomatitis, and type 2 (HSV 2) causes herpes progenitalis; however, there may be as much as 20% crossover in the syndromes caused by the two types.

Initial infection with HSV results in characteristic lesions accompanied by a viremia that produces systemic symptoms such as fever, joint and muscle tenderness, and meningitis-like symptoms, myalgias, arthralgias, and meningismus. Once the initial infection resolves, the virus persists in the nerve ganglia, with periodic reactivation of local lesions by stimuli such as stress, local trauma, or ultraviolet light.

The patient is not infectious between occurrences but is infectious from a few days before lesions appear until they are fully healed. In addition, women in particular can shed virus, frequently with occult reactivation of cervical lesions. Lesions will recur periodically. The characteristic lesions consist of clusters of tiny vesicles on an erythematous macular base. The vesicles become larger and more pustular over roughly 72 hours, eventually breaking down and leaving tiny, very shallow, clean, and tender ulcerations that gradually heal without scarring. The lesions last 7–10 days; secondary bacterial infection may occur. Roughly 50% of patients will stop having recurrences after about 2 years. The remainder will continue to have recurrences, some for life.

Intervention

1. Antiviral therapy is in the evolutionary stage. Acyclovir (Zovirax), which may be given topically, parenterally, and PO, is the drug of

choice for the first occurrence of HSV 2. Topical acyclovir does little to reduce recurrent episodes. Given PO, the drug has been found to decrease symptoms and reduce the rate of recurrence. Acyclovir, 200 mg PO 5 times daily, is prescribed for 7–10 days or may be given for a longer period of time to reduce recurrence.

2. When large areas are involved and painful, as with extensive vulvitis, the use of sitz baths and loose cotton underwear provides some relief. Topical anesthetics such as viscous lidocaine or benzocaine cream may help, as may aspirin and acetaminophen.

3. Patients with persistent anogenital herpetic infections should be evaluated for AIDS.

NONGONOCOCCAL URETHRITIS

Nongonococcal urethritis is a venereal infection caused by *Chlamydia trachomatis*. *Chylamydia* is being recognized increasingly as a cause of PID and cervicitis that is not readily distinguished from that caused by other organisms.

Patients of both sexes may contract both chlamydial and gonococcal urethritis simultaneously. Many will have been treated for gonorrhea with penicillin, leaving a persistent and less symptomatic chlamydial infection ("postgonococcal urethritis"). Chlamydial urethritis may cause acute epidydimitis and prostatitis.

Intervention

The treatment of choice is tetracycline, 1.5 gm PO as a loading dose, followed by 500 mg PO qid for 10 days, or doxycycline, 100 mg PO bid for 10 days (this is more expensive but may improve compliance).

An alternative therapy is erythromycin, 500 mg PO qid for 10 days. All asymptomatic sexual contacts should be treated.

SYPHILIS

Syphilis is a venereal infection caused by the spirochete *Treponema pallidum*. The infection may be lifelong and passes through several symptomatic and asymptomatic phases:

1. Incubation persists for 3–6 weeks after inoculation and is asymptomatic.

2. Primary syphilis encompasses the appearance and resolution of the chancre. Chancres are transient and painless, and patients can easily overlook them. The raised indurated margins and size of the lesion

serve to distinguish the chancre from a herpetic lesion, as herpetic ulcers are very small and nonpalpable. Chancres heal without scarring, but this may require 3–6 weeks, even with therapy. Patients are infectious when the chancre is present. Early secondary syphilis is arbitrarily designated as the first 2 years after infection and is characterized by a generalized, sometimes intermittent maculopapular rash associated with mild constitutional complaints and a low-grade fever. The rash is extremely infectious. Late secondary or latent syphilis is clinically silent.

3. Tertiary syphilis is neurologic, cardiovascular, or other systemic involvement that may occur decades after initial infection. Only one-third of all infected patients ever develop tertiary disease, even if untreated.

Intervention

1. For primary, symptomatic early secondary, or latent infection of less than 1 year's duration, the treatment of choice is benzathine penicillin, 2.4 million units IM. Penicillin-allergic patients can receive either tetracycline or erythromycin, 500 mg PO qid for 15 days.
2. For latent infection of more than 1 year's duration or infection of indeterminate duration, the treatment of choice is benzathine penicillin, 2.4 million units IM weekly for 3 successive weeks. Alternatives include tetracycline or erythromycin, 500 mg PO qid for 30 days.
3. For tertiary infections such as neurosyphilis, hospitalization and administration of high-dose IV aqueous penicillin, 20 million units IV every day for 10 days, is the treatment of choice. Patients suspected of having neurologic infection should all receive a lumbar puncture.

ED Discharge Planning

All patients who appear toxic, have disseminated gonoccocemia, tertiary signs, acute or recurrent PID or require IV therapy should be admitted.

ED Discharge Instructions
1. Treatment for all sexual contacts
2. Importance of continuing multiple-dose therapy, if prescribed
3. Abstinence from alcohol (alcohol irritates the urethra) for a specified period of time
4. Need for follow-up examination
5. Use of condoms and general hygiene measures to reduce recurrence and prevent the spread of infection during the treatment phase

CELLULITIS

Etiology

Cellulitis is a localized soft tissue infection that consists of a diffuse acute inflammation that may progress to necrosis and abscess formation. Cellulitis can occur in any area of the body. Its development is made possible by the following:

1. Trauma with secondary bacterial contamination
2. Altered local skin conditions with infection by normal skin flora
3. Contiguous spread from a nearby lesion
4. Metastatic infection from bacteria in blood or lymph

Given the appropriate conditions, almost any of the bacteria that comprise the normal skin flora can cause clinical infection. Most commonly, *Staphylococcus* and *Streptococcus* are the offending organisms. Gram-negative organisms may be seen in diabetics and immunocompromised patients. Anaerobic organisms (as well as certain aerobic organisms in diabetic patients) can cause gas-forming infections.

Assessment

History
The patient should be questioned about the time course of the infection and any precipitating factors, such as local trauma or nearby infections. A past medical history of diabetes, alcoholism, IV drug use, etc. should be obtained. Note any allergy to penicillin.

Physical Findings
Vital signs - Particularly temperature.
General appearance of site - The involved area will almost invariably demonstrate erythema, tenderness, heat, and swelling. The margins of the infection are often clearly demarcated. Red streaks extending proximally with tender nodes indicate lymphangitis. Check for cords indicating thrombophlebitis. Note any local wounds, cutaneous ulcers, and drainage. Examine for crepitus due to gas.
Facial cellulitis occurs secondary to infection of local structures—paranasal sinusitis, facial bone osteomyelitis, conjunctivitis—or dental infections, as well as skin lesions.

Diagnostic Tests
CBC - This may be helpful to establish leukocytosis.
Gram stain - A sample aspirated from the infected area after the injection of sterile saline may be Gram stained and cultured.

X-rays - Films of the affected area may be taken if a gas-forming infection or osteomyelitis is suspected.

Intervention

Most cellulitis will respond to warm soaks, elevation of the affected site, and antibiotic therapy with penicillinase-resistant penicillins. More serious infections with potentially mixed organisms may require combination antibiotic therapy. All abscesses must be surgically aspirated or incised for drainage. Puncture wounds may require tetanus toxoid. The presence of a gas-forming infection is a surgical emergency.

ED Discharge Planning

Patients with the following should be admitted:

1. Immunosuppression, septis, diabetes, and conditions requiring combination antibiotic therapy or surgical drainage
2. Orbital or facial (around the nose and mouth) cellulitis
3. Rapidly spreading infection requiring IV antibiotics
4. Evidence of gas-forming infections
5. Those unable to comply with outpatient therapy

ED Discharge Instructions
1. Provide wound care and dressing instructions.
2. Give medication information.
3. Provide outpatient referral for follow-up care.

SUGGESTED READINGS

Meningitis

Keroack MA. The patient with suspected meningitis. Emerg Med Clin North Am 1987; 5:807–826.

Paterson PY. Central nervous system infection: general considerations. In: Youmans GP, Paterson PY, Sommers HM, eds. The biologic and clinical basis of infectious disease. Philadelphia: WB Saunders, 1985:552–568.

Prendergast V. Bacterial meningitis update. J Neurosci Nurs 1987;19:95–99.

Roberts RB, Hartman BJ. Central nervous system infections. In: Roberts RB, ed. Infectious diseases: pathogenesis, diagnosis, and therapy. Chicago: Year Book Medical Publishers, 1986:42–58.

Endocarditis

Burden LL, Rodgers JC. Endocarditis. RN 1988;51:38–45.

Chadwick EG, Shulman ST. Prevention of infective endocarditis. Mod Concepts Cardiovasc Dis 1986;55:3.

Marrie TJ. Infective endocarditis: a serious and changing disease. Crit Care Nurs1987; 7:31–46.

Owens-Jones S, Hopp L. Viral myocarditis. Focus Crit Care 1988;15:25–37.

Roberts RB, Francicola P, Alonso DR. Infective endocarditis and other intravascular infections. In: Roberts RB, ed. Infectious diseases: pathogenesis, diagnosis, and therapy. Chicago: Year Book Medical Publishers, 1986:159–195.

Scrima DA. Infective endocarditis: nursing considerations. Crit Care Nurs 1987;7:47–56.

Pericarditis

Fowlers NO. The pericardium in health and disease. New York: Futura Publishing, 1985:153.

Kusiak V. Pericarditis, myocarditis, and endocarditis. In: Chung EK, ed. Cardiac emergency care. Philadelphia: Lea & Febiger, 1985:268–295.

Sokolow M, Mellroy MB. Clinical cardiology. Los Altos, California: Lange Medical Publications, 1986:573–585.

Sternbach GL. Pericarditis. Ann Emerg Med 1988;17:214–220.

Ear, Nose, and Throat Disorders

Gulya AJ, Wilson WR. Otitis media. In: Rakel RE, ed. Conn's current therapy. Philadelphia: WB Saunders, 1989:148–150.

Ramsey PG, Meymuller EA. Complications of bacterial infection of the ears, paranasal sinuses, and oropharynx in adults. Emerg Med Clin North Am 1985;3:143–160.

Slay RD. Sinusitis. In: Rosen P, Baker FJ, Barkin RM, Braen GR, Dailey RH, Levy RC, eds. Emergency medicine. 2nd ed. St Louis: CV Mosby, 1988:1091–1097.

Weinstein L. Diseases of the upper respiratory tract. In: Braunwald E, Isselbacher KJ, Petersdorf RG, Wilson JD, Martin JB, Fauci AS, eds. Harrison's principles of internal medicine. 11th ed. New York: McGraw-Hill, 1987:1111–1115.

Tetanus

Centers for Disease Control. Tetanus—United States, 1985–1986. MMWR 1987; 36:477–481.

Edlich RF, Silloway KA, Stark DR, Rodeheaver GT, Morgan RF. Tetanus. In: Edlich RF, Spyker DA, eds. Current emergency therapy. 3rd ed. Rockville, Maryland: Aspen Publishers, 1986:403–411.

Harmon AR. Wound management. In: Harmon AR, ed. Nursing care of the adult trauma patient. New York: John Wiley & Sons, 1985:225–259.

Acquired Immunodeficiency Syndrome

Flaskerud JH. Aids: psychosocial aspects. J Psychosoc Nurs Ment Health Serv 1987;25:8–16.

Halpern JS, ed. Precautions to prevent transmission of human immunodeficiency virus infections in emergency settings. J Emerg Nurs 1987;13:298–300.

Jackson MM, Lynch P, McPherson DC, Cummings MJ, Greenawalt NC. Why not treat all body substances as infectious? Am J Nurs 1987;87:1137–1139.

Jordan KS. Assessment of the person with acquired immunodeficiency syndrome in the emergency department. J Emerg Nurs 1987;13:342–345.

Moskowitz LD, Moskowitz SH. Acquired immunodefiency syndrome: legal issues in the emergency department. J Emerg Nurs 1986;12:297–300.

Nelson WJ. Nursing care of acutely ill person with AIDS. In: Durham JD, Cohen FL, eds. The person with AIDS nursing perspectives. New York: Springer Publishing, 1987:95–109.

Sexually Transmitted Diseases

Centers for Disease Control. Increases in primary and secondary syphilis. MMWR 1987;36:25.

Kaplan MH, Swenson PD. Herpes-virus infections. In: Sun T, ed. Sexually related infectious diseases: clinical and laboratory aspects. New York: Field, Rich & Associates, 1986:85–95.

Loucks A. Chlamydia, an unheralded epidemic. Am J Nurs 1987;87:920–922.

Treatment of Sexually Transmitted Diseases. Med Lett Drugs Ther 1986;28:708.

Wicher K, Wicher V. Syphilis. In: Sun T, ed. Sexually related infectious diseases: clinical and laboratory aspects. New York: Field, Rich & Associates, 1986:15-41.

Cellulitis

Rest JG, Goldstein EJC. Management of human and animal bite wounds. Emerg Med Clin North Am 1985;3:117–126.

Stone HH. Infection. In: Polk HC, Stone HH, Gardner B, eds. Basic surgery. 3rd ed. Norwalk, Connecticut: Appelton-Century-Crofts, 1987:140–154.

Chapter 10

GYNECOLOGIC AND OBSTETRIC EMERGENCIES

VAGINAL BLEEDING

Vaginal bleeding may be due to a wide variety of causes, from infection to trauma, to complications of pregnancy. The woman who comes to the ED* for vaginal bleeding may be frightened, embarrassed, and in pain. The nurse can decrease the traumatic nature of the situation by a careful, sensitive approach, by providing for the patient's privacy, and by providing support during the examination.

Assessment

History
Obtain vital signs before obtaining a complete history. Patients found to be orthostatic or hypotensive should be brought directly into the ED for initiation of emergency treatment. Obtain a gynecologic history including previous pregnancies, menstrual cycle, use of birth control, previous treatment for venereal disease, pelvic inflammatory disease, and medication taken. Note the date of the last menstrual period and, if the patient is pregnant, the expected date of confinement (EDC).

Abdominal pain, if present, should be described. An attempt should be made to quantitate the bleeding, either in relation to the patient's usual menses or by the number of pads or tampons used. Give the patient a new pad so that bleeding during time of ED treatment can be observed. If the patient is pregnant, be sure to note whether any tissue was passed, and if tissue was brought to the hospital by the patient, retain it for exami-

---

*See "Appendix A" for definition of common abbreviations used in the text.

nation. Always ask for symptoms of anemia or acute volume depletion, such as weakness, orthostasis, dizziness, or chest pain.

Physical Findings
Vital signs - Check for tachycardia, fever, and orthostatic hypotension.
General - Note pallor, bruising, or petechiae.
Pelvic signs - Observe for sources of bleeding: rectal, vaginal, urethral. Note signs of trauma, inflammation, or growths.

Diagnostic Tests
CBC - Do a spun Hct. Send for a CBC platelet count.
PT - Check for coagulopathy.
Type and cross-match - For all patients with significant bleeding a blood sample should be sent.
Pregnancy testing - A urine pregnancy test should be obtained in all premenopausal patients. A negative urine slide test does not absolutely rule out pregnancy; a serum test for the beta subunit of human chorionic gonadotropin (HCG) is more reliable.
Culdocentesis - A diagnostic culdocentesis should be considered if any suspicion of ruptured ectopic pregnancy is indicated by history or physical examination.
X-rays - Films are rarely helpful, but they should be avoided if the patient may be pregnant.
Sonography - A sonogram may detect an ectopic or intrauterine pregnancy.

Intervention

1. Hemodynamic instability should be treated with placement of a large-bore catheter (14 or 16 gauge) and administration of fluids or transfusions. On occasion, bleeding may be so severe as to require emergent surgical intervention, in which case a gynecologist should be consulted immediately. Take frequent vital signs and serial Hcts if bleeding continues. To assess the amount of bleeding, count the number of pads saturated.
2. An incomplete abortion will usually require a short stay, admission for observation, and treatment. Curettage to remove retained tissue from the uterus may, if necessary, be performed in the ED, but it is best done in the OR.
   a. For a completed abortion (tissue passed and the os now closed, with bleeding tapering off or stopped), the blood Rh group is determined, and the Rh-negative woman is treated with RhoGAM.
   b. Patients with an incomplete abortion (the os is still open) must be admitted for an oxytocin drip (10 units/ liter of D5/NS) and, if necessary, a D&C or suction curettage.

c. Patients with a threatened abortion (bleeding but no tissue passed and the os still closed) should be sent home on strict bed rest and advised to return immediately if bleeding becomes heavy or tissue is passed. Third-trimester patients should be examined in the delivery room.

d. Patients with a missed abortion (fetal death without passage) need to be admitted for D&C.

3. Patients who are having their normal menses should be reassured. Those with abnormally heavy or irregular menses without obvious cause and those with breakthrough bleeding who are on oral contraceptives should be referred for outpatient follow-up for further evaluation.

4. Patients with salpingitis or endometritis will require antibiotic therapy and may need admission (see "Pelvic Inflammatory Disease" in this chapter).

5. All patients with suspected ruptured ectopic pregnancy should be examined by a gynecologist, have culdocentesis performed, and be admitted for immediate surgical intervention, if necessary (see "Ectopic Pregnancy" in this chapter).

6. Patients with trauma should be questioned carefully about possible battering (see "Battered Woman" in Chapter 15).

ED Discharge Planning and Instructions

Plan for admission of patients with the following:

1. Ectopic pregnancy
2. Incomplete or missed abortions
3. Hemodynamic instability from vaginal bleeding
4. Severe trauma requiring surgical repair
5. Endometritis

Patient discharge instructions should include:

1. Information on the etiology of vaginal bleeding
2. Review of medication instructions
3. Referral for follow-up care

Patient discharge instructions after a D&C include:

1. Not having sexual intercourse or using douche or tampons for 2 weeks
2. Avoiding heavy lifting, and getting additional rest
3. Medication instructions for methylergonovine (Methergine), 0.2 mg PO every 6 hours

Discharge instructions for patients with threatened abortion include:

1. Bed rest until bleeding stops, then only light activity
2. Follow-up gynecologic examination within 1 week
3. No intercourse or use of tampons or douche until the next gynecologic examination

Patient should return to the ED for any of the following:

1. Increased bleeding
2. Passage of clots or tissue (bring material to the ED)
3. Increased pain or cramps
4. Signs of infection, e.g., temperature over 100°F or foul-smelling vaginal discharge

ECTOPIC PREGNANCY

Description

Ectopic pregnancy is the implantation of a fertilized ovum in an extrauterine site, usually the Fallopian tube. An ectopic pregnancy occurs once in every 150–200 deliveries. Ninety percent of these occur in the Fallopian tubes; the majority are right sided; and 80% are diagnosed within the first 2 weeks as having ruptured ectopic pregnancy.

An ectopic pregnancy may occur at any time from menarche to menopause, but 40% of ectopic pregnancies occur in women between the ages of 20 and 29. The incidence is higher in infertile women, and the frequency is greater in lower socioeconomic groups. Roughly 50% of ectopic pregnancies are caused by tubal inflammatory lesions or scarring, such as that occurring as a result of pelvic inflammatory disease. Risk factors for an ectopic pregnancy include:

1. History of pelvic inflammatory disease
2. Previous abdominal or pelvic surgery
3. Use of an IUD
4. History of previous ectopic pregnancy
5. History of peritonitis from any cause
6. Use of progesterone-containing birth control pills

Assessment

History
Ectopic pregnancy should be suspected whenever abdominal pain occurs within the first 6–8 weeks after a missed period. All female patients with lower abdominal pain should be questioned as to date and normalcy of their last period, as well as to history of previous pregnancies, abortions,

and deliveries. A history of pelvic inflammatory disease, use of an IUD, or previous ectopic pregnancy is very important.

Complaints of sharp, constant abdominal pain and backache are most common in acute tubal pregnancy. Shoulder pain, referred pain from intraperitoneal hemorrhage, is reported in approximately 15% of cases. About 80% of patients have scant persistent uterine bleeding. Roughly 60% will give a history of abnormal menstruation and infertility. However, as many as 25% will not report amenorrhea. Thus the diagnosis must be entertained regardless of the menstrual history.

Physical Findings

Vital signs - Check rectal temperature, pulse, and pressure. Do orthostatics (blood pressure with the patient in both the lying and the standing position). If the patient is too weak to stand, take the vital signs with the patient in the seated position with legs dangling over the stretcher. An increase in heart rate of 10 beats/min or more or a decrease in blood pressure of 10 mm Hg or more constitutes a positive test (see "Assessment of Vital Signs" in the "Introduction"). The presence of hypotension and a rapid pulse requires emergency intervention. Bring the patient immediately to the attention of the physician.

Abdomen - Listen for normal bowel sounds. Palpate for localized tenderness, rebound, or palpable masses.

Pelvic signs - Check for vaginal bleeding. Remember that any young female with lower abdominal pain and shock should be considered to have a ruptured ectopic until proven otherwise.

Diagnostic Tests

Pregnancy testing - Urine pregnancy test is not always sufficiently sensitive. A positive test may verify pregnancy but does not identify the site. A negative test does not exclude ectopic pregnancy. A serum assay for the beta subunit of human chorionic gonadotropin (HCG) is the most sensitive test of pregnancy. Any patient with an IUD and a positive pregnancy test must be considered to have an ectopic pregnancy until it is proven otherwise.

CBC - A spun Hct should be obtained immediately on any female patient with vaginal bleeding, suspected ectopic pregnancy, or unexplained shock. In the patient with a ruptured ectopic pregnancy with acute bleeding, it may take several hours for the Hct to fall.

Type and cross-match - This should be drawn on all patients suspected of having an ectopic pregnancy.

SMA - A serum amylase can be obtained and may be as high as 1600.

Culdocentesis - The diagnostic procedure of choice is culdocentesis (aspiration of peritoneal fluid through a needle inserted into the posterior vaginal fornix to the cul-de-sac). Culdocentesis is considered positive if the peritoneal fluid contains noncoagulable blood. A negative tap excludes a ruptured ectopic pregnancy.

Sonogram - May confirm clinical suspicion of ectopic pregnancy and can be very useful in the emergency care setting.

Intervention

1. Stabilize the patient's vital signs (see "Shock" in Chapter 1). Rapid volume replacement with blood and crystalloids, oxygen, MAST suit, and preparation for surgery are lifesaving measures.
2. Consult a gynecologist immediately. No time should be wasted, as a ruptured ectopic can lead to profound shock quite rapidly. Definitive therapy currently consists of surgical removal of the pregnancy, usually via unilateral salpingectomy.

Admission Criteria

All patients with ectopic pregnancies will require admission for surgery. Patients in whom ectopic pregnancy is suspected will often require admission for observation and possible intervention. Any patient discharged from the ED with a suspicion of an unruptured ectopic pregnancy must be brought back for a recheck. In such cases, a serum specimen for the beta subunit of HCG must be drawn, and the patient must be counselled to return immediately if she experiences pain or vaginal bleeding.

THIRD-TRIMESTER BLEEDING

Bleeding in the third trimester of pregnancy may be caused by trauma, placenta previa, abruptio placentae, uterine rupture, labor ("bloody show"), cervical erosion, polyps, or tumor. The most common cause is either placental abruption or placenta previa. Many of these causes of bleeding may bring on premature labor and are potentially life-threatening to the mother, fetus, or both.

Assessment

History
Determine the length of time and the amount of bleeding, as well as any previous episodes. A history of pain, trauma, or recent illness should be noted. The patient should be asked if any decrease in fetal activity has occurred. A brief obstetric history should include previous pregnancies and outcomes, including miscarriages and abortions. Previous obstetric

complications, as well as underlying medical illnesses, should be noted. Patients who have bright red vaginal bleeding, not mixed with mucus ("bloody show" or mucus plug) should be immediately triaged and examined by a physician. The obstetrical service should be immediately notified as well.

In abruptio placentae, there is usually no history of previous bleeding in the current pregnancy. Abruption occurs more often in hypertensive women. Patients with abruption describe the sudden onset of abdominal pain with bleeding; the pain may be severe and constant, depending on the extent of separation. Fetal movement may be decreased or absent. In severe cases, maternal shock, uterine tetany, and fetal distress or death can result. In placenta previa (low-lying placenta), there is often a history of previous bleeding in the current pregnancy. The incidence is greater in multiparous women and in women who have had placenta previa in previous pregnancies. There is often no pain, and the patient may be in labor with intermittent contractions. Fetal movement is usually present.

The woman who comes to the ED for third-trimester vaginal bleeding is often apprehensive and fearful. Provide reassurance and information during her examination and treatment.

Physical Findings
General - Note pallor or the appearance of shock.
Vital signs - Do orthostatics (blood pressure and pulse). Check for fever.
Abdomen - Palpate the uterus gently for size, tone, and tenderness. Listen for a fetal heartbeat. In abruption, the uterus may be tender and may be tense without relaxation if abruption is extensive; the fetal heart may be absent. In placenta previa, the abdomen is soft and contractions may be palpable; the fetal heart is usually audible. A fetal heart rate under 110 or over 160 suggests fetal distress.
Pelvic signs - An internal examination should not be done, as this can cause massive hemorrhage in placenta previa. Consult an obstetrician immediately. The pelvic examination is generally delayed by the obstetrician until a sonogram has ruled out placenta previa or, in an emergency situation, is performed under controlled conditions in the delivery room.

Diagnostic Tests
CBC - Spin a Hct immediately. Check the platelet count.
PT - Check for clotting abnormalities. (Acute disseminated coagulopathy is a possible complication of abruptio placentae.)
Type and cross-match - These should be drawn in anticipation.
Doppler ultrasound - A Doppler ultrasonogram, if necessary, will determine the location of fetal heartbeat.

Sonogram - A sonogram may be obtained to determine the location of the placenta.

Intervention

1. Fluid balance - Start an IV line with Ringer's lactate immediately if bleeding is significant or if the patient is hypotensive or tachycardic. Monitor for hemodynamic stability. Urine output per hour and Hct should each be at least 30.
2. Oxygenation - Give the mother oxygen if she is hypotensive or there is evidence of fetal distress.
3. Consult an obstetrician immediately - Further management will generally depend on results of sonography and fetal monitoring.
4. In the presence of hypotension and significant blood loss, type-specific (non-cross-matched) blood should be administered immediately (see Chapter 1 for the treatment of shock).

PELVIC INFLAMMATORY DISEASE

Etiology

Pelvic inflammatory disease (PID) or salpingitis usually occurs when infecting agents travel through the cervix past the endometrium to the salpingeal mucosa. It may involve the uterus, tubes, ovaries, and adjacent abdominal structures. PID may develop postpartum or following pelvic surgery. Transmission is by sexual contact, and PID is due to *Neisseria gonorrhoeae* in 40–60% of cases. Other bacterial pathogens include *Bacteroides* species and anaerobic Gram-positive cocci. *Chlamydia trachomatis* has been reported either alone or in combination with other pathogens in up to 30% of cases studied. *Mycoplasma hominis* has been implicated. *Actinomyces* species are an uncommon cause of PID associated with the use of an IUD.

Assessment

History

Ask the patient to give an accurate chronologic history of the present illness. Specifically elicit a description of the discharge, presence of fever, nausea, vomiting, diarrhea, dysuria, and lower back or abdominal pain. The date of the last menstrual period is important, not only to determine whether the patient is pregnant but also because symptoms of acute PID frequently begin during or shortly after menstruation. Important points to cover include parity, previous bouts of vaginal or pelvic infection, or recent sexual intercourse with partners known to be infected. The form of birth control is useful information (IUD, diaphragm, condom). Tuboovarian abscess may be associated with an IUD.

Physical Findings
General - Note if the patient appears toxic.
Vital signs - Check for fever and orthostasis.
Abdomen - Palpate for tenderness or masses.
Pelvic signs - Observe for presence of sores, vesicles, or chancres. Note the color and quantity of the vaginal discharge. The patient with PID commonly experiences pain on pelvic examination and movement of the cervix.

Diagnostic Tests
Gonococcal culture - Have proper culture tubes and slides available so that discharge may be cultured for gonorrhea. Slide examination may show white cells with Gram stain negative with diplococci (gonorrhea), hyphae (candidiasis), motile forms (*Trichomonas*), or "clue" cells (*Haemophilus vaginalis* and/or *Gardnerella vaginalis*). Dispose of all pads, gloves, etc. as required by the infection control protocol. Wash hands thoroughly.
CBC - PID can cause a leukocytosis of 15,000–20,000.
VDRL - All patients thought to have any sexually transmitted disease, including PID, should have a VDRL done.

Intervention (Outpatient Antibiotic Therapy)

Nonpenicillin-allergic patients - Aqueous procaine penicillin G, 4.8 million units IM (or ampicillin, 3.5 gm PO, or amoxicillin, 3 gm PO, or cefoxitin, 2 gm IM), with probenicid, 1 gm PO. Ceftriaxone, 250 mg IM, can also be used. Any of these options should be followed by doxycycline, 100 mg PO bid for 10 days, or tetracycline, 500 mg qid for 14 days.
Penicillin-allergic patients - Spectinomycin, 2 gm IM, followed by doxycycline or tetracycline in above doses.
Penicillinase-producing *N. gonorrhoeae* (PPNG) - If PPNG is suspected, cefoxitin, ceftriaxone, or spectinomycin in the above doses is given.

Note: PID in the presence of an IUD may or may not require removal of the IUD, as per consultation with a gynecologist.

ED Discharge Planning and Instructions

Hospital admission is recommended for patients with the following:

1. Severe PID (toxic or temperature over 100.4°F)
2. Complicated PID (pregnancy, adnexal mass, or abscess)
3. Recurrent PID (may be predominantly anaerobic infection)
4. Noncompliant patient
5. Nausea and vomiting, unable to take medication PO

Patients with mild PID may be treated as outpatients with close follow-up, although many consultants prefer to admit all patients with PID for parenteral antibiotic therapy because of the risk of tubal scarring, which can result in infertility and ectopic pregnancy. Patients treated as outpatients should be reexamined in 24–48 hours. If they are not responding to treatment at that time, they should be admitted for IV antibiotics.

Discharge instructions should include:

1. Patient should follow the treatment plan—antibiotics and follow-up examination.
2. Patient should feel significantly improved after 2–3 days of antibiotics; she should return to the ED if symptoms persist or increase after 3 days of antibiotics.
3. To avoid reinfection, sexual contacts should be examined.
4. Suggest the use of condoms or spermicide to reduce the risk of future infection.

SEXUAL ASSAULT

Description

Rape is not a sexual act; it is an act of violence with sexual intercourse as the weapon. Victims of sexual assault are assaulted both physically and emotionally and require emergency medical care that focuses on their psychologic, medical, and legal needs. Ideally, every ED that deals with rape victims should have a team of nurses, counsellors, and physicians working in conjunction with the local police department. Many emergency services have developed useful protocols for sexual assault victim management, including collection and handling of evidence.

Practitioners are often uncomfortable in treating rape victims. Some staff members may erroneously interpret rape in sexual terms and may blame the victim. Others may feel awkward or frightened, as the situation evokes their own anxieties or sense of vulnerability. Many fear involvement in a potential court case. Note that rape is a legal, not a medical, term and should not be used in front of the patient. In order to provide good medical care, ED staff must be gentle and nonjudgmental toward all rape victims. A thorough and sensitive history and examination are essential. If legal action is taken, both the patient and clinician will benefit from an assessment and intervention that is complete and well documented.

Victims of sexual assault are emergencies. The triage nurse should bring the patient directly into a private gynecologic examining room. Have a telephone available for patients who want to call a friend or family member. Assess the patient for signs of serious injury that may require immediate intervention, e.g., fractures, bleeding. The nurse should facilitate and monitor the patient's treatment by streamlining the registration process, notifying the victim's services counsellor and/or social worker, and encouraging prompt medical evaluation.

Review the treatment plan with the patient; notification of police, collection of evidence, and turning the rape kit over to police require the patient's consent. Support the patient's decision making; it is vital that she (or he) feels in control of herself (or himself) and the circumstances. Instruct the patient not to wash, eat, drink, or change clothes until after the examination.

The patient may want to initiate legal proceedings or may be too distraught to decide about filing charges. Impress upon the patient that evidence, to be valid, must be collected as soon after the assault as possible. Some state laws permit and/or require the collection (with consent) and securing of evidence by the hospital for a specified period of time until the patient makes a decision about filing legal charges.

Ninety-five percent of rape victims are women. A nurse or counsellor (preferably of the same sex) should remain with the victim throughout the ED stay.

Assessment

History
Determine the chronology of events and how recent the rape occurred relative to the current examination. Note if the patient bathed or douched since the assault. Obtain details concerning use of instruments, weapons, or force and the location of injuries and circumstances under which they were sustained. Question the victim in common terminology about oral and anal as well as vaginal penetration. Determine whether and when ejaculation occurred. Record the statement of events, whenever possible, in the patient's own words.

A general gynecologic history should also be obtained. This includes last menstrual period, current pregnancy, contraceptive use, and prior history of sexually transmitted disease. Note drug allergies, such as to penicillin, and any general medical problems.

Physical Findings

General - Note the patient's appearance (e.g., disheveled, agitated, bloody).

Skin - Look for bruises and lacerations.

Pelvic - Examine the external genitalia for ecchymoses, dried semen, laceration, or perineal injuries.

Rectal examination - May be performed if clinically indicated, in order to find any tenderness or lacerations.

Diagnostic Tests

NS wet mount - Smears of the cervix and vaginal vault will be taken to establish whether sperm are present.

Pap smear - This may provide later identification of sperm by laboratory.

Acid phosphatase strips - These can be tested immediately or saved. They will test for presence of semen in secretions collected from the vagina and the external genitalia or any suspicious location.

Pubic hair combings and material scraped from fingernails - These may be placed in an envelope for laboratory analysis by police.

VDRL - A VDRL should always be performed.

Intervention

1. Manage any serious physical injuries immediately - Although these are not usual, their treatment takes precedence.
2. Provide reassurance and support - If the patient needs to ventilate feelings of anger, fear, guilt, or embarrassment, he or she should be allowed to do so. Many patients will blame themselves in some way for their handling of the assault; these patients may need to be reassured that their actions were appropriate because they prevented worse brutality. One of the most important and therapeutic functions of the staff is simply to listen.
3. Documentation and collection of potential evidence - Provide the gynecologist with a rape kit and sexual assault form and assist with evidence collection. The following specimens are collected, labelled, and placed in paper (not plastic) containers: scrapings from under fingernails; vaginal, oral, rectal, and urethral aspirant or scrapings; pubic hair combings; and torn, bloody, or soiled clothing (underwear). Because lubricant will interfere with the forensic test, only water can be used on the speculum. All labelled specimens and a copy of the sexual assault form are placed in the kit, sealed, and given over to the police or other designated official. Polaroid pictures of bruises and other injuries may be taken with the patient's consent. Do not leave kit unsecured; maintain the "chain of evidence." After examination, assist the patient to wash and change clothing.

4. Medication
   a. Pregnancy prevention - The physician will discuss the options for pregnancy prevention if pregnancy is a possibility. High-dose estrogens may prevent pregnancy, and possible regimens include:
      i. Ethinyl estradiol, 5 mg daily for 5 days
      ii. Diethylstilbestrol, 25 mg bid for 5 days
      iii. Conjugated estrogens (Premarin), 25 mg daily for 5 days
      Frequent side effects of estrogen therapy include nausea and vomiting. An antiemetic given orally or rectally can be prescribed. Estrogen therapy is not given if the patient is currently pregnant (if her current status is unclear, blood pregnancy tests are generally available within 24–48 hours). The patient should be informed that withdrawal bleeding will occur after estrogen therapy is stopped and that should estrogen therapy fail and pregnancy ensue, there is an increased potential for birth defects.
   b. Prevent gonorrhea - Gonorrhea may develop in 3–4% of rape victims. Treatment is as for a known contact according to the guidelines discussed under "Sexually Transmitted Diseases" in Chapter 9.
   c. Tetanus prophylaxis is indicated for any open wounds.

ED Discharge Planning and Instructions

The crisis counsellor or nurse should assist in contacting a family member or friend to accompany the patient home. Consult the physician concerning a psychiatric evaluation for patients who display an unstable emotional status.

At discharge, the nurse should

1. Encourage follow-up within 6 weeks on laboratory tests—veneral disease and pregnancy–as indicated.
2. Review medication instructions.
3. Arrange (with the patient's permission) for follow-up crisis counselling.

CHILDBIRTH—EMERGENCY DELIVERY

The ED staff is often called upon to evaluate patients in labor prior to transport to the delivery room. Although obviously every effort has to be made to get the patient in labor to the delivery room, the ED needs to be equipped for emergency deliveries. Have a transport Isolette and an ED delivery/obstetric pack available that should include sterile towels, clamps, scissor, basin, sterile gloves, umbilical cord clamp, bulb syringe,

DeLee suction, and numbered identification bands for mother and baby. An infant radiant warmer and scale must be available upon request.

Assessment

History
Ascertain the following (time permitting):

1. Time that labor started
2. Frequency, duration, and strength of contractions
3. Whether the water has broken
4. Number of children - Labor time is shorter for women with two or more children (multipara) than for those who have had one (primipara) or no (nullipara) previous deliveries
5. Prenatal care and estimated delivery date
6. Complications during pregnancy
7. Medical conditions, allergies, medications

Examine the patient for signs of imminent delivery, including:

1. Bulging perineum
2. Crowning
3. Patient feels she has to bear down or push

Listen for a fetal heart. The normal range is 120–160.

Intervention

1. Support the mother - Convey a sense of controlled urgency—that all needed equipment and personnel are available, that her doctor and pediatrician are being notified, and that you will stay will stay with her during the delivery.
2. Delivery in the ED - When it is deemed that the delivery is imminent, the triage nurse will notify the physician and bring the patient to a private, equipped room for delivery. The obstetric pack, transport Isolette, and infant resuscitation equipment should be quickly assembled. Notify the pediatrician that a delivery is in progress. As the infant's head becomes more visible, slight pressure with the palm of one hand is placed against the head to control the speed of delivery and to prevent complications. When the head is delivered, wipe the nose and mouth of secretions. If meconium is present, suction the infant's nose and mouth with DeLee suction prior to delivery of the chest in order to prevent aspiration of meconium on the first breath. Observe that the umbilical cord is not wrapped around the baby's neck. Delivery of the shoulders will be assisted by a slight downward traction for

delivery of the anterior shoulder and by slight upward movement for delivery of the posterior shoulder. Support the infant's head and body during delivery. Keep the head lower than the body to allow for gravity drainage of secretions. Record time of delivery and initial Apgar score. The infant can be placed on the mother's abdomen while the placenta is being delivered. This immediate mother-infant contact will reassure the mother and promote bonding, and the pressure will stimulate uterine contractions. Once the placenta is delivered (do not pull on the cord) and the cord stops pulsating, clamp the cord several inches from infant's abdomen and cut with sterile scissors.

3. Care of the mother - Assess the mother for bleeding and vital signs. If fundus is boggy or bleeding persists, massage the fundus with a gentle circular motion. As soon as the mother's condition permits, transport her to the obstetric department. If bleeding is fulminant, call the obstetrical consult STAT and administer oxytocin (pitocin).

4. Infant care - The first priority is airway and breathing. Suction the infant's nose and mouth with a bulb syringe and rub the soles of the feet and the back to stimulate crying. Keep the baby in a head-down position to prevent aspiration. Have oxygen and an infant bag/mask device on standby. Prevent hypothermia by wrapping the infant in a warm blanket, keeping the head covered, and placing the infant in a warm transport Isolette. Infants should have an identification band with number and mother's name and be evaluated by the physician/pediatrician before transport to the isolation area of the nursery. The Apgar score should be documented at 1 and 5 minutes following delivery. A rating of 0, 1, or 2 is given for heart rate, respirations, muscle tone, reflex irritability, and color.

Apgar Scoring System

Sign	0	1	2
Heart rate	Absent	<100/min	>100/min
Respiratory effort	Absent	Slow, irregular	Good cry
Muscle tone	Flaccid	Flexion of extremities	Active, well-flexed extremities
Reflex irritability and color	No response, blue, pale	Grimace, body pink, extremities blue	Vigorous cry, fully pink

An infant needing resuscitation will have an overall score of 0–3, while an infant with a score of 10 can be described as completely pink, with a good vigorous cry, active movements, and a heart rate over 100/min. If the infant is underweight or premature or shows signs of respiratory distress, call a pediatric consult STAT.

SUGGESTED READINGS

Vaginal Bleeding

Bland EH. Uterine curettage in the emergency department. J Emerg Nurs 1986;12: 41–43.

Brennan DM, Caldwell M. Dilatation and evacuation performed in the emergency department for miscarriage. J Emerg Nurs 1987;13:144–148.

Dwyer JM. Manual of gynecologic nursing. Boston: Little, Brown, 1986.

Gibbons H, Shaffer M. Management of patients with vaginal bleeding. Top Emerg Med 1985;7:67–72.

Williamson HO. Dysfunctional uterine bleeding. In: Edlich RF, Spyker DA, eds. Current emergency therapy. 3rd ed. Rockville, Maryland: Aspen Publishers, 1986:546–549.

Ectopic Pregnancy

Devone N, Baldwin K. Ectopic pregnancy on the rise. AJN 1986;86:674–678.

Hockberger RS. Ectopic pregnancy. Emerg Med Clin North Am 1987;5:481–491.

Quilligan EJ. Ectopic pregnancy. In: Quilligan EJ, ed. Current therapy in obstetrics and gynecology 2. Philadelphia: WB Saunders, 1983:34–35.

Rothberg L. The frightening cost of ectopic pregnancy. RN 1985:48–52.

Weckstein LN. Clinical diagnosis of ectopic pregnancy. Clin Obstet Gynecol 1987;30: 236–244.

Third-Trimester Bleeding

Hayashi RH. Third trimester bleeding. In: Quilligan EJ, ed. Current therapy in obstetrics and gynecology 2. Philadelphia: WB Saunders, 1983:9–11.

Rayburn WF, Lavin J Jr. Obstetrics for the house officer. 2nd ed. Baltimore: Williams & Wilkins, 1988:94–98.

Pelvic Inflammatory Disease

Hemsell DL, Cunningham FG, Wendel GD. Pelvic infections & sexually transmitted diseases. In: Martin ML, Benson RC. eds. Current obstetric & gynecologic diagnosis & treatment. 6th ed. Norwalk, Connecticut: Appleton & Lange, 1987:715–741.

Labadie LL, Rhule RL. Management of genital infections. Emerg Med Clin North Am 1987;5:443–480.

McElhose P. The "other" STDs as dangerous as ever. RN 1988;51:52–58.

Mickal A, Faro S, Pastorek JG. Emergency care. In: Nichols DH, Evrard JR, eds. Ambulatory gynecology. Philadelphia: Harper & Row, 1985:445–460.

Nesse RE. Office management of sexually transmitted disease and management of pelvic inflammatory disease in the ambulatory patient. Primary Care 1988;15:489–515.

United States Dept of Health and Human Services: Pelvic inflammatory disease. MMWR Suppl 1982;31(25):435–445.

Sexual Assault

Foley TS, Grimes BA. Nursing interventions with sexual assault and rape victims. In: Stuart

GW, Sundeen SJ, eds. Principles and practices of psychiatric nursing. St Louis: CV Mosby, 1987:971–1010.

Hicks DJ. Sexual assault. In: Nichols DH, Evrard JR, eds. Ambulatory gynecology. Philadelphia: Harper & Row, 1985:473–487.

Hochbaum SR. The evaluation and treatment of the sexually assaulted patient. Emerg Med Clin North Am 1987;5:601–622.

Childbirth—Emergency Delivery

Albarran-Sotelo R, et al. Textbook of advanced cardiac life support. Dallas, Texas: American Heart Association, 1987.

Bock SF, Brengman SL. A delivery room you can set up anywhere. RN 1986:28–30.

Krzyston D. Nursing assessment and general care of the gynecological patient. Emerg Med Clin North Am 1987;5: 399–404.

Roberts J, McGowan N. Emergency birth. J Emerg Nurs 1985;11:125–131.

Williams C. Emergency childbirth. Nursing 1986;16:33.

Chapter 11

UROLOGIC EMERGENCIES

TESTICULAR TORSION

Description

Testicular torsion is a twist in the spermatic cord that interferes with blood supply to the testis. It occurs almost exclusively in adolescents and young adults. The exact cause is not known, but underlying anatomic abnormalities are usually present. Testicular torsion is a surgical emergency, in that absence of blood flow to the testis for more than several hours will result in gangrene and loss of the testis.

Assessment

History
The patient will usually describe the sudden onset of severe testicular pain, which may radiate to the abdomen and is accompanied by scrotal swelling. In young adolescents, there may be a history of previous attacks. Less commonly, torsion may be accompanied by nausea, vomiting, fever, or urinary symptoms. Important points to include in the history are recent trauma, the presence of a penile discharge or lesions, fever, or previous episodes of sexually transmitted disease.

Physical Findings
Vital signs - Check for fever.
Genitalia - In torsion the testis is usually swollen, tender, and retracted, and the cord above the swelling is normal. Elevation of the testis causes an increase in pain.

Diagnostic Tests
Doppler ultrasound - This will evaluate blood flow to the testis by compar-

ing blood flow through the testicular (internal spermatic) artery on each side. Diminished or absent arterial pulse on the affected side is considered positive. This test is not totally reliable as there may be false positive as well as false negative results.

Nuclear scan - Another method of evaluating blood flow to the testis; however, in cases of acute torsion it may be too time-consuming to be worthwhile. Surgical exploration is indicated in a clear-cut case of torsion, especially if a scan is not immediately available.

Laboratory tests - CBC* and urinalysis.

Note: In acute torsion, it is often necessary to go immediately to surgery without awaiting results of diagnostic tests.

Intervention

Attempts to relieve the torsion manually in the ED are appropriate. However, should such maneuvers fail, the treatment is immediate surgical intervention and orchiopexy (suturing the testicle in the scrotum). Unless the testis is clearly gangrenous and intervention was significantly delayed, every attempt should be made to save the testis. Orchiopexy is often performed bilaterally because of the common incidences of bilateral congenital anomaly and the possibility that torsion might occur on the other side at some time in the future.

Patients who have intermittent, spontaneously resolving or manually treated torsion should be referred to a urologist for follow-up evaluation because of the high rate of recurrence.

ACUTE URINARY RETENTION

Difficulty in voiding may be caused by a variety of conditions including prostatic and urethral trauma, tumor, or infection, neurologic events (multiple sclerosis, spinal cord injury), drug intake (narcotics, anticholinergic agents, diazepam), and psychologic disturbance.

Assessment

History
Patients may complain of acute onset of complete inability to urinate, accompanied by suprapubic pain, which may be mild to severe. Determine whether there is any prior history of urinary hesitancy or retention, re-

---

*See "Appendix A" for definition of common abbreviations used in the text.

cent trauma or instrumentation, and underlying systemic or neurologic disease. Obtain a thorough history of drug use, including psychotropics, anticholinergics, opiates, tranquilizers, decongestants, or ethanol.

Physical Findings
Vital signs - Take a rectal temperature of the patient.
Abdomen - Palpate and percuss the suprapubic area to determine bladder size.
Neurologic signs - Note any sensory or motor impairment.
Rectal examination - Examine the prostate, and note any tenderness, enlargement, or hard or boggy consistency.

Diagnostic Tests
CBC - Check the WBC and differential if acute infection is suspected.
Urinalysis - If urinalysis is available, send a specimen for RBC and WBC and a Gram stain. Urine culture may also be ordered if there is significant dysuria or bacteriuria.
Laboratory tests - SMA including BUN, creatinine, and acid phosphatase which may be elevated in renal and prostatic disease.

Intervention

1. Intervention should be prompt, since prolonged distention of the bladder can permanently damage the detrusor muscles.
2. Inadequate urinary output - If the patient is able to void but complaining of decreased urinary stream or incomplete voiding, assist the patient to stand to void; provide the patient with privacy if conditions permit. Consult with the physician concerning placement of a Foley catheter. According to the patient's history a urology consult and catheterization may be indicated. A catheterization should not be attempted in patients with a history or signs of urethral trauma (a urethral tear can be iatrogenically extended by catheterization). If the catheter passes, clamp the tubing after drainage of 500–750 ml (within 1 hour). Sudden removal of a large amount of urine may cause shock. After treatment and relief of distention, monitor urine output every hour initially. Consider the need for increased or supplemental fluid intake.
3. Retrograde urethrogram is performed if there is a history or signs of urethral trauma or if the catheter cannot be passed, in order to determine whether the urethra is patent. If the urethra is partially occluded, a urologist may be called to catheterize the bladder (with a filiform and follower) or to attempt urethral dilatation. If the urethra is completely occluded, a suprapubic puncture or cystostomy should be performed by an experienced physician.

4. Monitor urine output for postobstructive diuresis. Maintain hydration.
5. Further treatment depends on the specific cause.

ED Discharge Planning and Instructions

In general, patients with acute urinary retention will require admission for a diagnostic workup, further treatment, or observation for post-obstructive diuresis. Patients with repeated occurrences of urinary retention or chronic urinary retention may not require admission.

If the patient is to be discharged, review prescriptions and needed follow-up medical care. The patient and his or her family should be knowledgeable about maintaining adequate fluid intake and about signs of infection.

RENAL COLIC

DESCRIPTION

Renal colic is excruciating pain produced by partial or complete obstruction of the urinary outflow tract by one or more calculi (stones), blood clots, or sloughed papillae. The pain is frequently described as the worst ever experienced, even comparable to labor pains. It may be associated with hematuria, urgency, nausea, vomiting, or ileus.

Nephrolithiasis (stone formation) affects an estimated 0.1–1% of the population, and its principal manifestation is renal colic. Calcium stones, in addition to being the most common type, are also the most likely to cause colic. Other types (cystine, uric acid, struvite, and magnesium ammonium phosphate) can also produce colic.

Assessment

History
A typical episode of colic begins abruptly during the night or early in the morning when the patient is at rest. Stones obstructing the renal pelvis and proximal ureter cause severe flank pain. As the stone passes downward, pain may migrate anteriorly around the abdomen to the testes, labia minora, or round ligament. Bladder stones may produce symptoms mimicking cystitis or urethritis. High fever, diaphoresis, and chills suggest coexistent urosepsis.

Include in history taking the timing of symptoms, pattern of pain, associated symptoms, and personal and family history of calculi. A family history of calculi may indicate an inherited disorder. Ask the patient about conditions associated with renal lithiasis, surgery, and hyperparathyroidism. Take a complete medication history.

In contrast to the patient with peritoneal pain, the patient with renal colic is usually thrashing about trying to find a comfortable position.

Physical Findings

Vital signs - Low-grade fever may rarely result from colic alone, but high fever (>102°F) is indicative of an underlying infection. Blood pressure and pulse may be elevated because of pain and agitation.

Abdomen - Palpation will reveal tenderness over the location of the calculus but no guarding, rebound, or point tenderness.

Diagnostic Tests

Urinalysis - Usually shows red cells, with trace protein found if many red cells are present. In the presence of total unilateral obstruction, the urine may contain no red cells. As many as 10–15% of patients with nephrolithiasis will not have hematuria. The diagnosis can be confirmed, but not excluded, with a urinalysis. For cloudy urine containing pus and white blood cells, a Gram stain and culture and sensitivity should be done. Microscopic examination of the urine can result in identification of the type of crystal (urate, cystine, calcium oxalate). All urine collected while the patient is in the ED should be poured through a 4 × 4-inch gauge pad in an attempt to identify the stone.

CBC - A slight elevation in the WBC may be observed with colic, but a WBC over 15,000 suggests infection.

X-rays - A KUB x-ray should be obtained if renal colic is suspected. Since the majority of stones contain calcium, many calculi (calcium phosphate, calcium oxalate, struvite) are radiopaque and will be evident on plain film. An IVP should be done stat on patients with uncertain diagnosis, those thought to have nonradiopaque stones, and those thought to have ureteric obstruction.

Sonography - A sonogram may be useful to confirm the diagnosis in those patients for whom an IVP is contraindicated, i.e., pregnant patients, those with renal failure, and those with only one kidney.

Intervention

1. Provide for patient comfort - Administration of analgesia is commonly delayed until a relatively certain diagnosis is reached. However, the patient with classical colicky pain or hematuria and a benign abdominal examination should not be left unmedicated because of an unjustified fear of "obscuring" the diagnosis. Thereafter, meperidine, 75–100 mg IM or IV, can be given as prescribed. Patients who are in refractory pain should be assessed by a urologist and may need an IVP. Moist

heat to the flank area may make the patient feel more comfortable.
2. Hydration - A fluid intake of 200–300 ml/hr/day is recommended unless the patient has cardiac or renal failure. If the patient is unable to take an adequate amount of fluid PO, start an IV.

ED Discharge Planning

Expect patients with the following to be admitted:

1. Presence of infection or a fever of >101°F
2. Refractory pain
3. Obstruction indicated by an IVP

Most renal calculi are smaller than 4–5 mm in diameter and will pass spontaneously. Calculi that are larger than 10 mm in size are more likely to obstruct and necessitate an IVP.

ED Discharge Instructions
1. Review use of and precautions when taking analgesics.
2. Stress the need for 3000 ml of fluid intake per day.
3. Exercise between attacks is beneficial.
4. All urine should be strained through gauze or a fine sieve (fish tank scoop), and any strained stones should be brought to the hospital for analysis.
5. If the composition of the stone has been determined, review specific diet:
   a. Uric acid stones - Increase alkanization of urine and decrease purines in diet, i.e., avoid sardines, herring, liver, kidneys, goose.
   b. Calcium stones - Decrease oxalates in diet, i.e., spinach, rhubarb, parsley, chocolate, cocoa, instant coffee, tea. Dietary calcium may need to be reduced. The patient should consult his or her physician before taking calcium supplements and vitamins A and D.
6. Follow-up appointment to a urologist within a week is essential.

PYELONEPHRITIS AND CYSTITIS

Etiology

Pyelonephritis is an inflammatory bacterial infection of the kidney. It is often the result of the spread of a bladder infection and is usually caused by the same organisms including *Escherichia coli* (90%), *Proteus* (3%), *Klebsiella* (2%), and enterococci (2%).

Bacterial ascent from the urethra to the bladder or kidney accounts for over 95% of UTIs; hematogenous spread secondary to bacteremia occurs in <5%. A UTI in women is usually caused by enteric bacteria from feces colonizing the vaginal vestibule and subsequently ascending the urethra.

Although infection may be limited to the bladder (cystitis), ascent of infection through the ureter to the kidney (pyelonephritis) occurs in roughly 30–50% of cases. Preexisting vesicoureteral reflux may play a role in development of some upper tract infections; however, cystitis alone may produce reflux. Although the majority of patients who develop pyelonephritis have no demonstrable functional or anatomic defects, other factors that favor ascent to kidney infection include impaired bladder function, ureteral obstruction, and the presence of a foreign body, such as a stone, catheter, tumor, or sloughed papilla. Pregnant patients are prone to develop pyelonephritis.

Assessment

History

Cystitis - Patients with cystitis (bacterial and symptomatic abacteriuria) will complain of dysuria, urgency, frequency, nocturia, suprapubic tenderness, cloudy urine, and sometimes hematuria. Important facts to be elicited include a previous history of cystitis and the presence of symptoms of pyelonephritis. In symptomatic abacteriuria there may be a history of recent trauma or local irritation. Sexual activity may be an important factor.

Pyelonephritis - Patients with pyelonephritis are usually febrile and toxic in appearance. In addition to symptoms of cystitis, they may complain of shaking chills, nausea and vomiting, and low back pain. However, complaints may be no more severe than in cystitis. Pyelonephritis associated with ureteral obstruction, as in nephrolithiasis (renal stones), may present primarily with renal colic. High fever (>102°F) usually signifies a pyelonephritis.

Physical Findings

General - Note if the patient appears toxic.

Vital signs - Always check a rectal temperature. Check for orthostatic changes if the patient seems dehydrated.

Abdomen - Check for localized tenderness or rebound. Listen for bowel sounds. Palpate to elicit bladder tenderness or fullness in the suprapubic area. Check for percussion tenderness in the flanks.

Diagnostic Tests

Urinalysis - Obtain a clean-catch (midstream) urine sample. Urine should be sent for routine analysis and culture. Chemstrips, which are tests for leukocyte esterase and nitrites, are useful in the ED for screening urine for infection. Microscopic examination may show red and white cells;

white cell casts are seen in pyelonephritis. The presence of bacteria on Gram stain of an unspun sample of urine is indicative of an infection (colony count of 100,000/ml).

Laboratory tests - SMA may show an elevated BUN in volume depletion secondary to vomiting and in parenchymal renal disease. The WBC is usually elevated.

X-rays - A KUB should be done in patients with renal colic. If obstruction is suspected, an emergency IVP should be performed to detect a surgically treatable cause.

Sonography - Pregnant women will require sonography for the location of stones.

Intervention

1. Antibiotic therapy - Many women with acute uncomplicated UTI can be treated successfully with single large doses of antibiotics including amoxicillin, kanamycin, sulfisoxazole (Gantrisin), or trimethoprim-sulfamethoxazole (Bactrim or Septra). Single-dose therapy is not recommended for patients with upper tract disease, for any male, for pregnant women, or for patients who may not be available for follow-up cultures. Conventional therapy for cystitis includes sulfisoxazole, ampicillin, tetracycline, or cephalosporins given for 10–14 days. Patients who may have acquired the infection in an institution (e.g., hospital, nursing home) where resistant organisms are common or patients who have chronic UTI often require treatment with IM or IV aminoglycosides. Patients thought to have chlamydial urethritis are placed on prolonged therapy of up to 4 weeks, and treatment of sexual partners may be necessary. Treatment is doxycycline, 100 mg PO bid. Pyridium, a urinary tract anesthetic, 50 mg PO qid, may be ordered to ease discomfort.

2. Young, ambulatory patients who have uncomplicated pyelonephritis and do not appear toxic may be treated with the same outpatient regimens as is used for patients with cystitis. However, most patients will require IV therapy.

3. Hydration and support measures - If vomiting or dehydration are present, IV fluid replacement should be started. Medicate the patient for pain and give an antipyretic for elevated temperature.

ED Discharge Planning

Patients with pyelonephritis and any of the following need to be admitted:

1. Toxic appearance

2. Inability to keep oral medications down
3. Immunosuppression (e.g., elderly, diabetics, drug addicts, sicklers, alcoholics)
4. Urologic obstruction (e.g., prostatitis, tumor, renal stone, sloughed papilla)
5. Probable resistant organism (e.g., recent hospital discharge, chronic catheter, institutional resident, chronic UTI)
6. Pregnancy (an obstetric consultation is needed)
7. Unreliable, noncompliant patients

ED Discharge Instructions
Discharge instructions should include:

1. Encouraging the patient to maintain a fluid intake of 3000 ml/day
2. Follow-up examination with repeat urine culture in 7–10 days
3. Hygiene measures to prevent cystitis, i.e., avoidance of use of bath salts and vaginal sprays
4. Telling the patient to void more frequently, i.e., every 2–3 hours
5. Signs and symptoms of UTI, including burning and frequency of urination, cloudy urine, blood in urine, and flank pain
6. Warning the patient that phenazopyridine (Pyridium), if ordered, will turn urine a reddish-orange color and can stain clothes

EPIDIDYMITIS AND PROSTATITIS

Infections and inflammation of the prostate gland and the epididymis may be caused by bacteria such as *Chlamydia trachomatis*, *E. coli*, and *Neisseria gonorrhoeae*. In young males they are most often caused by sexually transmitted organisms.

Assessment

History
Acute epididymitis - This condition is marked by the sudden onset of scrotal pain with rapid unilateral scrotal enlargement. There is exquisite tenderness extending over the spermatic cord, which is relieved by elevation of the testes. Acute infection may be associated with urethral discharge. Patients with chronic epididymitis usually have minimal local tenderness and pain, have no urethral discharge, and may have an associated hydrocele.
Prostatitis - Patients should be questioned about acute local symptoms including frequency, urgency, dysuria, hematuria, pain in defecation,

fever, chills, and recent onset of chronic enlargement of the gland. The patient should be questioned about any recent penile discharge, genital lesions, or new sexual partners. A past history of previous UTI or prostatitis is important. Recent urinary catheterization may suggest iatrogenic infection.

Physical Findings
Vital signs - Check for fever.
Genitalia - Examine the genitalia for scrotal enlargement and tenderness. Determine whether pain is relieved by elevation of the testes (relief is seen in the epididymis, in contrast to torsion) (see earlier discussion under "Testicular Torsion"). Note penile lesions, urethral discharge, and adenopathy suggestive of sexually acquired infections.
Rectal examination - A tender, boggy prostate is found in acute prostatitis.
Urinalysis - Send a routine analysis and culture. Bacteriuria and leukocytosis are common. A Gram stain of urine and urethral discharge is often done.
CBC - Commonly shows an elevated WBC.

Intervention

1. Antibiotic therapy - Both acute prostatitis and epididymitis can be treated with tetracycline, 500 mg PO qid for 10–14 days, or trimethoprim-sulfamethoxazole (Bactrim, Septra) for 2 weeks or more. Since younger men are more sexually active and therefore more prone to sexually transmitted disease, tetracycline is the drug of choice. In older men, trimethoprim-sulfamethoxazole therapy is favored due to the frequency of Gram-negative organisms. Epididymitis due to gonococcal infection may be treated as is gonococcal urethritis (see "Sexually Transmitted Diseases" in Chapter 9).
2. Supportive and comfort measures - Analgesics are commonly prescribed. Sitz baths and limited activity (bed rest) for 1–2 days will ease discomfort. Patients with epididymitis should use a scrotal support.

ED Discharge Planning

Patients who appear toxic, those who have underlying immunocompromise (e.g., diabetes, the elderly), and those who require IV antibiotics (high fever, toxic appearance) should be admitted.

ED Discharge Instructions
1. Review the use and method of sitz bath with the patient.
2. Review medication instructions; be sure to inform the patient that

food, milk products, and antacids interfere with the absorption of tetracycline. The drug should be taken at least 1 hour before or 2 hours after meals.
3. Sexual partners, if this is a sexually transmitted disease, should be treated.

SUGGESTED READINGS

Testicular Torsion

Haynes BE, Bessen HA, Haynes VE. The diagnosis of testicular torsion. JAMA 1983; 249:2522

Nagler NH, White RD. A clinical approach to testicular torsion. In: Kaufman JJ, ed. Current urology therapy. 2nd ed. Philadelphia: WB Saunders, 1986:423–425.

Son KA, Koff SA. Evaluation and management of the acute scrotum. Primary Care 1985;12:637–646.

Acute Urinary Retention

Mills J, McAninch JW. Genitourinary emergencies. In: Mills J, Ho MT, Salber PR, Trunkey DD, eds. Current emergency diagnosis and treatment. Los Altos, California: Lange Medical Publications, 1985:607–611.

Tanagho EA. Urinary obstruction and stasis. In: Smith DR, ed. General urology. 11th ed. Los Altos, California: Lange Medical Publications, 1984:149–161.

Renal Colic

Crowley AR, Smith AD. Percutaneous ultrasonic lithotripsy. Postgrad Med 1986;79:57–64.

Greene C. Urinary tract. In: Handbook of adult primary care. New York: John Wiley & Sons, 1987:491–539.

LaValle S. Infectious and obstructive diseases of the kidney. In: Richard CJ, ed. Comprehensive nephrology nursing. Boston: Little, Brown, 1986:85–98.

Spirnak JP, Resnick MI. Urinary stones. Primary Care 1985;12:735–759.

Pyelonephritis and Cystitis

Hart CC, Weisholtz SJ. Urinary tract infections. In: Roberts RB, ed. Infectious diseases: pathogenesis, diagnosis, and therapy. Chicago: Year Book Medical Publishers, 1986:73–92.

Mulholland SG. Female urinary tract infection. Primary Care 1985;12:661–673.

Schaeffer AJ. Cystitis and pyelonephritis. In: Youmans GP, Paterson PY, Sommers HM, eds. The biologic and clinical basis of infectious diseases. 3rd ed. Philadelphia: WB Saunders, 1985:418–435.

Epididymitis and Prostatitis

Ball TP. Epididymitis. In: Kaufman JJ, ed. Current urologic therapy. Philadelphia: WB Saunders, 1986:429–432.

Guze PA, Nagami PH. Infectious disease emergencies. In: Mills J, Ho MT, Salber PR, Trunkey DD, eds. Current emergency diagnosis and treatment. Los Altos, California: Lange Medical Publications, 1985:645–646.

Chapter 12

HEMATOLOGIC EMERGENCIES

SICKLE CELL CRISIS

Etiology

Sickle cell anemia is an inherited disorder of abnormal hemoglobin synthesis. Deoxygenated hemoglobin S (HbS) forms aggregates that damage the red cell membrane, eventually causing irreversible elongation or "sickling," dehydration, and rigidity of the erythrocyte. The sickling cells form multiple small thromboses, clogging small vessels. This vaso-occlusion can lead to tissue ischemia and necrosis including pulmonary infarction, hepatic infarctions, renal and bone marrow infarcts, priapism, painful crisis, and neurologic events. Painful thrombotic crisis should be responded to without delay. Other forms of crisis in sickle cell anemia (aplasia, hemolysis, splenic pooling) are seen less commonly.

Chronic complications of sickle cell disease include hepatomegaly, osteoporosis, joint pain, nerve palsies, and chronic leg ulcers.

Crisis may occur spontaneously without an identifiable cause or may be precipitated by factors that result in decreased supply or increased utilization, such as infection, high altitude, trauma, or emotional stress.

In patients with sickle trait (HbAS), red blood cells will only sickle when oxygen saturation is <20%. These patients are therefore asymptomatic and are not considered to have sickle cell disease. They may have hematuria from a small papillary infarct and may have 1½ times the incidence of pulmonary infarction found in the normal population.

Assessment

History
The disease is usually diagnosed during infancy or early childhood. Determine when the present crisis started and possible precipitating factors,

such as illness, physical or emotional stress, dehydration, cold, or pregnancy. Ask the patient about his or her condition and symptoms prior to crisis, including medication (narcotics, pneumococcal polysaccharide vaccine (Pneumovax), folate therapy), medical care, hospital admissions, and any history of allergy or antibodies to morphine or aspirin. Be aware that many patients with sickle cell take strong analgesics regularly and may show tolerance.

Physical Findings
General - Note the severity of discomfort and degree of pain.
Vital signs - Take the patient's rectal temperature at least twice in the first hours before giving aspirin or acetaminophen. Check the patient's sitting and supine BPs,* respiratory rate, and pulse rate. Tachycardia and tachypnea are common.
Lungs - Note rales, rub, decreased sounds, and splinting.
Skin - Skin may be pale, jaundiced, or dehydrated, with decreased skin turgor.
Extremities - Look for active cellulitis, leg ulcers, swollen joints, and osteomyelitis. Check peripheral pulses.
Neurologic signs - Look carefully for focal deficits. Assess level of consciousness.

Diagnostic Tests
CBC - Send specimen for reticulocyte count and WBC. Both tests will usually show elevated values in sickle cell anemia. If the reticulocyte count is low (<6–7%), think of aplastic anemia.
Chemistry - Check electrolytes, BUN, and creatinine. Results may aid in evaluation of fluid status. Obtain urine for analysis of specific gravity and a Chemstrip to test for hematuria.

Intervention

1. Oxygenation - Administer oxygen by mask or cannula to enhance oxygenation. A quiet atmosphere and rest will decrease oxygen utilization.
2. Hydration - Adequate fluid intake will decrease blood viscosity and improve perfusion. Fluids should be given PO, if possible, to avoid the loss of venous access that often results after frequent hospitalizations.
3. Provide comfort and pain relief - In order to avoid complications of multiple IM or IV injection sites, morphine sulfate and other potent analgesics can be given PO. Morphine (Roxanol) given PO requires 30 minutes for absorption and therefore must be given immediately on entry to the ED. Prophylactic prochlorperazine (Compazine) to relieve nausea may be needed. If a painful crisis is complicated by associated

---

*See "Appendix A" for definition of common abbreviations used in the text.

illness prohibiting oral intake, morphine may be given via the IV line used for hydration. IM injection is contraindicated. An initial dose of morphine, 60 mg PO, should be given with frequent reassessment of BP, respirations, level of sedation and pain relief. After 30 minutes, if there are no signs of sedation or pain relief, morphine, 15 mg PO, may be prescribed every 20 minutes until either sedation or analgesia is achieved.

Analgesic Potency for Severe Pain

	Dosage (mg)	Duration (hr)
Morphine IM[a]	10	4–6
Morphine PO	60	4–7
Hydromorphone IM	1.5	3–5
(Dilaudid) PO	7.5	4–6
Merperidine IM	75	2–4
(Demerol) PO	300[b]	4–6
Methadone IM	10	4–6
(Dolophine) PO	20	4–6
Oxymorphone IM	0.5–1.5	4–6
(Numorphan)		

[a]Standard for comparison.
[b]Recommended starting dose is 50–100 mg. Oral-to-parenteral efficacy ratio is 4:1.

Analgesic Potency for Mild to Moderate Pain

	Dosage (mg)	Duration (hr)
Aspirin[a] PO	650	4–6
Acetaminophen PO	650	4–6
Codeine PO	50	4–6
Meperidine PO	50	4–6

[a] Standard for comparison.

4. Transfusion - Administration of blood (non-sickle trait) may be necessary in patients with life-threatening complications and in patients in crisis who are unresponsive to conventional therapy.

ED Discharge Planning

Patients with the following should be admitted:

1. Inadequate response to ED treatment, i.e., a patient unable to manage with codeine and oral hydration at home
2. Evidence of infection

3. Severe complications, i.e., liver, renal, cardiac, or pulmonary illness
4. Severe anemia

ED Discharge Instructions
1. Use of analgesics such as acetaminophen or aspirin in synergy with codeine
2. Regular use of folate
3. Caution against misuse of strong analgesics
4. Maintenance of good oral intake
5. Adequate rest periods, i.e., a decrease in physical and emotional stress
6. Avoidance of factors that can precipitate crisis (high altitudes, and physical or emotional stress)
7. Encouragement of regular medical follow-up and prompt treatment of infections
8. Consideration of the need for social work intervention

CLOTTING DISORDERS

ETIOLOGY

Clotting disorders may be generally viewed as due to the following qualitative and quantitative abnormalities: platelets, blood vessels, and plasma coagulation factors. Etiologies for bleeding disorders commonly seen in the ED are discussed below.

Platelet Abnormalities
1. Thrombocytopenia
   a. Decreased production (bone marrow dysfunction)
   b. Decreased platelet survival (drugs, infection, DIC)
   c. Platelet sequestration (splenomegaly)
2. Abnormal platelet function (drug-induced, uremia, cirrhosis, lupus)

Blood Vessel Wall Abnormalities
1. Purpura (senile, drug-induced, Henoch-Schönlein)
2. Dysproteinemias (multiple myeloma, cryoglobulinemia)
3. Cushing's syndrome
4. Scurvy
5. Hereditary connective tissue disorders (Marfan's syndrome)

Coagulopathies
1. Acquired (liver disease, Coumadin, DIC)
2. Congenital (hemophilia, von Willebrand's disease)

Assessment

History
Ascertain whether a clotting or bleeding disorder has been previously diagnosed. A family history of clotting disorders is commonly found in hemophiliacs and in patients with von Willebrand's disease. Previous bleeding episodes, frequency, and treatment should be noted. There is often a history of spontaneous hematuria, melena, and excessive bleeding after dental extraction.

History of liver disease, ethanol abuse, or anticoagulant use is most significant. DIC is seen in the setting of shock, sepsis, severe burns, or obstetrical complications.

Physical Findings
Vital signs - Check orthostatic BP and pulse. No rectal temperature should be taken.
HEENT - Look for signs of head trauma. Note hemotympanum. Look for gingival bleeding.
Lungs - Listen for rales or wheezes (pulmonary hemorrhage).
Pelvic - Note vaginal bleeding.
Rectal examination - Check stool for blood.
Extremities - Note prolonged bleeding at venipuncture sites. A swollen thigh may contain a large hematoma. Joint pain and decreased range of motion may be seen at sites of joint bleeding.
Neurologic signs - Check pupils carefully. Look for focal deficits (subdural hematoma). Assess level of consciousness.
Skin - Note ecchymoses. Note any petechiae that appear after placement of a tourniquet.

Note: Bleeding into the retroperitoneum or the thigh may result in significant blood loss and shock without obvious external bleeding.

Diagnostic Tests
CBC - Do a spun Hct. Check the platelet count. A reduction below 150,000/μl is considered thrombocytopenia, but bleeding is uncommon until the platelet count falls below 50,000/μl.
PT - PT is elevated in liver disease, vitamin K deficiency, warfarin use, and DIC but is normal in von Willebrand's disease and classic hemophilia.
PTT - If the PT is elevated, the PTT is usually also increased. If the PT is normal, the PTT may be elevated in heparin abuse, von Willebrand's disease, and classic hemophilia.
Rumpel-Leede test - Inflate a BP cuff midway between the patient's systolic and diastolic pressure. Maintain this pressure for several minutes.

Look on the patient's volar forearm 4 cm distal to the antecubital crease
and count the number of petechiae in a circle with a 2.5-cm diameter
(the size of a quarter). The finding of more than 5 petechiae in men
or more than 10 in women is abnormal and indicates platelet abnormalities or vascular fragility.

Intervention

1. Obtain venous access - Prepare for clotting factor and/or blood administration.
   a. O-negative blood transfusion may be required if the patient is hem-
      orrhaging and in shock. Obtain the type and cross-match as soon
      as possible.
   b. Factor VIII concentrate is used for treatment of hemophilia A.
   c. Cryoprecipitate contains fibrinogen and factor VIII and should be
      withdrawn from bags and given by slow IV push through a filter.
   d. Fresh frozen plasma (FFP) is used to treat clotting factor deficiency
      of an unknown cause, a deficiency resulting from hepatic disease,
      and a factor V deficiency. Administer FFP via a standard blood ad-
      ministration set and filter.
   Request a hematology consult immediately.
2. Warfarin-induced hemorrhage or liver disease - Vitamin K (Aqua-
   mephyton) in a dosage of 30–50 mg is given SC or by slow IV drip
   (<1 mg/min).
3. Prevent further bleeding. Avoid any unnecessary trauma, IM injections, etc. Immobilize bleeding joints, and apply ice if bleeding is recent.

Disseminated Intravascular Coagulation

DIC is a hypercoagulable clinical state in which both clotting and bleeding
occur. In DIC a critical physiologic disturbance triggers a systemic coagulation response in which clots line the body's capillaries. DIC may be precipitated by a variety of critical conditions including septicemia, hypoxemia, carcinoma, septic abortion, hypoxemia, and heat stroke. Bleeding
occurs as clotting factors are consumed. Coagulation studies (PT, PTT,
platelet count) will be abnormal, and treatment includes correction of hypovolemia, hypoxia, acidosis, hypotension, and restoration of clotting ho-
meostasis with heparin and administration of clotting factors. Patients will
require admission to the ICU for treatment of the underlying condition
and critical monitoring. Nursing intervention in the ICU includes:

1. Monitor the patient for bleeding, both overt and occult. Test urine,
   stool, and gastric secretions for blood.
2. Avoid trauma during treatments, turning, bathing, etc.

3. Assess tissue perfusion. Check the patient for cyanosis, skin color, and peripheral pulses.
4. Monitor fluid balance including urine output, hypotension, and urine-specific gravity.
5. Monitor cardiopulmonary functions—cardiac monitoring, CVP, lung auscultation for rales, and pulmonary capillary wedge pressure.

ED Discharge Planning

Any patient with a significant bleeding disorder or a Hct low enough to require transfusion will need to be admitted. Patients with drug-induced bleeding will usually require admission to readjust medication dosages.

ED Discharge Instructions
1. Provide for a follow-up hematology consult.
2. Ensure that the patient and his or her family knows when and where to seek emergency care.

SUGGESTED READINGS

Sickle Cell Crisis

Anonymous. Sudden death in sickle cell carriers. Emerg Med 1988;20:125–126.

Friedman E, Webber A. Protocol for the oral treatment of painful sickle cell crisis. New York, North Central Bronx Hospital, October 1981.

Rosenthal DS, Younger WB. Hematologic emergencies. In: May HL, ed. Emegency medicine. New York: John Wiley & Sons, 1984:767–769.

Clotting Disorders

Griffin JP. The bleeding patient. Nursing 1986;16:34–40.

Ives J. Disseminated intravascular coagulation syndrome (DIC). In: Hudak CM, Gallo BM, Lohr T, eds. Critical care nursing. Philadelphia: JB Lippincott, 1986:233–241.

Chapter 13

OPHTHALMOLOGIC EMERGENCIES

RED EYE

Etiology

Conjunctivitis is the most common cause of red eye. Frequently encountered causes include bacterial or viral infection, allergic reactions, exposure to irritants, and some systemic diseases. Conjunctivitis is generally gradual in onset and typically causes vague ocular discomfort, burning, itching, tearing, and mild photophobia. Visual acuity is not altered. A discharge is often present. Prior exposure to family members or others with "pink eye," an associated upper respiratory tract infection, or recent history of swimming is suggestive of an infectious conjunctivitis. Patients with allergic conjunctivitis often have a history of asthma or hay fever. An occupational history will identify chemical exposures. A history of systemic illness should be sought, particularly inflammatory disease (Behçet's syndrome, collagen vascular disease, etc.).

Iritis is a somewhat less common cause of a red eye, but it may be difficult to differentiate from acute conjunctivitis. Associated pain is moderate; there may be photophobia, and vision is slightly blurred. When a light is shined in the good eye, the consensual light reflex will cause pain in the affected eye. Causes include collagen vascular diseases such as rheumatoid arthritis.

Acute angle-closure glaucoma is an uncommon cause of red eye, but it requires immediate diagnosis and treatment to prevent ocular damage. The onset is sudden and often occurs at night. Pain is extreme, vision is blurred, and there is no associated discharge. The patient may complain of nausea, vomiting, and headache and may describe halos around lights. A history of previous episodes in recent weeks of self- limited ocular pain and blurred vision may be obtained.

Assessment

Physical Findings

External eye - Examine the periorbital area and eyelids for signs of trauma or cellulitis. To examine the lower lid, place a finger over the patient's cheek bone and pull down. If it is necessary to evert the upper lid, place an applicator in the upper lid crease, have the patient look down, and while holding the lashes, pull the lid over the applicator. Observe for edema, redness, ulceration of eyelid, and follicle (cavity) formation. Viral infection or toxic effects of pilocarpine are frequent causes of follicular conjunctivitis in the lower lid. Trachoma (a *Chlamydia* infection common in Asia but rare in the United States) results in follicle formation in the upper lid. Chemosis or edema is seen with allergy and gonococcal or orbital infections. Discharge is seen in conjunctivitis but is not commonly seen in iritis or glaucoma. Purulent exudate is seen in gonococcus, meningococcus, *Pseudomonas*, and other pyogenic bacterial infections.

Conjunctiva - In conjunctivitis, dilation of small blood vessels (injection) is suggestive of infectious conjunctivitis, whereas a whitish pale conjunctiva is seen with allergic conjunctivitis.

Cornea - Using a flashlight, look at the cornea from the side; it should be clear, but acute glaucoma, cataracts, and abrasions will cause opacities.

Anterior chamber - Examine the anterior chamber in the same manner as for the cornea; using lateral light, observe for a clear anterior chamber with a flat, nonbulging iris. Because of the increased intraocular pressure the anterior chamber is virtually absent in acute angle-closure glaucoma.

Pupil - Examine the pupil for size and reaction to light. To test for consensual reaction, shine a light into one pupil and observe the other pupil. It should promptly constrict but to a lesser degree than with the direct reaction. Iritis causes reduced size of the pupil on the involved side and pain in the involved side upon eliciting the consensual light reflex in the other eye. In acute glaucoma the pupil is often in a dilated midposition.

Diagnostic Tests

Stains of discharge - Gram stain may aid in identification of the predominant organism in bacterial conjunctivitis.

Tonometer - An instrument used to measure intraocular pressure. A low reading indicates a hard eyeball and high intraocular pressure. Normal reading is 11–22 mm Hg.* Intraocular pressure is normal in conjuncti-

---

*See "Appendix A" for definition of common abbreviations used in the text.

vitis, usually normal in acute iritis, and markedly elevated in acute glaucoma.

Slitlamp - Used to examine anterior chamber, iris, and cornea.

Fluorescein staining of the cornea - Fluorescein strip is moistened with normal saline and touched against the inner lower eyelid. The stain solution is spread as the patient blinks. Staining pattern will provide diagnostic information in herpes simplex (dendritic ulcers), conjunctivitis, and corneal abrasion.

Differential Diagnostic Features

	Conjunctivitis	Iritis	Glaucoma
Incidence	Very common	Common	Uncommon
Onset	Gradual	Gradual	Sudden
Pain	Mild	Moderate	Severe visual
Acuity	Normal	Slight blurring	Marked blurring
Conjunctival injection	Present	Present	Present
Pupil size	Normal	Small, irregular	Midsize, dilated
Pupil reflex	Normal	Sluggish	Minimal
Consensual reflex (affected eye)	Normal	Painful	Normal
Cornea	Clear	Clear	Steamy
Discharge	Watery to purulent	None	None

Intervention

1. Prevent further injury - Place the patient in a supine or mid-Fowler's position. Decrease room light and apply an eye patch if indicated. An ophthalmologist should be consulted for any red eye that is not clearly a case of conjunctivitis.
2. Conjunctivitis - Bacterial conjunctivitis should be treated with a broad-spectrum antibiotic such as sulfisoxazole (Gantrisin) eye drops given every 2–4 hours to both eyes for the first 48 hours and then qid for 5–7 days. Viral conjunctivitis is usually treated with broad-spectrum antibiotics as well, not to hasten recovery but to prevent secondary bacterial infection. Clear-cut cases of allergic conjunctivitis may be treated with cold compresses and removal of the allergen, if possible. Severe allergic reactions may require systemic antihistamines (not local).
3. Iritis - The patient with eye pain, blurred vision, and small irregular pupils should be referred to the physician from triage. Immediate dilation of the pupil is necessary to prevent adhesions to the lens, with

subsequent glaucoma or cataracts. Topical corticosteroid drops can be administered subsequently in order to decrease the inflammatory response. Warm compresses and analgesics will increase patient comfort.

4. Acute angle-closure glaucoma - Immediate treatment is aimed at promoting aqueous humor drainage. Blindness can result in a few hours if not promptly treated. Pilocarpine 4% solution is given every 5 minutes for 30 minutes and then hourly until a clinical response is seen. In addition, acetazolamide (Diamox), 500 mg PO along with 500 mg IV, is given to decrease intraocular pressure. If these maneuvers do not produce a clinical response rapidly, IV mannitol may be necessary. Provide analgesia, usually morphine sulfate.

5. Other eye emergencies
   a. Orbital cellulitis - An extremely dangerous infection because extension may result in cavernous sinus thrombosis. Serious orbital cellulitis is marked by entrapment of the involved eye with loss of movement. These patients should be admitted, started on IV antibiotics, and seen by an ophthalmologist immediately. See "Cellulitis" in Chapter 9 for further details.
   b. Central retinal artery occlusion - Suggested by an abrupt, painless loss of vision in one eye. Immediate treatment is aimed at moving the blockage to a more peripheral vessel and consists of gentle digital massage on the closed eye to lower intraocular pressure, acetazolamide at 500 mg PO along with 500 mg IV, and having the patient breathe into a paper bag to increase pCO_2 and dilate retinal arterioles. An ophthalmologist should be consulted immediately, as every minute counts.

ED Discharge Planning

Expect patients with the following diagnosis to be admitted:

1. Orbital cellulitis
2. Acute glaucoma
3. Retinal artery occlusion

ED Discharge Instructions
1. Review diagnosis and specific instructions.
   a. Conjunctivitis - Infection is highly contagious. Patient should avoid direct contact with family and friends by use of separate towels, hand washing, etc.
   b. Acute iritis - Patient has photophobia. Advise cold compresses and dark glasses or an eye patch. Caution the patient about loss of depth perception with the use of an eye patch.

2. Arrange a follow-up examination with the ophthalmologist, if indicated.

EYE TRAUMA

If general or facial trauma is present, life-threatening injuries must be given priority. Immediate action is indicated if the patient complains of sparks, flashes of light, or moving spots in the visual field. These symptoms are suggestive of a detached retina, and the nurse should place the patient on a stretcher with the head immobilized. Apply bilateral eye patches and notify the physician. The eye patch will decrease discomfort by decreasing eye movement. To apply the patch, have the patient close both eyes, then fold the pad in half, cover the eye with an open pad, and tape it in place. Provide reassurance. Eye injury and the fear of blindness can cause a near panic state. The patient with chemical injury to the eye requires immediate eye irrigation with large amounts of water or saline to remove injurious substances. Notify the physician that irrigation is in progress.

Assessment

History
Determine how, when, and where the trauma occurred. Establish the condition of the eye prior to injury and any treatment given prior to the patient's presentation to the ED. Note any history of previous injury, infection, or surgery, as well as whether the patient wears or has ever worn glasses. Ask about a history of strabismus. Inquire about any history of systemic disease, allergies, or current medications. Ask about tetanus immunization, when appropriate.

Physical Findings
External eye - Observe the lids and lashes, conjunctiva, and cornea for
    swelling, laceration, penetration, and foreign bodies. Blood in the anterior chamber (hyphema) is more easily seen in blue eyes than in darker eyes. Check for contact lenses. Assist the physician to do a slitlamp examination of the anterior chamber for normal depth, signs of inflammation, hyphema (blood), or hypopyon (pus). The lens is examined for effects of trauma; note if lens implant is present. If a penetrating or perforating injury is suspected, shield the eye. An immediate ophthalmology consult is indicated. If the lids are very swollen, lid retractors (which may be fashioned with a paper clip) can be used to examine the eye. Corneal stains with fluorescein and examination under cobalt blue

light will identify keratitides, ulcers, or abrasions. In cases of blunt trauma, palpate the orbital rim for gross defects and crepitus.

Pupils - The pupils should be equal, round, and reactive to light. Pupillary abnormalities should be evaluated by a physician or ophthalmologist.

Visual acuity - Assess visual acuity via a Snellen chart, if available. Test each eye separately with the patient using her or his glasses.

Intervention

Prevent further injury. Institute emergency measures, i.e., immobilization and eye patch or eye irrigation, if indicated. Place the patient in a mid-Fowler's position, with the side rails of the bed up, and consult a physician concerning further treatment.

Specific Injuries

Corneal abrasion - A corneal abrasion is the traumatic removal of corneal epithelium. Abrasions may be caused by such things as foreign bodies, twigs, and fingers. Poorly fitted or overworn contact lenses are a common cause. A foreign body may be lodged between the contact lens and cornea, or the corneal epithelium may be damaged upon manipulation of the lens. The chief complaint may be a foreign body sensation. Abrasions may produce severe pain, tearing, blepharospasm, and blinking. Photophobia may occur, and the conjunctiva is generally hyperemic. Visual acuity may be normal or decreased. Diagnosis involves ruling out a foreign body under the lids and identifying the abrasion, which is easily identified when fluorescein dye is instilled into the lower fornix. A vertical abrasion may indicate a foreign body under one of the lids. The dye will stain the abraded area and fluoresce a bright yellow-green when examined with a cobalt blue light. On occasion, examination will be difficult, and instillation of a topical anesthetic eye drop will facilitate the examination. However, continued use of topical anesthetic drops will delay healing and may mask symptoms of infection. Treatment should include a short-acting, eye muscle-paralyzing agent (cycloplegic), topical antibiotics, and modified pressure patching. Any patched eye should be examined daily, with instillation of antibiotics until the abrasion is healed. Small abrasions with minimal discomfort do not require patching.

Foreign bodies - Foreign material (e.g., wood, glass, or metal) may be propelled into the eye and become adherent to or embedded in the cornea, causing chronic irritation. The patient will complain of foreign body sensation, pain, and tearing. Visual acuity may be normal or decreased, and the conjunctiva will be hyperemic. Photophobia may be observed.

A slitlamp should be used to determine the depth and extent of corneal injury. The aim of treatment is to remove the foreign body, relieve pain, prevent infection, and minimize scarring. Administration of a topical anesthetic is required to remove a superficial foreign body. First, attempt to remove the foreign body by irrigation. If this is inadequate, a moistened cotton swab may be used to gently wipe away a superficial foreign body. An embedded foreign body may be removed by using a 25-gauge needle stabilized on a cotton-tip applicator or tuberculin syringe. An embedded foreign body should be removed via a slitlamp. A metallic foreign body is surrounded by a rust ring within a relatively short time, and the rust ring should be removed along with the foreign body, if possible. Deep corneal foreign bodies that may be penetrating the anterior chamber should be removed only by an experienced ophthalmologist. After removal of the foreign body, fluorescein staining will show the extent of the injury. As in corneal abrasion, a short-acting muscle-paralyzing agent, a topical antibiotic, and a moderate-pressure eye patch are applied. Patched eyes should be examined daily and treated with antibiotics until reepithelialization has occurred.

Chemical injuries - Chemical burns may be alkali or acid in origin. Generally, the eyelids and surrounding skin, as well as the conjunctiva and cornea, are involved. The conjunctiva, if severely injured, may be pale secondary to ischemia. Pain may be severe or minimal, depending on the extent of damage to corneal nerve endings. Strong alkalis cause a liquefaction injury, and penetration of the cornea into the anterior chamber is immediate. Therefore, prompt irrigation is crucial. Acids cause a coagulation necrosis and are thus less penetrating than alkalis. However, prompt therapy is still indicated. The prognosis worsens directly with the amount of time elapsed from injury to removal of the offending substance. Do not wait for sterile or physiologic solutions to begin irrigation. Begin to wash immediately with tap water. The fornices of the conjunctiva should be cleared with wet cotton-tip applicators, the eyelids should be everted and washed, and any foreign particles should be removed. Prolonged irrigation may not be necessary for acid burns. However, it is wise to treat all chemical exposures aggressively. The initial washing should be followed by continuous irrigation with 1–2 liters of normal saline for at least 1 hour. Therapy can be monitored by using litmus paper. This is best done by anesthetizing the eye with a topical anesthetic and then providing continuous irrigation with a liter bag of normal saline and IV tubing aimed at the eye. An ophthalmologist should be called to manage patients with evidence of serious chemical injuries, as these patients may require hospital admission.

Burns - Burns may also be thermal, radiation-induced, or electrical. Rapid reflex lid closure usually protects the globe from flame burns. Contact burns from molten metal are more likely to cause corneal damage. Ultraviolet radiation injuries from the sun, sun lamps, or welding arcs are relatively common. The corneal epithelium is highly susceptible to injury by ultraviolet radiation. Symptoms usually occur several hours after exposure when the injured epithelial cells are shed. Treatment consists of cycloplegic agents, topical antibiotics, and application of a pressure patch. The patient should be followed daily until the keratitis (inflammation) resolves. This is usually within 24–48 hours. An eclipse burn of the retina should be referred to an ophthalmologist. Infrared radiation may produce a superficial keratitis that may be treated with a topical antibiotic for 4–5 days.

Blunt trauma to the globe - Blunt trauma can be classified as a contusion (i.e., direct contact with the eye) or a concussion (i.e., an indirect injury due to tissue or air conduction). These may cause damage to the anterior or posterior segment. Some of the injuries that may be caused by blunt trauma include ecchymosis, subconjunctival hemorrhage, corneal abrasions or penetrations, hyphema, subluxation or dislocation of the lens and cataract, retinal hemorrhage, retinal detachment, or a ruptured globe. Subconjunctival hemorrhage and ecchymosis require no special treatment. Signs of a ruptured globe (corneal perforation) may include decreased visual acuity, a soft eye (i.e., decreased intraocular pressure), and a shallow or flattened anterior chamber. Any injuries secondary to blunt trauma that are suspected to be more complex than ecchymosis, subconjunctival hemorrhage, or corneal abrasion should be evaluated by an ophthalmologist.

Orbital fractures - An orbital fracture should be suspected whenever there is significant blunt trauma to the orbit. Clinical signs vary with the site of the fracture. Orbital x-rays (not skull films) will aid in making the diagnosis. Associated signs include:

1. Decreased sensation and numbness of teeth or lip, diplopia on upward gaze (orbital floor or blow-out fracture)
2. Cerebrospinal fluid rhinorrhea; test suspicious nasal discharge for glucose (orbital roof fracture)
3. Downward displacement of the affected eye, orbital crepitus, diplopia on lateral gaze (medial wall fracture)
4. Flattening of the cheek bone, trismus (trimalar zygomatic fractures)

Closed reduction or surgical intervention may be required.

Lid lacerations - Lid lacerations may occur in isolation or be associated with injury to the eye. Evert the lids to rule out a penetration or perforation of the globe. With a medial laceration, damage to the lacrimal duct must be ruled out. Immediate treatment consists of irrigation, little to no debridement, and early precise suturing to avoid any deformity.

Consultation Criteria

The majority of cases of ocular trauma are treatable in the ED with a follow-up referral to an ophthalmologist. The following require immediate consultation by an ophthalmologist:

1. Significant nonrefractive decrease in visual acuity
2. Pupillary abnormalities
3. Limitation of extraocular movements
4. Complicated lid lacerations (e.g., involving the lid margin, the lacrimal glands, or the entire thickness of the lid)
5. Severe corneal abrasions, ulcers, or foreign bodies
6. Severe chemical injuries, particularly alkali burns
7. Eclipse burns of the retina
8. Penetrating or perforating injuries of the eye
9. Dislocation of the lens
10. Traumatic cataract
11. Retinal abnormalities

ED Discharge Planning

Expect patients with the following conditions to be admitted:

1. Orbital cellulitis
2. Entrapment syndrome
3. Orbital fracture, which requires operative treatment
4. Perforation of the globe
5. Severe corneal abrasion, corneal ulcer, or penetration
6. Retinal detachment
7. Lenticular dislocation
8. Hyphema (blood in anterior chamber)
9. Hypopyon (pus in anterior chamber)

ED Discharge Instructions
1. Review physician's instructions on activity and follow-up care.
2. Caution the patient about loss of depth perception with the use of an eye patch.
3. Patient should not drive while eye is patched.

SUGGESTED READINGS

Red Eye

Budassi SA, ed. Ophthalmic examinations. J Emerg Nurs 1984; 10:112–114.

Garcia GE. Ophthalmology for the nonophthalmologist. Emerg Med 1987:63–76.

Howes DS. The red eye. Emerg Med Clin North Am 1988;6:43–56.

Lawlor MC. Common ocular injuries and disorders, Part II: red eye. J Emerg Nurs 1989;15:36–41.

Yanofsky NN. The acute painful eye. Emerg Med Clin North Am 1988;6:21–42.

Eye Trauma

Lawlor MC. Common ocular injuries and disorders, Part I: acute loss of vision. J Emerg Nurs 1989;15:32–36.

McDonald K, Norton MS. Facial injuries. In: Harmon AR, ed. Nursing care of the adult trauma patient. New York: John Wiley & Sons, 1985:71–132.

Pavan-Langston D. Manual of ocular diagnosis and therapy. Boston: Little, Brown, 1980.

Chapter 14

PSYCHIATRIC EMERGENCIES

VIOLENT PATIENT

Description

Violent patients are encountered with regularity in the ED.* Some are brought in by family or police because of acts or threats of violence outside the hospital, and others become violent during the course of treatment. ED staff members need to be attuned to the signs of impending violent behavior and be prepared to respond in a planned, organized manner to prevent physical harm to the patient, staff, or other patients.

Etiology

The following problems or disorders may cause a patient to become violent:

Drug intoxication - Alcohol, phencyclidine, amphetamines, etc.
Drug withdrawal - Delirium induced by withdrawal or manipulative hostility aimed at securing more drugs
Acute psychosis - Schizophrenia, acute mania, paranoid states, etc.
Borderline or antisocial personalities, often also with intoxication
Seizure disorders - Postictal combativeness or temporal lobe epilepsy
Drug reactions - Idiosyncratic reactions to medication
Metabolic disorders - Hypoxia, acidosis, hypoglycemia, hypercalcemia, hypercapnea
Intracranial bleeding, often associated with head trauma
Central nervous system infection - Meningitis or encephalitis

---

*See "Appendix A" for definition of common abbreviations used in the text.

283

Assessment

History

A past history of violence is a relatively reliable, although not an absolute, indicator of violent behavior. Patients who have exhibited poor impulse control or a low tolerance for frustration in the past are more likely to become acutely violent when dissatisfied.

Observe some rules of caution when speaking with a violent or potentially violent patient. Introduce yourself and explain what the patient can expect in a direct and straightforward manner. Focus initially on non-threatening topics to allow the patient a chance to relax and establish some rapport with you. Offering the patient juice or food, if appropriate, often has a calming effect. Speaking softly to a patient who is yelling or speaking loudly may force him to lower his or her voice so he or she can hear. It is generally accepted that the violent patient is fearful and trying to regain control by using loud, aggressive behavior. Do not get into a shouting match with the patient. An interviewer who is out of control will only increase the patient's agitation.

Place yourself so you can escape the patient quickly, if necessary. Never put the patient between you and the door. Other safety measures include leaving the door open or having other staff members present during the interview. Never turn your back on a potentially violent patient while you are within the patient's reach.

If the patient is armed, either have the patient surrender the weapons voluntarily or have the security guards search and remove any weapons. If the patient is willing to surrender the weapons, do not take them directly; have him or her place them on the table or floor where they can be removed safely.

If a combative patient makes you feel unusually anxious, have another staff member perform the interview and examination. Otherwise, the patient will sense your anxiety and respond negatively.

Physical Findings

General - Note the patient's physical appearance and affect. Observe the patient's posture for tension, i.e., pacing, clenched fist. Examine the clothes for signs of incontinence.

Vital signs - Vital signs including temperature are exceedingly important and are often the only clue to serious illness in these patients. There is never a reason not to take a complete set of vital signs once the patient is restrained.

HEENT - Check for evidence of head trauma. Examine the pupils and extraocular movements. Check for nystagmus. Examination of the fundi may show signs of increased intracranial pressure. Check the mouth for tongue lacerations (which usually indicate a seizure).

Extremities - Note track marks. Check for cyanosis.

Neurologic signs - Note the patient's level of consciousness and quality of speech (calm, regular speech pattern versus strident, pressured speech). Be alert to excessive motor activity, such as restlessness or pacing, which presages more violent activity. Check for focal neurologic deficits.

Diagnostic Tests

SMA - Do a Dextrostix for blood glucose in the agitated patient.

ABGs - ABG analysis is indicated in the patient who might be acutely hypoxic or acidotic.

Toxicologies - Drug levels should be drawn as clinically indicated.

CAT scan - This should be performed in patients suspected of having serious intracranial pathology (see "Head Trauma" in Chapter 4 for indications for a CAT scan).

Lumbar puncture - This should be performed emergently if meningitis is suspected and there is no evidence of increased intracranial pressure (see "Meningitis" in Chapter 9 for details).

Intervention

1. Assess the patient's need for immediate medical attention.
2. Provide reassurance and a supportive atmosphere - Speak calmly and positively. Use the assistance of any available person who has rapport with the patient. Provide a quiet environment; e.g., turn the lights down, and move noisy patients away. Give the patient simple directions, and set limits on the patient's behavior. Avoid use of angry or threatening behavior or language, i.e., hands on hips, arms folded across chest.
3. Call the security guards when necessary - Sometimes just their presence will quiet the patient who is going out of control. Many patients with personality disorders will respond to a show of force.
4. Medication - If the Dextrostix is low or normal, administer 50 ml of D50W. Patients with acute psychiatric disorders may require tranquilizing medication. Drug concentrates in orange juice are readily absorbed and may be given to willing patients. Patients who resist medication may require IM administration. Effective medications include haloperidol (Haldol), 5–10 mg, trifluoperazine (Stelazine) or thiothixene (Navane), 10–15 mg, or chlorpromazine (Thorazine) or thioridazine (Mellaril), 25–50 mg, all of which can be given PO or IM every 30 minutes until the patient is symptomatically improved. Usually 1–3 doses will induce tranquilization without sedation. Haloperidol has a lower incidence of cardiovascular side effects than many other neuroleptics, while thioridazine has the least effect on seizure

threshold. If the patient cannot be given neuroleptics, an alternative is sodium amytal, 250 mg IM, or diazepam (Valium), 5–10 mg IV.

5. Use restraints as a last resort - The patient who refuses medication and becomes increasingly agitated will need to be restrained. Once the decision is made, the security guards should act quickly, as negotiation is generally of little use at this point. Remember that agitated patients have five extremities—the arms, legs, and head—that must be restrained, as patients will punch, kick, and bite, if possible. At least five people are needed to restrain a violent patient, one for each extremity and one to apply restraints. Have additional staff on standby. If hospital security personnel are called to assist, give them specific instructions. In general, it is advisable to restrain patients on their side by using gauze, stocking net, and chest restraints, but never handcuffs. Tie restraints to the bed or stretcher frame—never to the side rails. If the patient has not been completely undressed prior to application of restraints, search the patient's clothing and pockets for weapons, matches, etc. The restraints must be checked periodically to make sure that the circulation is maintained. After the patient is restrained, he or she should be tranquilized rapidly, provided with supportive therapy, and observed closely. When the patient's condition warrants, begin to release the restraints and continue to monitor the patient closely. Removing an opposite arm and ankle (right arm and left ankle) restraint will provide maximum safety. Do not remove both restraints on one side or all but one extremity, as it will allow the patient to throw himself or herself over the side rail. A physician's written order and a progress note should be completed as soon as the situation permits. The note should include a specific description of the patient's behavior, what other attempts were made to calm the patient, the type, method of restraint, and who applied them. Circulation checks, restraint rotation, and range-of-motion exercises also need to be documented.

SUICIDAL PATIENT

Description

Suicidal patients are generally evaluated in the ED prior to referral to a psychiatrist. Patients may present in a variety of ways, and the evaluating staff must be sensitive to their needs and fears. The suicidal patient should never be taken lightly. Many successful suicides are preceded by unsuccessful attempts or "gestures." Also be sensitive to the patient who presents one or more times to the ED with vague complaints and a depressed affect. A majority of those who commit suicide present to a doctor for some reason prior to the act.

Etiology

The risk of suicide is higher in the following groups: white males, elderly, unemployed, patients with chronic physical illness, those who live alone, patients with a history of drug or alcohol abuse, those with a family or personal history of suicide attempts, and those with a personal or family history of manic-depressive illness. Although the elderly more commonly commit suicide, the rate of suicide is rising among adolescents, causing the average age of suicide to fall in recent years.

Assessment

History
Obtain the patient's description of why he or she is seeking treatment. If an accurate history is not obtainable from the patient or the information is inconsistent or incomplete, consult the patient's family or significant others. Patients who describe suicidal thoughts, plans, or recent attempts should be placed on one-to-one observation until a further evaluation is made by a psychiatrist. The patient history should also include recent life changes or crises, drug or alcohol use, prior treatment for medical or psychiatric illness, medications taken, and family history of suicide, alcoholism, and manic-depressive illness.

Although some suicide attempts appear to be major attempts (e.g., gunshots, hanging, jumps), while others are viewed as suicide gestures in which there was no real intention of success, all must be taken seriously.

Physical Findings
General - Note the patient's appearance and ability to answer questions. Describe the patient's affect or behavior—withdrawn, angry, loud, rambling speech.
Skin - Look for ecchymoses and signs of trauma. Examine wounds.
Extremities - Check for track marks.
Neurologic signs - Note mental status, orientation, memory, and any focal deficits.

Diagnostic Tests
CBC - Check a Hct in the wounded patient.
Toxicologies - Draw specimens for drug and/or alcohol levels as ordered by a physician.
X-rays - Films of areas of local trauma may be needed.

Intervention

1. Stabilize the patient's medical condition - See Chapter 7 under "Drug Overdose: A General Approach" and Chapter 4 on the treatment of trauma.
2. Protect the patient from self-inflicted injury - Never leave him or her alone. The suicidal patient must be observed closely at all times while in the ED. Remove any potentially harmful equipment from the patient's reach (thermometer, liquids, restraint ties), and obtain a "hold" order, pending medical or psychiatric evaluation. Notify hospital security to be on standby.
3. Be nonjudgmental and concerned - Do not reprimand the patient for his or her behavior. Try to get the patient to focus on the positive aspects of life. Emphasize that family and friends as well as the medical staff are supportive. Have family and friends come to the ED to speak with the patient. Allow the patient to ventilate feelings of unhappiness, as this may defuse suicidal energy. Inform the patient of the treatment plan and measures being taken to provide for his or her safety.
4. Medication - No sedatives should be given to patients with drug overdose or intoxication. On rare occasions, it may be necessary to give patients with acute situational disturbances some mild tranquilization. Psychotic patients may benefit from treatment with neuroleptics (haloperidol, 5–10 mg PO, or thiothixene, 10–15 mg PO, every 30 minutes until symptomatic relief is obtained).
5. Psychiatric evaluation - No patient should leave the ED without having been seen by a psychiatrist. Escort the patient to a psychiatric treatment area. If the patient requires further medical treatment, follow-up appointment, etc., inform a member of the psychiatry nursing staff to escort the patient back to the medical emergency area.

ED Discharge Planning

The decision to admit a suicidal patient is usually made by a psychiatrist. However, on occasion a suicidal patient will need to be admitted to the medical or surgical service because of complications of the suicide attempt. These patients should be carefully evaluated by a psychiatrist for suicidal potential prior to leaving the ED. Patients who are judged to be seriously suicidal or whose suicidal risk cannot be judged with certainty (e.g., comatose patients) should have arrangements made for continuous observation at all times while in the hospital.

For patients who are discharged, help the patient obtain the support of family or friends, arrange for outpatient counselling, and review medications and available community emergency resources.

SUGGESTED READINGS

Violent Patient

Antai-otong D. When your patient is angry. Nursing 1988;18:44.

Braverman BG, Shook J. Spotting the borderline personality. Am J Nurs 1987;87:200–203.

Cousins A, ed. Management of the ED patient with a borderline personality disorder. J Emerg Nurs 1984;10:94–96.

Fauman BJ, Fauman MA. Emergency psychiatry for the house officer. Baltimore: Williams & Wilkins, 1981.

Morton PG. Managing assault. Am J Nurs 1986;86:1114–1116.

Navis ES. Controlling violent patients before they control you. Nursing 1987;17:52–54.

Tavani-Petrone C. Psychiatric emergencies. Primary Care 1986;13:157–167.

Suicidal Patient

Cavanaugh S. Psychiatric emergencies. Med Clin North Am 1986;70:1185–1202.

Lesseig DZ. Home care for psych problems. Am J Nurs 1987;87:1317–1320.

Lewis S, McDowell WA, Gregory RJ. Saving the suicidal patient from himself. RN 1986: 26–28.

Pellitier LR, Cousins A. Clinical assessment of the suicidal patient in the emergency department. J Emerg Nurs 1984; 10:40–43.

Schmidt T. Psychiatric evaluation of self-poisoning. In: Bayer MJ, Rumack BH, eds. Poisoning and overdose. Rockville, Maryland: Aspen Publishers, 1983:121–127.

Chapter 15

SOCIAL AND LEGAL CONCERNS

VICTIMS OF DOMESTIC VIOLENCE— THE BATTERED WOMAN

Description

The extent and seriousness of domestic violence has only recently been recognized by health care providers. In 1980 in the United States alone, approximately 8 million women were involved in abusive relationships, and more than 1 million of these turned to emergency services. Battering is a common complaint in divorce cases. It occurs in all classes and cultural groups. The violence is often severe and may even be fatal; spouse murders account for up to one-fifth of all homicides.

In recent years, law enforcement agencies, the courts, and social services have made great progress in identifying battering as a significant social issue. Unfortunately, the ED* medical and nursing staffs frequently fail to recognize or act on battering. It is estimated that only 1 in 30 battered women is identified during treatment in the ED. The battered woman is often given symptomatic treatment because her complaints are taken at face value and causal factors are not considered.

Assessment

History
The victims of domestic violence are overwhelmingly women. They often have a pattern of repeated ED visits. ED nurses often become aware of

---

*See "Appendix A" for definition of common abbreviations used in the text.

290

the patients because of repeated visits and injuries or history that generate suspicion. The nurses' support and sensitivity will aid the patient in her decision to seek counselling and, possibly, legal intervention.

, A battered woman coming to the ED has just been severely traumatized and is in physical and emotional pain. She often feels ashamed and fears ridicule and humiliation if she admits to being beaten by her husband or boyfriend. She may feel guilty, believing that she was responsible for the beating (dinner wasn't ready, the kids were crying, etc.). She may have been threatened with further violence if she tells the truth. All of these feelings may prevent her from telling her true story. As a consequence, the ED staff not only must maintain a high index of suspicion but also must question the patient gently. The following information obtained during triage history will raise the suspicion that the patient is battered:

1. Frequency of ED visits - Ask the patient if she has used other emergency treatment facilities and request the patient's medical record.
2. Injury and history that are incongruous, i.e., multiple injury sites from a fall, black eye from walking into a door.
3. Depression and/or previous suicide attempts - The woman feels hopeless, trapped. She may give reasons for her depression, e.g., she has been going through some hard times, or her husband lost his job; or her delay in seeking treatment; i.e., the patient may have been too fearful or may actually have been prevented from seeking treatment.
4. Vague somatic complaints such as muscle aches, headaches, insomnia, dysphagia, hyperventilation, and palpitations - These signs of fear and stress are all too easily passed over in a busy ED. The patient may be seen as a hypochondriac.
5. Pregnancy - Battering often starts or is escalated during pregnancy. The abuser sees the prospect of an infant as a threat to his control and having his needs met. The battering may focus on the abdomen with the pregnant patient complaining of abdominal pain and bleeding. Battered women have a higher frequency of spontaneous abortion than do other women.
6. Multiple trauma to the trunk - Most accidental trauma involves the extremities. In addition, there are very few ways other than assault to sustain injuries to multiple sites, particularly bilateral injuries.

Physical Findings
General - The woman may be agitated, hysterical, or fearful.
Vital signs - Note hyperventilation or tachycardia.
Skin - Note location and size of traumatic lesions and signs of old or healing injuries.
Trauma signs - Do a complete physical examination with the patient disrobed, and look for signs of trauma.

Intervention

1. Provide a safe, supportive environment. Interview and examine the patient in a private treatment area. The battered woman is often brought to the hospital by an aggressive, seemingly overprotective male companion who is frightened that he may have seriously injured her or that she may implicate him. This situation should add to the staff's suspicion that the patient is battered. Stay with the patient, acknowledge the male companion's concern, but inform him he has to wait outside the treatment area. If necessary, call hospital security officers to assist. Approach the patient with empathy and concern. Avoid being judgmental if the patient denies being battered or if she sees herself as the cause of the abuse. Consider the following nursing diagnosis in planning interventions: ineffective individual coping, ineffective family coping, anxiety, fear, potential for injury, hopelessness, powerlessness, spiritual distress, social isolation, posttrauma response, potential for violence.

2. Documentation of injuries - Carefully describe the patient's injuries by using a body chart, if available. Use the patient's own words to document how the injury took place. If the patient's explanation is inconsistent with the injury, ask her in a direct, caring manner if at home she is ever hit or if her boyfriend or husband loses his temper, etc. Photographs can be taken after the woman signs consent; many hospitals have a Polaroid camera available in the ED for this purpose. Assure the patient that the pictures will be sealed, secured, and retained by the hospital until she requests that they be released to the legal authorities. Date and label the pictures. Other evidence of the beating, such as bloody or torn clothing, should be collected in a paper (not plastic) bag and labelled. The battered woman will need all of this as evidence when she goes to court.

3. Counselling and crisis intervention - Once the patient has been examined and has received medical treatment, the physician or nurse seeing the patient should inform the social worker assigned to the ED. The social worker should assume responsibility for crisis intervention, act as a patient advocate, and arrange for future counselling. When no social worker is available, it is the responsibility of the physician or nurse to see that a safe disposition is arranged. If the woman feels that she can return home, she should be given literature about facilities available to assist battered women, as well as any phone numbers that might be of assistance in the future. She should be informed of her legal options for protection of herself and her children, as well as her right to request a copy of her chart and any photographs.

4. Protective services - If she cannot go home, she should be assisted in

finding shelter or in locating a friend or relative with whom she and her children can stay temporarily. She should be advised not to leave any children behind (a neglect charge may be brought against her, and she may lose custody) and not to stay with a nonrelated male (construed as adultery). If she has no place to go, she should be held in the ED until a social worker is available.

Ask the patient if she wants you to call the police. The police are required by law to take down her complaint if she wishes to press criminal charges. If she has an order of protection from family or criminal court, they must make an arrest upon her request. She has a right to police escort to her house to pick up children, clothes, etc. Find out what precinct she lives in before calling the police. Hospital security officers can be helpful in this regard.

Patients should not be sent home with tranquilizers or sedating pain medication. A battered woman's survival may depend on her ability to think and react quickly.

If a battered woman is admitted to the hospital, the medical and nursing staff should be informed that she is a battered woman. This is essential so that her personal safety in the hospital can be assured and adequate discharge planning can be done.

ED Discharge Planning

One of the most frustrating aspects of caring for battered women is that many of them will return to their batterers after leaving the ED. The problems these women face are complex and often involve emotional or financial ties to the batterer, fear of retaliation, or feelings of guilt. Many women will return to the home in the hope that improved behavior on their part or on the part of the batterer will help them avoid future episodes of violence. Medical personnel must maintain a sense of perspective when confronted with this situation and must avoid blaming the battered woman for her victimization. Providing an atmosphere that preserves a woman's dignity and respects her capacity for self-determination is the main goal. The supportive treatment she receives during one ED visit may give her the ability to seek further protective and/or legal intervention in the future.

The discharge plan should be a collaborative effort by the physician, nurse, and social worker. Prior to discharge, the patient should:

1. Be given a list of counselling services available in the hospital and community.
2. Be given the number for an emergency hotline:
   Domestic Violence Hotline - 1-800-942-6906

Spanish Domestic Violence Hotline - 1-800-942-6908
Local Department of Social Services Protective Services for Adults
Child Abuse and Maltreatment Reporting Center - 1-800-342-3720
Victims' Service Agency
3. Be encouraged to develop resources she may need in the future, e.g., extra keys, driver's license, identification, birth certificate, social security card, money, friend/family she can go to in an emergency.
4. Know to go to any ED, and call an ambulance or the police, if injured.

HOMELESS PATIENT

Description

The "homeless" currently constitute one of our nation's most urgent social, medical, and mental health problems. Their number has reached epidemic proportions (up to 2 million), and these individuals appear with increasing frequency in the ED. Many are homeless because of the "deinstitutionalization" of the state mental hospitals that has occurred over the past decade. Others are homeless because of the shortage of inexpensive, accessible housing in a time when many are unable to find work. The homeless population in the 1980s is composed of a higher number of young adults (30–35 years), women, children, and adolescents than in previous years. As a group, the homeless have many individual as well as shared public health problems.

In addition to medical diseases associated with aging, the homeless person must additionally suffer the stresses of malnutrition, trauma, exposure, and social isolation. Common medical problems encountered include:

1. Hypothermia
2. Frostbite
3. Seizures
4. Trauma
5. Food poisoning
6. Drug overdose
7. Alcohol abuse and its complications
8. Tuberculosis (TB)
9. Viral hepatitis
10. Lice and scabies
11. Leg ulcers
12. Diabetes and its complications
13. Congestive heart failure
14. Pregnancy

Many of these patients suffer some mental impairment (one study estimated up to 85% are impaired), ranging from psychiatric disorders to organic neurologic deficits. Prolonged exposure to the stress of being homeless encourages development of psychiatric disorders. A frequent problem is that of noncompliance—the homeless person may not be able or willing to follow the necessary medical regimen to maintain or regain a state of health.

Assessment

History

When taking a history from a homeless person, the practitioner must be sensitive to the possibility that the person may be chronically confused, may be intimidated or angered by the medical bureaucracy, or may be reluctant or ashamed to reveal details. It is the role of the practitioner to be gentle and nonjudgmental while eliciting the history of the present illness. Previous medical history should focus on major disease, such as heart, lung, or kidney disease. A history of drug or alcohol abuse should be quantified.

Physical Findings

General - Note mental status, gait, and signs of nutritional deficiency (cachexia, bloating).

Vital signs - Always check a temperature in addition to blood pressure, pulse, and respirations.

Head - Check for signs of trauma. Look for nits or scalp lesions suggestive of lice.

Extremities - Look carefully for skin ulcers. Note pedal edema or track marks. Look for the burrows of scabies.

Intervention

Facilitating entry into the health care system - The homeless, who often suffer from feelings of powerlessness, isolation, distrust, and fear, may have limited ability to cope with or comply with the bureaucracy of the health care system. Payment for care, long waiting time, disinterest and disrespect of hospital staff, and limited hospital resources and beds all impede care of the homeless. Community health clinics, which also furnish shelter, clothing, and social services, are an effective alternative to ED care for many patients. Clinics operated in shelters, such as that conducted by Elmhurst Hospital Center at a women's shelter in New York City, has a record of improved patient compliance and the availability of all hospital resources. Homeless patients suffer from many of the medical and psychiatric problems listed elsewhere in this text. However, several disorders warrant brief mention here.

Frostbite - Damage to the hands, feet, and face can be caused by exposure to cold. Dampness and wind accelerate frostbite even when the temperature outside is not below freezing. Black patients are more severely affected. People whose judgment and mentation are impaired by alcohol or other drugs are at increased risk. Edema, anemia, malnutrition, poor local circulation, cigarette smoking, alcohol, or other drugs (psychotropic agents) increase the risks and complications of hypothermia. The first effects of cold exposure are pallor and numbness of the skin. Mild frostbite turns the skin a reddish or bluish color; blisters may be seen, but the underlying tissue retains resiliency. Severe frostbite causes loss of both sensation and movement, and the underlying tissue has a hard wooden consistency. Mild frostbite may be treated by immersing the affected area in water no warmer than body temperature. Rubbing or exposure to greater heat or cold may cause more damage and should not be performed. Severe frostbite may be treated by immersion in warm water (104–107°F) for 15–20 minutes. The patient should not attempt to use the affected parts. Restriction of cigarettes and good nutrition will enhance recovery. Treatment with antiprostaglandin preparations and those containing aloe vera is now advised. Follow-up is essential, as the degree of damage may be difficult to assess initially. Common complications include gangrene, severe infection, and loss of substantial amounts of tissue.

Lice - Lice can be found on the head or body or in pubic area. Head lice deposit white eggs called nits, which are attached closely to the base of the hair. The lice bite the scalp and cause itching. On examination, tiny bite marks and nits are often seen. Remember that dandruff will shake off; nits will not. Body lice are small black or brown insects that live in clothing, particularly in the seams. They are not adherent to the body and can be brushed off. Pubic lice are found in the short hairs of the trunk and thighs. Lice are readily spread by exchange of clothing, combs, hats, and close physical contact. Treatment for lice is either pyrethrins (A-200 or RID) or lindane or gammabenzene hexachloride (Kwell). Because Kwell, if used incorrectly, is potentially toxic, the pyrethrins are preferable in these patients. The hair should be shampooed and then combed out with a fine-tooth comb to get out the nits. If the hair is too matted to comb, it must be cut. Eyelashes or brows can be treated with Vaseline applied thickly twice daily for 8 days. Body lice can be killed with pyrethrin cream or lotion applied diffusely during a shower; the lather is left on for 15 minutes and then rinsed off. Contaminated clothing must be washed in hot water and then placed in a dryer or ironed; the heat will kill the lice.

Scabies - Scabies is caused by mites that burrow under the skin and cause itching and small, linear, gray-white marks where they burrow. Look for scabies between the fingers, on the wrists, behind the knees, on the elbows, and on the borders of the buttocks and waist. Treatment is with Kwell applied diffusely after a shower; the medicine should be left on for 24 hours and then removed completely. Pregnant or nursing women or their infants should not be treated with Kwell. Alternative therapies include precipitated sulfur in petrolatum applied nightly for 3 nights and crotamiton cream (Eurax) applied twice in 48 hours.

TB - Any homeless person suspected of having active TB will require in-patient antibiotic treatment. Patients previously diagnosed with TB who have been discharged are frequently noncompliant with their medications. In some cities (e.g., New York), the Bureau of Tuberculosis Control provides all treatment free, and such bureaus may need to be contacted. Patients who have been noncompliant should be examined carefully to determine whether they are contagious. TB is often the presenting illness in AIDS patients, so HIV testing should be performed.

Admission Criteria

Any homeless patient with acute disease or an acute exacerbation of chronic disease will probably require inpatient hospitalization. Homeless patients who might be released to follow complex or rigorous outpatient regimens should generally be admitted. ED staff must not be afraid to admit patients for social reasons. A large number of homeless or socially disadvantaged patients turn out to have significant medical illness when properly evaluated. Hospitalization may offer the homeless person the opportunity not only to regain health but also to make contact with necessary social services.

Unfortunately, some of these patients may refuse hospitalization. Unless the homeless person has been judged incompetent in a court of law or he or she constitutes an immediate threat to himself or herself or to others, the person has the right to refuse medical treatment or hospital admission. The legality of public policies on the mandatory sheltering of homeless persons during hazardous environmental conditions and for markedly asocial behavior is still being challenged in the courts.

SUGGESTED READINGS

Victims of Domestic Violence—The Battered Woman

Campbell JC, Sheridan DJ. Emergency nursing interventions with battered women. J Emerg Nurs 1989;15:12–17.

Helton A. Battering during pregnancy. Am J Nurs 1986;86:910–913.

Lifflander A, McMurray J, Siegel G, Smith AR, Osborn H. The battered woman: an unrecognized medical emergency. Hosp Physician 1983;10–25.

Loeb L. Spouse abuse. NY State J Med 1989;89:141–142.

Moehling KS. Battered women and abusive partners: treatment issues and strategies. J Psychosoc Nurs Ment Health Serv 1988;26:9–16.

Homeless Patient

Brider P. Too poor to pay: the scandal of patient dumping. Am J Nurs 1987;87:1447–1449.

Danis DM. Bringing nursing care to homeless guests: Barbara McInnis and the Pine Street Inn's Nurses Clinic. J Emerg Nurs 1987;13:26A–30A.

Gilligan ME, Lyman A. Management of lice and scabies. In: Rafferty M, et al, eds. The shelter worker's handbook. New York: Coalition for the Homeless,1983:38–52.

Goldfrank L. Exposure: thermoregulatory disorders in the homeless patient. In: Brickner PW, Scharer LK, Conanan B, Elvy A, Savarese M, eds. Health care of homeless people. New York: Springer Publishing, 1985:57–75.

Chapter 16

EMERGENCY PROCEDURES

PERIPHERAL VENOUS ACCESS

Preparation

1. Inform the patient of the need for an IV* line.
2. Select an IV site and type of catheter. Consider patient preference, movement, type and duration of solution. The cephalic, basilic, and antecubital veins and the dorsal veins of the hand are most commonly used. Because of a higher rate of complications, do not use leg and foot veins unless you consult the physician.
   a. Butterfly or scalp vein needles are best for short-term therapy. This needle has a lower rate of infection but can be easily dislodged and infiltrated. It should not be used for vasopressors, blood, or drugs that can cause tissue necrosis if infiltrated.
   b. Catheter within needle is used for long-term IV infusions. It has a higher rate of infection, and care must be taken to prevent shearing of the catheter against the needle.
   c. Catheter over needle is for long-term therapy. It provides a secure, relatively low infiltration rate but is associated with a higher rate of phlebitis than is the butterfly needle.
3. Assemble equipment including tourniquet, needle/catheter, solution tubing and bag, alcohol/povidone-iodine, antibiotic ointment, 4 × 4-inch gauze, and tape. Set up infusion and prime the tubing. Choose the smallest gauge IV catheter appropriate: 14–16 gauge for hypotension, 18–20 gauge for hydration.

---

*See "Appendix A" for definition of common abbreviations used in the text.

Procedure

1. Wash hands and wear gloves as indicated by hospital policy and the patient's condition.
2. Apply the tourniquet a few inches above the selected site; the arterial pulse should still be palpable.
3. Palpate the vein. If the vein is not sufficiently dilated, tap lightly or have the patient open and close his or her fist several times.
4. Prep the skin and hold the skin taut.
5. Puncture the skin slightly below and to the side of the vein, at a 15° angle, with the bevel of the needle upward (Fig. 16.1).
6. Blood return indicates the needle is within the vein.
7. According to the type of IV device, advance the needle or catheter into the vein. Be cautious not to damage or bend the catheter during insertion.
8. Connect the IV tubing to the needle/catheter and regulate the flow.
9. Tape the IV needle/catheter and short loop of tubing in place. Apply a small sterile gauze or clear dressing over the IV site. Do not obscure or overly tape the insertion site, so infiltration can be easily detected. If the patient is restless or uncooperative, apply an IV board.
10. Label the IV site (date, time, size of IV device), and document the procedure in the patient's record.

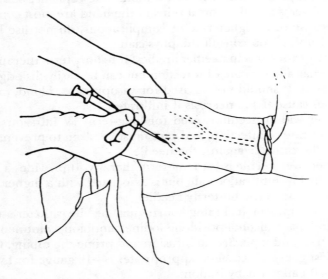

Figure 16.1. Peripheral vein cannulation. (From Simon RR, Brenner BE. Procedures and techniques in emergency medicine. Baltimore: Williams & Wilkins, 1982.)

MILITARY ANTISHOCK TROUSERS (MAST) SUIT

The MAST suit is an inflatable suit that, when placed around the abdomen and/or legs, will increase peripheral resistance (afterload) and elevate the blood pressure (Fig. 16.2). This autotransfusion effect will increase the patient's preload and augment perfusion of the heart, lungs, and brain. The MAST suit is used to treat patients in hypovolemic and/or hemorrhagic shock (see "Shock" in Chapter 1 for further discussion). In addition to the effects on blood pressure, the MAST suit can aid in the control of abdominal and lower extremity bleeding by pressure tamponade. The MAST suit also provides increased stabilization for pelvic and extremity fractures.

The MAST suit is contraindicated in conditions in which increased venous return would be detrimental, such as, increased intracranial pressure, congestive heart failure, pulmonary edema, tension pneumothorax, and possible pregnancy.

Procedure

1. If the patient is alert, explain what you are about to do.
2. Take baseline vital signs.
3. Remove any sharp objects that could injure the patient or puncture the suit.
4. Place the patient on the suit by log rolling or lifting the patient and sliding the suit under the patient. Position the suit so the upper edge is just below the rib cage; any higher placement could interfere with respirations.
5. Fasten the suit around both legs and abdomen, check that all valves are open, and connect the foot pump.
6. Inflate the suit to the desired level, usually 100 mm Hg. Start with one leg, then the other, followed by the abdominal compartment. If the suit is overinflated, the pressure release valve will cause air to escape.
7. Close the valve stopcocks and monitor the patient's blood pressure.
8. Continue monitoring vital signs while administering prescribed therapies for shock.
9. Have suction available; inflation of the abdominal compartment may precipitate vomiting.
10. Once the physician has determined that the patient's condition is sufficiently stable, gradual deflation can begin.
11. Deflate the abdominl compartment first. Slowly release air while monitoring the patient's blood pressure at frequent intervals. If blood pressure drops 5 mm Hg, stop deflation, increase fluid, and/or wait until blood pressure stabilizes at the predeflation level. Continue

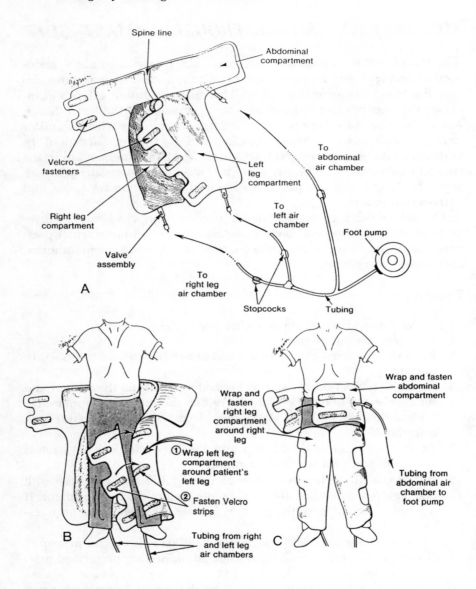

Figure 16.2. *A:* The garment is opened and spread with the left leg overlying the right, ready to receive the patient. Place the patient on the garment, supine, with the top of the abdominal section resting just below the lowest rib. *B:* Individual compartments are wrapped and secured with Velcro strips, beginning with the left leg, and the tubing is connected to the foot pump. *C:* After all indicated compartments are closed, the valves are opened and the garment is inflated, again beginning with the legs. A pop-off valve or needle gauge regulate the final pressure attained. (From Wilkins EW, et al, eds. MGH textbook of emergency medicine. 2nd ed. Baltimore: Williams & Wilkins, 1983).

to deflate the suit's abdominal compartment, then deflate one leg at a time according to the 5-mm Hg precaution.

EMERGENCY AIRWAY MANAGEMENT: CRICOTHYROIDOTOMY

A cricothyroidotomy is a surgical opening or puncture through the cricothyroid membrane into the trachea. Since the procedure is performed under emergency circumstances, preparation time is at a minimum. A tracheostomy tray (scalpel, tracheal dilator, 4 × 4-inch gauze, Jackson tracheostomy tubes) plus povidone-iodine and a large-gauge (11–12-gauge) needle in catheter is assembled, if available.

Assist the physician with the procedure:

1. Position the patient supine with head and back extended (in the absence of cervical trauma).
2. The patient should be closely monitored for blood pressure, pulse, and cardiac rhythm.
3. Administer oxygen by any means possible.
4. After the neck is prepped, the physician will locate the thyroid and cricoid cartilages as shown (Fig. 16.3). The narrow space between the cartilages is the cricothyroid membrane, the midline of which will be the puncture site. Have local anesthetic available.
5. A large-gauge needle puncture or incision is made in the cricothyroid membrane. A cricothyroidotomy permits the placement of a small (4–5-French) tracheostomy tube (Fig. 16.4).
6. Once properly positioned, the catheter or tracheostomy tube is se-

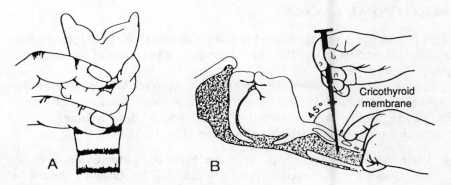

Figure 16.3. Needle cricothyroidotomy. (*B* is from Simon RR, Brenner BE. Procedures and techniques in emergency medicine. Baltimore: Williams & Wilkins, 1982.)

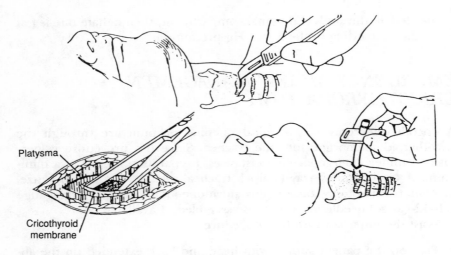

Platysma

Cricothyroid
membrane

Figure 16.4.   Cricothyrotomy. (From Rosen P, Sternbach GL. Atlas of emergency medicine. Baltimore: Williams & Wilkins, 1980.)

cured, and oxygen is administered by bag, high-frequency jet apparatus, or manually controlled oxygen valve.
7. Auscultate the patient bilaterally for breath sounds, and check vital signs.
8. Monitor the patient for possible complications of the procedure, including bleeding and subcutaneous emphysema.

ABDOMINAL AND PELVIC PROCEDURES

PERITONEAL LAVAGE

This procedure is primarily performed on patients with multiple or blunt abdominal trauma in an effort to determine the presence of bleeding into the peritoneal cavity.

Assemble the equipment, i.e., an abdominal tap set, lavage catheter, lidocaine 1% with epinephrine, povidone-iodine, normal saline or Ringer's lactate, IV tubing (without backflow valve), and a 50-ml syringe.

Assist the physician with the procedure (Fig. 16.5):

1. Place the patient in a supine position. Have the patient void, if possible. Consult the physician about whether a Foley catheter should be inserted.
2. The area immediately below the umbilicus is prepped, draped, and infiltrated with a local anesthetic containing epinephrine (to minimize local bleeding).

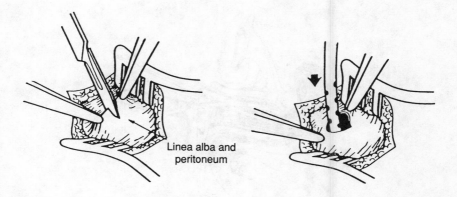

Linea alba and
peritoneum

Figure 16.5. Peritoneal lavage. (From Simon RR, Brenner BE. Procedures and techniques in emergency medicine. Baltimore: Williams & Wilkins, 1982.)

3. A 2–3-cm incision is made through the skin, subcutaneous tissue, and fascia. A small cut is then made in the peritoneum, and the dialysis catheter is inserted through the opening.
4. A 50-ml syringe is then attached to the catheter and aspirated for blood. More than 20 ml of frank blood is considered a positive result. If less than 20 ml of blood is aspirated, a liter of IV solution will be instilled through the catheter. If condition permits, gently move the patient from side to side to disperse the solution. To drain, lower the tubing and bag below the abdomen and open the clamp (glass IV bottles will need to be vented). Aspirant may be analyzed for RBC, WBC, bile, amylase, and Gram stain/culture. A RBC of >100,000/ml, a WBC of >500/ml, or the presence of bile is considered positive.
5. The wound is sutured closed, and a sterile dressing is applied. The catheter may be left indwelling, if properly secured, for repeat lavage later.

CULDOCENTESIS

This procedure is performed to determine the presence of blood in the posterior cul-de-sac of the pelvic cavity.

Assemble the equipment needed, i.e., a vaginal speculum and a 20-ml syringe with a long, 18-gauge needle.

Assist the physician with the procedure (Fig. 16.6):

1. Have the patient void before the procedure. Ask the physician about whether a Foley catheter should be inserted.
2. Assist the patient into the lithotomy position. Give a brief explanation of the procedure.

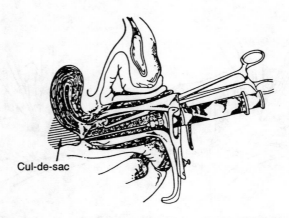

Cul-de-sac

Figure 16.6. Culdocentesis. (From Wilkins EW, et al, eds. MGH textbook of emergency medicine. 2nd ed. Baltimore: Williams & Wilkins, 1983.)

3. With a speculum in the vagina, the cervix is displaced anteriorly via a tenaculum.
4. The vaginal mucosa of the posterior cul-de-sac is punctured with a long, 18-gauge needle on a 16- or 20-ml syringe and aspirated as shown (Fig. 16.6).
5. A positive result is usually considered to be more than 2 ml of nonclotting blood for ruptured ectopic pregnancy. Pus indicates pelvic infection. Serosanguineous fluid suggests a ruptured ovarian cyst.

ELECTRICAL DEFIBRILLATION AND SYNCHRONIZED CARDIOVERSION

ELECTRICAL DEFIBRILLATION

Defibrillation is an emerency procedure. It is considered the most effective modality to treat ventricular fibrillation.

Preparation

The defibrillator as well as all emergency equipment should be checked for proper operation and needed supplies on a regular basis (every tour of duty). An ED needs at least two defibrillators, one of which should be battery operated and can be used for transport of critical patients. The ED defibrillator should contain an oscilloscope, pediatric (8.0-cm) and adult paddles (internal as well as external), and synchronizing capacity.

Procedure

Once the decision has been made to defibrillate the patient:

1. Apply conductive jelly or commercial pads to defibrillator paddles. Be sure to use only enough jelly to cover the paddles; excess jelly on the chest can cause some of the current to be misdirected.
2. Turn on the machine and set the energy level (i.e., 200 watt-sec or J initially, to 360 watt-sec maximum), and press the button to charge the paddles. Announce that the paddles are charged.
3. Place the paddles on the patient's chest: one just below the right clavicle, the other paddle at the fifth intercostal level at the anterior axillary line. Hold the paddles firmly in place, using approximately 25 pounds of pressure.
4. Survey the area to ensure that no staff member is in direct or indirect contact with the patient. Remove the oxygen source from immediate vicinity of defibrillation. Call out "all clear."
5. Deliver the charge by pressing both discharge buttons simultaneously.
6. Assess the patient for rhythm and pulse, and be prepared to repeat defibrillation.

SYNCHRONIZED CARDIOVERSION

Electrical cardioversion is used under urgent circumstances to treat hemodynamically unstable ventricular and supraventricular arrhythmias. Remember that the patient is awake; provide reassurance and support during the procedure.

Procedure

1. If condition permits, explain the procedure to the patient, and obtain written consent.
2. In addition to the defibrillator with synchronizing capacity, assemble emergency cardiac equipment and drugs, and notify the anesthesiologist to be on standby.
3. Check the IV line for patency, and administer a sedative (diazepam, brevital) as ordered.
4. Turn on the machine and attach the patient monitoring cable to the patient. Check operation of synchronization circuit. Make sure that the indicator light or beeper corresponds to each QRS complex.
5. Set the energy level desired, i.e., low settings initially (50 watt-sec for atrial fibrillation, SVT, and ventricular tachycardia), and increase the energy level, if necessary, in 50-watt-sec increments.
6. Place the paddles, observe for safety precautions, and deliver the cur-

rent as for defibrillation. The charge is delivered during the QRS complex by the synchronization circuit of the defibrillator.
7. If this is not successful, the energy level can be increased, and cardioversion can be repeated.
8. When the procedure is concluded, turn the synchronization switch back to defibrillate.

AUTOTRANSFUSION

Autotransfusion provides a system by which the patient's own blood can be collected, filtered, and reinfused. Used intraoperatively and in the ED during trauma resuscitation, it is primarily performed for hemothorax. Many manufacturers of chest drainage systems have inexpensive, easily set up autotransfusion attachments (Fig. 16.7).

Assemble the equipment needed, i.e., a chest tube, chest drainage set, autotransfusion collection bottle, and blood filter.

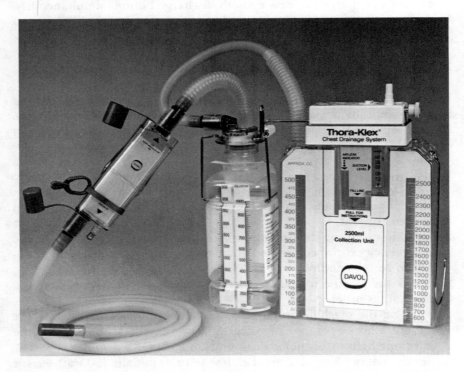

Figure 16.7. Chest drainage system with autotransfusion setup. (Reprinted with permission of Davol Corporation.)

Procedure

1. Prepare the chest drainage system, and set the vacuum pressure between 15 and 30 mm Hg to reduce hemolysis.
2. Blood obtained from a hemothorax does not require the addition of an anticoagulant. If the source of blood is uncertain, a regional anticoagulant, commonly citrate phosphate dextrose (CPD), is added before and during the blood collection.
3. Once the chest tube is inserted and is draining blood, the autotransfusion collection bottle with in-line filter can be attached. (Consult the manufacturer's instructions.)
4. To reinfuse the blood, the chest tube is clamped, and the collection bottle is detached from the chest drainage system.
5. An infusion filter and tubing is attached, the collection bottle is inverted, and the blood is ready for administration.
6. Whenever the collection bottle is attached to the chest drainage system, the chest tube must be clamped to avoid loss of vacuum, and when the collection bottle is removed, the chest tube must be reconnected to the underwater seal.

ARTERIAL PRESSURE MONITORING

Initiation of arterial pressure monitoring provides the constant display of the patient's systolic, diastolic, and mean pressures. The monitor will also provide a visual and audio alarm when pressures deviate from preset limits. The arterial catheter provides easy access to blood samples. Assemble the equipment needed, i.e., a pressure monitoring kit (containing pressure tubing, transducer, dome, flush device, and three-way stopcocks), pressure infusor bag, transducer mount, 500-ml bag of normal saline (with 500–1000 units of heparin, if ordered).

Preparation

1. Wash hands and assemble all equipment.
2. Open the pressure monitoring kit, and check all connections. Insert the IV tubing spike into the 500-ml normal saline and invert the bag. Squeeze the bag until all air is removed, and close the tubing clamp.
3. Place the saline bag in the pressure infusor, and hang it from the IV pole.
4. If tubing, transducer, and monitoring cable must be assembled, see the manufacturer's instructions.
5. Using a continuous flush device, flush all pressure tubing, including stopcock ports. Hold the port upright to remove air when flushing,

and replace open-end caps with dead-end caps. Flush tubing slowly under minimal pressure, as rapid flushing causes turbulence and air bubbles. Tapping the tubing or dome can displace air bubbles.

6. Check all tubing for the absence of air bubbles, and inflate the pressure infusor bag to 300 mm Hg.
7. The pressure monitor system is connected to the cardiac monitor via a transducer cable. The end of the pressure tubing can be connected to the arterial catheter, once inserted.

NURSING CONSIDERATIONS

1. Equipment assembly and catheter insertion must be done under aseptic conditions. Mishandling with consequent contamination of stopcock ports and caps is a frequent source of infection.
2. The patient's arterial blood supply to the hand should be checked by the Allen test prior to insertion of a radial artery catheter to ensure that collateral circulation is adequate. During monitoring, check the involved site and distal extremity for color, temperature, and movement.
3. Check the system for leaks, air bubbles, and infuser pump pressure (300 mm Hg).
4. Zero and calibrate to the monitor (according to the manufacturer's instructions) at least once every 8 hours and whenever there has been a disruption in the system.
5. To zero, check that the transducer is at the height of the right atrium, close the stopcock nearest the patient, open the stopcock nearest the transducer to air, and press the zero button on the monitor. When the zeroing and calibration are complete, close the stopcock near the transducer, open the stopcock to the patient, and pull the flush device. Check the wave form.
6. Keep the arterial catheter site in view so that any disconnections or bleeding will be promptly noticed.
7. Secure the arm to an IV board, if needed, but do not obscure the insertion site.
8. Observe the wave form for loss of pressure or decreased acuity (damping) of the wave form. If this is present, assess the patient, and take a cuff blood pressure; if the wave form remains unchanged, check the pressure monitoring system for leaks and air or blood in the tubing. If the wave form remains depressed, notify the physician; the arterial catheter may be displaced.

EXTERNAL PACING

With the advent of new technology, external electric pacing has proven to be a safe and easily employed technique. External pacemakers have many features in common with temporary transvenous pacemakers. External pacers consist of two large pacing electrode pads, an ECG monitor scope, a strip recorder, and a battery power pack. The pacemakers can be used for up to a few hours on conscious or unconscious patients. External pacing may cause varying degrees of discomfort which may limit its use in some conscious patients.

Procedure

1. Connect the external pacemaker monitoring electrodes to the patient. Consult the manufacturer's instructions prior to use.
2. Turn on the monitor and adjust the size of the wave form. Verify that the QRS indicator shows detection of each QRS complex.
3. Apply back and front electrode pads before connection of the pacing output cable (Fig. 16.8).
4. Set the pacer to the 1:1 (pacing) or 4:1 (temporary testing) mode.
5. Set the pacemaker rate. The usual setting is 10–20 beats/min above the patient's intrinsic rate.
6. Turn on the pacer power switch.
7. Observe the pacing artifact on the ECG monitor/tracing and verify that it is occurring during mid to late diastole.
8. Slowly increase the pacer output. Range: 0–140 milliamps (mA).
9. Determine the milliamps at which capture occurs. Capture is noted when the pacer artifact is followed by an ectopic QRS complex (Fig.

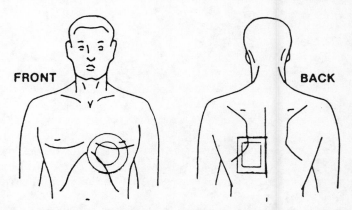

FRONT   BACK

Figure 16.8. Electrode placement. (Reproduced with permission of ZMI Corporation.)

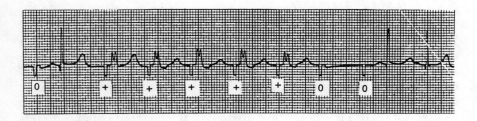

Figure 16.9. External pacing rhythm strip. The negative deflection is the transcutaneous pacing artifact. As the milliamps are adjusted higher, the ineffective pacing (0) stimuli will be replaced with effective pacing (+) beats. Note that paced beats have a wide aberrant ORS. (Reproduced with permission of ZMI Corporation.)

    16.9). The pacer output is commonly set at 10% above the capture threshold. The usual pacemaker output setting is between 40 and 60 mA. Electrode placement will effect patient comfort as well as the output current required to achieve capture.

10. Avoid touching the gelled electrode area while pacing.
11. Set high and low alarm limits and activate the alarm.

APPENDICES

Appendix A
Common Abbreviations

a	Before
A–a	Alveolar-arterial
ab	Abortion
Ab	Antibody
abd	Abdomen
ABG	Arterial blood gas
ABO	Blood types
ac	Before meals
ADH	Antidiuretic hormone
ad lib	As desired
AFB	Acid-fast bacillus
Ag	Antigen
A/G ratio	Albumin/globulin ratio
AIDS	Acquired immunodeficiency syndrome
AK	Above knee
ALT	Alanine aminotransferase (SGPT)
AP	Anteroposterior, appendectomy
ARDS	Adult respiratory distress syndrome
ARF	Acute renal failure
ASA	Aspirin
ASHD	Arteriosclerotic heart disease
AST	Aspartate aminotransferase (SGOT)
AV	Atrioventricular
AVM	Arteriovenous malformation
bid	Twice daily
BK	Below knee
BMR	Basal metabolism rate
BP	Blood pressure
BPH	Benign prostatic hypertrophy
BRP	Bathroom privileges
BS	Bowel sounds
BSA	Body surface area
BUN	Blood urea nitrogen
Bx	Biopsy
c	With
Ca	Calcium
CA	Cancer
CABG	Coronary artery bypass graft
CAD	Coronary artery disease
CAT	Computerized axial tomography

CBC	Complete blood count
cc	Cubic centemeter(s)
CC	Chief complaint
CCU	Coronary care unit
CDC	Centers for Disease Control
CHF	Congestive heart failure
Cl	Chloride
cm	Centimeter(s)
CNS	Central nervous system
c/o	Complained of
CO_2	Carbon dioxide
COPD	Chronic obstructive pulmonary disease
CP	Cerebral palsy
CPAP	Continuous positive airway pressure
CPK	Creatine phosphokinase
CPR	Cardiopulmonary resuscitation
C&S	Culture and sensitivities
CSF	Cerebrospinal fluid
CVA	Cerebrovascular accident
CVAT	Costovertebral angle tenderness
CVP	Central venous pressure
Cx	Cervix
CXR	Chest x-ray
Cysto	Cystoscopy
D5W	5% dextrose in water
D50W	50% dextrose in water
D/C	Discontinue
D&C	Dilation and curettage
DI	Diabetes insipidus
DIC	Disseminated intravascular coagulopathy
Diff	Differential white blood cell count
dl	Deciliter(s) (one-tenth of a liter)
DM	Diabetes mellitus
DOA	Dead on arrival
DOE	Dyspnea on exertion
dPT	Diphtheria, pertussis, tetanus toxoid (pediatrics)
DR	Delivery room
dT	Diphtheria-tetanus toxoid (adults)
DVT	Deep vein thrombosis
Dx	Diagnosis
ECG	Electrocardiogram
ED	Emergency department
EDTA	Ethylenediaminetetraacetic acid
EEG	Electroencephalogram

EENT	Eye, ear, nose, and throat
EMD	Electromechanical dissociation
EMG	Electromyogram
EMT	Emergency medical technician
ENT	Ear, nose, and throat
EOM	Extraocular movements
Epi	Epinephrine
ER	Emergency room
ESR	Erythrocyte sedimentation rate
ETOH	Ethanol
FB	Foreign body
FBS	Fasting blood sugar
FH	Family history
F_IO_2	Forced inspiratory oxygen (concentration of O_2)
FUO	Fever of unknown origin
Fx	Fracture
GC	Gonococcus (gonorrhea)
GI	Gastrointestinal
glu	Glucose
gm	Gram(s)
gr	Grain(s)
GSW	Gunshot wound
GTT	Glucose tolerance test
gtts	Drops
GU	Genitourinary
HAA	Hepatitis-associated antigen
HAV	Hepatitis A virus
Hb	Hemoglobin
HBsAb	Hepatitis B surface antibody
HBsAg	Hepatitis B surface antigen
HBV	Hepatitis B virus
HCO_3	Bicarbonate
H_2CO_3	Carbonic acid
Hct	Hematocrit
HCTZ	Hydrochlorothiazide
HCVD	Hypertensive cardiovascular disease
HDL	High-density lipoprotein
HEENT	Head, eyes, ears, nose, and throat
Hg	Mercury
Hgb	Hemoglobin
HIV	Human immunodeficiency virus
HMO	Health maintenance organization
H/O	History of
HPI	History of present illness

hr	Hour(s)
HTN	Hypertension
hs	At bedtime
Hx	History
IABP	Intraaortic balloon counterpulsation
ICP	Intracranial pressure
ICS	Intercostal space
ICU	Intensive care unit
I&D	Incision and drainage
IDDM	Insulin-dependent diabetes mellitus
IgG	Immunoglobulin G
IgM	Immunoglobulin M
IHSS	Idiopathic hypertrophic subaortic stenosis
IM	Intramuscular(ly)
IMB	Intermenstrual bleeding
IMV	Intermittent mandatory ventilation
INH	Isoniazid (Nydrazid)
I&O	Intake and output
IPPB	Intermittent positive pressure breathing
IU	International unit(s)
IV	Intravenous(ly)
IVC	Intravenous cholangiogram, inferior vena cava
IVP	Intravenous pyelogram
J	Joule(s) (watt-sec)
K	Potassium
Kg	Kilogram(s)
KUB	Kidney, ureter, and bladder (an x-ray view)
KVO	Keep vein open
lb	Pound(s)
LBBB	Left bundle branch block
LBP	Low back pain
L/D	Labor and delivery
LDH	Lactic dehydrogenase
LDL	Low-density lipoproteins
LE prep	Lupus erythematosus prep
LFT	Liver function tests
LLL	Left lower lobe
LLQ	Left lower quadrant
LMP	Last menstrual period
LOC	Level of consciousness, loss of consciousness
LP	Lumbar puncture
LS	Lumbosacral
LVEDP	Left ventricular end-diastolic pressure
L&W	Living and well

lytes	Electrolytes
µg	Microgram(s)
m	Murmur
MAST suit	Military antishock trousers suit
mcg	Microgram(s)
MCH	Mean corpuscular hemoglobin
MCHC	Mean corpuscular hemoglobin concentration
MCP	Metacarpophalangeal joint
MCV	Mean corpuscular volume
MD	Medical doctor
mEq	Milliequivalent(s)
mg	Milligram(s)
MI	Myocardial infarction
mIU	Milli-international unit(s)
ml	Milliliter(s)
mm	Millimeter(s)
mOsm	Milliosmole(s)
MS	Multiple sclerosis
MST	Mean survival time
MVR	Mitral valve replacement
Na	Sodium
NAD	No acute distress
neb	Nebulized
NIDDM	Non-insulin-dependent diabetes mellitus
NKA	No known allergies
NMR	Nuclear magnetic resonance
NPO	Nothing by mouth
NS	Normal saline
NSR	Normal sinus rhythm
NTG	Nitroglycerin
N&V	Nausea and vomiting
NVD	Neck vein distention
O_2	Oxygen
OD	Overdose, right eye
OM	Otitis media
OOB	Out of bed
O&P	Ova and parasites
OPD	Outpatient department
OR	Operating room
ORIF	Open reduction internal fixation
OS	Left eye
OT	Occupational therapy
OU	Both eyes
p	After

PA	Posteroanterior
P&A	Percussion and auscultation
PAEDP	Pulmonary artery end-diastolic pressure
Pap	Papanicolaou smear
PAP	Pulmonary artery pressure
PBI	Protein-bound iodine
pc	After meals
Pcn	Penicillin
pCO_2	Partial pressure (tension) of carbon dioxide
P_aO_2	Partial arterial pressure of oxygen
P_AO_2	Partial alveolar pressure of oxygen
PCWP	Pulmonary capillary wedge pressure
PD	Postural drainage
PE	Physical examination
PEEP	Positive end-expiratory pressure
PERRLA	Pupils equal, round, reactive to light and accommodation
PFT	Pulmonary function test
pH	Hydrogen ion concentration
PH	Past history
PI	Present illness
Plt	Platelet
PMD	Private medical doctor
PMI	Point of maximal impulse
PMN	Polymorphonuclear leukocyte
PMP	Past menstrual period
PN	Pneumonia
PND	Paroxysmal nocturnal dyspnea
PNS	Peripheral nervous system
PO	By mouth, oral(ly)
POD	Postoperative day
PPD	Postpartum day, purified protein derivative (TB test)
prn	According to necessity
Pro time	Prothrombin time
PSP	Phenolsulfonphthalein
PSRO	Professional standards review organization
PSVT	Paroxysmal supraventricular tachycardia
PT	Prothrombin time, physical therapy
PTA	Prior to admission
PTT	Partial thromboplastin time
PVC	Premature ventricular contraction
PVD	Peripheral vascular disease
PZI	Protamine zinc insulin
qd	Every day
qh	Every hour

qhs	At bedtime
qid	Four times a day
qns	Quantity not sufficient
qod	Every other day
qoh	Every other hour
qpr	At earliest convenience
qs	As much as necessary
RA	Rheumatoid arthritis
RBBB	Right bundle branch block
RBC	Red blood count
RHD	Rheumatic heart disease
RIND	Reversible ischemic neurologic deficit
RLL	Right lower lobe
RLQ	Right lower quadrant
R/O	Rule out
ROS	Review of symptoms
RSR	Regular sinus rhythm
RUQ	Right upper quadrant
Rx	Treatment
s	Without
S&A	Sugar and acetone
SBE	Subacute bacterial endocarditis
SC	Subcutaneous(ly)
Sed rate	Sedimentation rate
SGOT	Serum glutamic oxaloacetic transaminase
SGPT	Serum glutamic pyruvic transaminase
SL	Sublingual(ly)
SLE	Systemic lupus erythematosus
SMA	Biochemical profiles done by an automatic analyzer (SMA6, SMA12, SMA18)
SOB	Short of breath
sos	Administer once if necessary
S/P	Status post (occurred in past)
SpG	Specific gravity
SR	Systems review
SSE	Soapsuds enema
stat	At once
STD	Sexually transmitted disease
STS	Serologic test for syphilis
SVT	Supraventricular tachycardia
Sx	Signs
T_3	Triiodothyronine
T_4	Thyroxine
tab	Tablet(s)

TB	Tuberculosis
TBG	Thyroxine-binding globulin
Tbsp	Tablespoon(s)
T&C	Type and cross-match
TENS	Transcutaneous electrical nerve stimulator
TIA	Transient ischemic attack
tid	Three times a day
TKO	To keep open
TM	Tympanic membrane
TP	Total protein
TPN	Total parenteral nutrition (hyperalimentation)
TPR	Temperature, pulse, respiration
T&R	Treated and released
TSP	Total serum protein
TSS	Toxic shock syndrome
TURP	Transurethral resection of prostate
Tx	Traction
u	Unit(s)
UA	Urinalysis
ung	Ointment
URI	Upper respiratory infection
US	Ultrasound
UTI	Urinary tract infection
UV	Ultraviolet
VC	Vital capacity
VDRL	Venereal disease research laboratory test
VF	Ventricular fibrillation
VNA	Visiting nurse association
VS	Vital signs
VT	Ventricular tachycardia
WBC	White blood count
WC	Wheel chair
WNL	Within normal limits
wt	Weight
w/u	Work-up
<	Less than
>	More than
#	Number

Appendix B
Classification of Patients by Acuity Level

	Emergent	Urgent	Nonurgent
Abdomen	Hypotension/orthostasis Penetrating trauma Upper or lower GI bleed Pain and fever > 102°F Moderate to severe tenderness Very severe pain	Moderate to severe pain Significant nausea/vomiting, diarrhea < 24 hours, or frequency once per hour; or dehydration Known diabetic, ulcer, jaundiced, alcoholic	Pain > 24 hours Mild to moderate nausea/vomiting/diarrhea without dehydration Hemorrhoids Abscesses
Allergies	Airway distress (wheeze, stridor, etc.) Moderate to severe facial or tongue swelling Altered mental status Hypotension	Urticaria with intense itching	Other
Back	Focal signs or paralysis < 72 hours, if nontraumatic Penetrating trauma Suspected rib Fx with abnormal VS or dyspnea	Backache with H/O direct trauma but no focal signs Fever > 101°F Uncomplicated rib Fx	Ache without history of direct trauma UTI symptoms or Sx
Breast		Mass or abscess with fever > 101°F	Mass or abscess Discharge from nipple

323

	Emergent	Urgent	Nonurgent
Burns	Airway involvement (singed nasal hair, carbonaceous sputum, involvement of mouth or throat, stridor, etc.)	Electrical shock without LOC	Partial thickness < 20% BSA
	H/O loss of consciousness (LOC)	Partial thickness > 20% BSA	
	H/O altered mental status at scene or now	Hands	
	Smoke inhalation		
	Wheezing, dyspnea, chest pain		
	Full thickness > 25% BSA		
	Caustic eye burns		
	Electrical shock with LOC		
Cardiac	Cardiac arrest	Mild to moderate CHF	Medication refill
	Chest pain	H/O heart disease with dyspnea, CHF	
	Arrhythmia	Palpitations	
	Heart rate (HR) > 140, < 50		
	Hypotension		
	BP > 120 diastolic with chest pain, dyspnea, CHF, altered mental status		
	Pulmonary edema		

Chest/respiratory	Airway distress (wheeze, stridor, can't talk) Altered mental status Respiratory rate (RR) > 30 or < 6 Penetrating trauma Cyanosis Decompensated COPD or asthma Hemoptysis > 1 teaspoon Foreign body	SOB with normal VS and mental status Cough with fever > 101°F AIDS Hx Rib Fx without SOB Hemoptysis < 1 teaspoon Difficulty swallowing	URIs Productive cough
Child abuse or battered woman	As per trauma	All others[a]	
Drug abuse/ETOH	Altered mental status[b] Coma Suicidal/homicidal[b] Ingestion of immediately life-threatening substances (e.g., cyanide, caustic agent, hydrocarbon) Delirium tremens (DTs) Respiratory depression	Fever > 101°F ETOH or sedative hypnotic withdrawal OD with normal VS and normal mental status	Narcotic withdrawal Mild intoxication without Sx or trauma Requesting detoxification

	Emergent	Urgent	Nonurgent
Ear	Battle's sign Otorrhea	Avulsion or severe laceration Trauma Earache with fever > 101°F Perforation of tympanic membrane	Tinnitus, vertigo, earache, wax, decreased hearing, otitis externa or otitis media
Extremities	Hypotension Uncontrolled bleeding Pelvic/hip Fx Neurovascular compromise Open Fx Traumatic amputation (excluding fingers/toes)	Long bone Fx Shoulder dislocation Displaced Fx Fx/dislocation Amputation of finger/toe involving a joint	Uncomplicated Fx Sprains Joint pain or swelling Simple laceration
Eye	Laceration or penetration of globe Glaucoma with headache (known case) Sudden blindness Raccoon's eyes Trauma with abnormal EOM Severe pain	Foreign body (should patch eye) Herpes Blurred vision External trauma (lids, etc.)	Conjunctivitis Stye

Genitourinary	Testicular pain with H/O trauma Testicular pain with temperature > 101°F Urinary retention	Temperature > 101°F with flank pain or CVAT, nausea/vomiting Gross hematuria Shaking chills	Dysuria, frequency Discharge, polyuria, nocturia, hematuria Other complaints
Gynecologic	Lower abdominal pain or vaginal bleeding with hypotension Missed period with abnormal VS R/O ectopic Sexual assault	Moderate to severe pain Temperature > 101°F Missed period with abdominal pain Vaginal bleeding with pain or >8 pads/day, but stable HR and BP	Vaginal discharge Vaginal bleed < 8 pads/day Missed period Request for pregnancy test (send to clinic)
Head Epistaxis	Airway distress Hypotension On anticoagulants	Significant (doesn't stop) with pressure for 10 minutes	Minor
Headache	H/O LOC or abnormal mental status Focal deficits BP of 130 diastolic Known migraine with severe pain	Sudden onset and most severe of life	Recurrent Sx for 24 hours

	Emergent	Urgent	Nonurgent
Head trauma	Altered mental status R/O skull Fx Focal deficits Neck pain/tenderness[c]	H/O LOC Facial laceration of 2 inches or involving eyelids/brows/mouth	Other
Pharyngitis	Airway distress Drooling	Difficulty swallowing	All others
Hematologic	Severe bleeding in patient with known clotting disorder or on anticoagulants Sickle cell crisis	Petechiae and/or ecchymosis Hemarthrosis	Check of clotting studies Medication refill
Neurologic	Altered mental status[d] Focal signs CVA Seizures Headache with any of above with temperature	Sx for 48–72 hours Headache for 48 hours	Sx for 72 hours Headache for 48 hours

Pain	Severe migraine Headache with abnormal mental status or focal signs Abdominal pain with peritoneal signs Sickle cell crisis with moderate to severe pain Pain with abnormal VS	Moderate to severe with normal VS	Mild to moderate Sore throat (without drooling)
Pediatrics	Convulsions Airway distress Altered mental status Stiff neck Drooling Temperature > 105°F Dehydration > 10% Trauma^e	Fever > 103°F Lethargy Dehydration < 10%	Temperature < 103°F Alert child
Psychiatric	Suicidal/homicidal^f Extreme agitation, hallucinations^f Disorientation, altered mental status, abnormal VS^g	Situational crisis Moderate to severe depression Grief	Medication refill Feeling nervous

	Emergent	Urgent	Nonurgent
Rash	Wheezing, SOB, hypotension Airway compromise Meningeal signs	Chickenpox (should be isolated)[h] Measles (should be isolated)[h] Herpes of eye Immunosuppressed Temperature of 101°F Urticaria of face	Simple urticaria and other rashes Uncomplicated zoster Athlete's foot
Skin	Urticaria with wheezes, SOB, airway compromise, hypotension	Urticaria without wheezes or SOB	Other
Trauma	Penetrating to trunk, abdomen, head Altered mental status Hypotension < 100 systolic or 60 diastolic HR > 120 Cervical spine or back trauma[i] Uncontrolled bleeding	Blunt trauma to torso or abdomen, without abnormal VS Laceration > 3 inches or involving flexor tendons	Other Laceration < 3 inches

Vital signs

Temperature	>105°F, <95°F		All other
	>101°F with altered mental status or stiff neck	>103°F with dyspnea or cough	
BP	<90 systolic or <50 diastolic >200 systolic or >130 diastolic, with CHF, chest pain, altered mental status		Hypertension (HTN) without Sx HTN with epistaxis
HR	>140, <50		
RR	>30, <8		

[a] Social Services needs to be notified, and the case needs to be presented to the attending in charge.

[b] Consider placement of mental health hold.

[c] All patients with suspected cervical spine injury must be evaluated immediately. A rigid collar and tape should be applied, if not already done. No collar should be removed prior to patient examination.

[d] All patients with altered mental status must have a "fingerstick" for blood glucose immediately; be placed on a 100% non-rebreathing mask; be seen by a MD immediately; and be given naloxone, 2 mg IVP, and thiamine, 100 mg IV. Dextrose at 50%, 50 gm IVP, should be given for "fingerstick" of 75 mg% or less, or if the "fingerstick" is not available.

[e] Joint response by trauma team and pediatric consultant.

[f] Place on mental health hold.

[g] Requires medical evaluation.

[h] Isolation may be in any room without another patient. The triage nurse should inform the head nurse of possible contagious disease so that the staff and other patients can be protected.

[i] See cervical spine protocol under "Head."

Appendix C
Triage Algorithms

ABDOMINAL PAIN

History - Pain characteristic and duration, precipitating event, trauma, bleeding, previous medical history and treatment, last menstrual period

Assessment - VS, color, skin temperature, abdominal tenderness, rigidity, rebound, amount of bleeding (pads/day); for female patients of childbearing age, obtain urine for stat pregnancy test

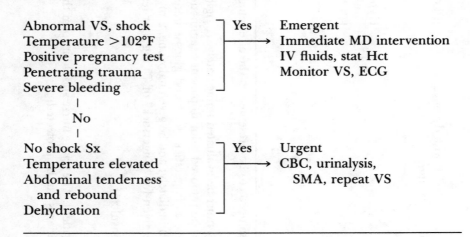

Abnormal VS, shock
Temperature >102°F
Positive pregnancy test
Penetrating trauma
Severe bleeding
    |
    No
    |
Yes → Emergent
Immediate MD intervention
IV fluids, stat Hct
Monitor VS, ECG

No shock Sx
Temperature elevated
Abdominal tenderness
   and rebound
Dehydration
Yes → Urgent
CBC, urinalysis,
   SMA, repeat VS

BACK PAIN

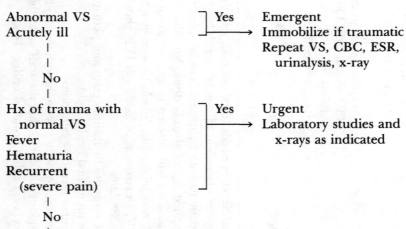

Abnormal VS
Acutely ill
    |
    |
    No
    |
Yes → Emergent
Immobilize if traumatic
Repeat VS, CBC, ESR,
   urinalysis, x-ray

Hx of trauma with
   normal VS
Fever
Hematuria
Recurrent
   (severe pain)
    |
    No
    |
Yes → Urgent
Laboratory studies and
   x-rays as indicated

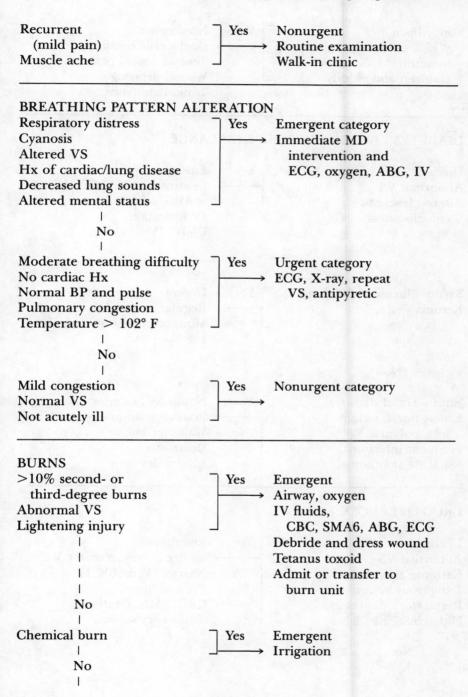

Recurrent
  (mild pain)   ] Yes   Nonurgent
Muscle ache   → Routine examination
                              Walk-in clinic

BREATHING PATTERN ALTERATION

Respiratory distress   ] Yes   Emergent category
Cyanosis   → Immediate MD
Altered VS   intervention and
Hx of cardiac/lung disease   ECG, oxygen, ABG, IV
Decreased lung sounds
Altered mental status
        |
       No
        |

Moderate breathing difficulty   ] Yes   Urgent category
No cardiac Hx   → ECG, X-ray, repeat
Normal BP and pulse   VS, antipyretic
Pulmonary congestion
Temperature > 102° F
        |
       No
        |

Mild congestion   ] Yes   Nonurgent category
Normal VS   →
Not acutely ill

BURNS

>10% second- or   ] Yes   Emergent
  third-degree burns   → Airway, oxygen
Abnormal VS   IV fluids,
Lightening injury   CBC, SMA6, ABG, ECG
        | Debride and dress wound
        | Tetanus toxoid
        | Admit or transfer to
        | burn unit
       No
        |

Chemical burn   ] Yes   Emergent
      | → Irrigation
       No
        |

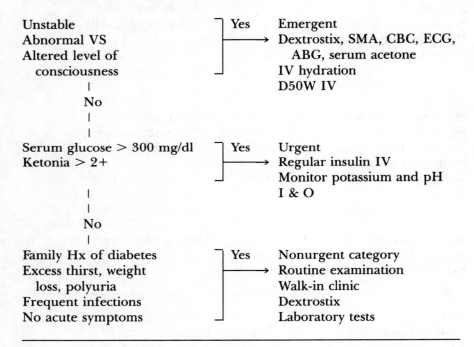

Minor burn ⎤ Yes   Nonurgent
  <15% partial thickness ⎟ ────→ Cool sterile compress
  in adult, <10% in ⎟   Tetanus toxoid prn
  children and elderly ⎦   Wound dressing
                                Topical antibiotic

DIABETES - BLOOD GLUCOSE IMBALANCE

Unstable ⎤ Yes   Emergent
Abnormal VS ⎟ ────→ Dextrostix, SMA, CBC, ECG,
Altered level of ⎟   ABG, serum acetone
  consciousness ⎦   IV hydration
  | D50W IV
  No
  |
  |
Serum glucose > 300 mg/dl ⎤ Yes   Urgent
Ketonia > 2+ ⎦ ────→ Regular insulin IV
                     Monitor potassium and pH
  | I & O
  |
  No
  |
Family Hx of diabetes ⎤ Yes   Nonurgent category
Excess thirst, weight ⎟ ────→ Routine examination
  loss, polyuria ⎟   Walk-in clinic
Frequent infections ⎟   Dextrostix
No acute symptoms ⎦   Laboratory tests

DRUG OVERDOSE

Unconscious ⎤ Yes   Emergent
Abnormal VS ⎟ ────→ Secure airway, monitor VS
Extreme agitation ⎟   Narcan IV, D50W IV
Dangerous behavior ⎟   Prevent injury
Respiratory depression ⎟   CBC, SMA, Dextrostix
Hallucinations ⎦   Toxicology screen
  |
  No
  |

Conscious	⎤ Yes	Urgent
Tremors	→	Laboratory studies
Mild withdrawal/		Ipecac/gastric lavage
symptoms		IV, specific therapy
Altered mental	⎦	
status		

EYE COMPLAINTS

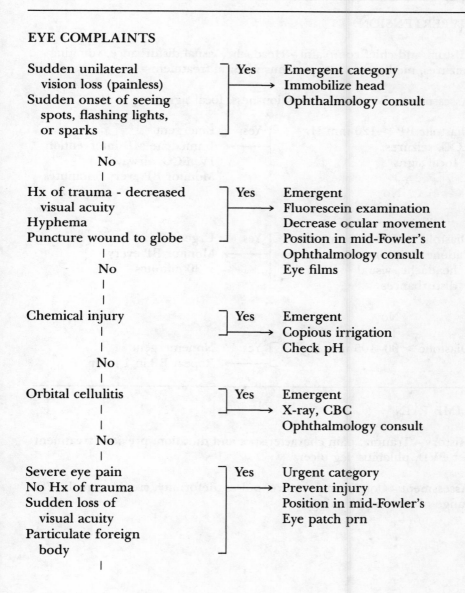

Sudden unilateral	⎤ Yes	Emergent category
vision loss (painless)	→	Immobilize head
Sudden onset of seeing		Ophthalmology consult
spots, flashing lights,		
or sparks	⎦	

No

Hx of trauma - decreased	⎤ Yes	Emergent
visual acuity	→	Fluorescein examination
Hyphema		Decrease ocular movement
Puncture wound to globe	⎦	Position in mid-Fowler's
		Ophthalmology consult
No		Eye films

Chemical injury	⎤ Yes	Emergent
	→	Copious irrigation
		Check pH
No		

Orbital cellulitis	⎤ Yes	Emergent
	→	X-ray, CBC
		Ophthalmology consult
No		

Severe eye pain	⎤ Yes	Urgent category
No Hx of trauma	→	Prevent injury
Sudden loss of		Position in mid-Fowler's
visual acuity		Eye patch prn
Particulate foreign	⎦	
body		

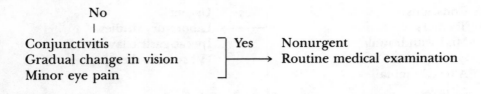

```
            No
             |
Conjunctivitis              ] Yes    Nonurgent
Gradual change in vision    ├──────→ Routine medical examination
Minor eye pain              ]
```

HYPERTENSION

History and chief complaint - Headache, visual disturbance, vomiting, seizures, medication and previous medical treatment

Assessment - BP, level of consciousness, focal signs

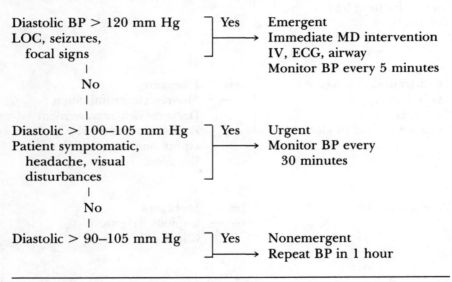

```
Diastolic BP > 120 mm Hg    ] Yes    Emergent
LOC, seizures,              ├──────→ Immediate MD intervention
    focal signs             ]        IV, ECG, airway
        |                            Monitor BP every 5 minutes
       No
        |
        |
Diastolic > 100–105 mm Hg   ] Yes    Urgent
Patient symptomatic,        ├──────→ Monitor BP every
    headache, visual        ]            30 minutes
    disturbances
        |
       No
        |
Diastolic > 90–105 mm Hg    ] Yes    Nonemergent
                            ┴──────→ Repeat BP in 1 hour
```

LIMB PAIN

History - Trauma, pain characteristics and duration, previous treatment for PVD, phlebitis, leg ulcers

Assessment - Color, temperature, pulses, deformity, crepitus, girth, VS, range of motion, bleeding.

Limb pain/trauma   ] Yes   Emergent
Abnormal VS, cold, color   → Immediate MD intervention
  (blue, blanched),   Pressure for bleeding,
  crepitus   IV fluids, and immobilize
Pulseless, open Fx   _| Monitor VS
      |
      |
      No
      |
Swelling, pain, and   ] Yes   Urgent
  positive pulses   → Immobilize (wheelchair,
Mobility   _| sling)
                                X-ray (trauma)

MULTIPLE TRAUMA

Abnormal VS   ] Yes   Emergent
Unconscious   → Secure airway, O_2
Severe injury   _| Protect cervical spine
      | Monitor VS and ECG
      | Surgical evaluation
      | Hct (spun), ABG, T&C,
      | 2 IV lines
      No   Urinalysis,
      | Lateral cervical spine
      | x-ray
Head injury   ] Yes   Urgent
Hx of loss of   → Immobilize neck
  consciousness   _| Monitor VS
      | Cervical spine and skull
      No   films
      | Slow IV fluid
      |
Extremity injury   ] Yes   Urgent
Lacerations   → Pressure for bleeding
                                Splint
                                Distal pulses
                                CBC
                                Surgery consult

SEIZURE DISORDER

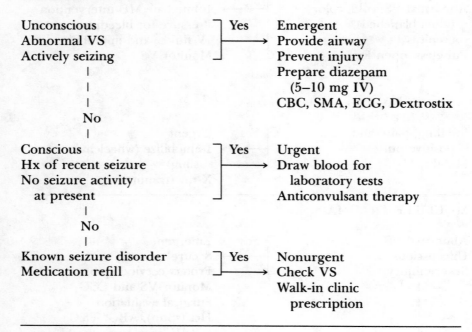

Unconscious
Abnormal VS
Actively seizing
    ]—→ Yes Emergent
    Provide airway
    Prevent injury
    Prepare diazepam
      (5–10 mg IV)
    CBC, SMA, ECG, Dextrostix

No

Conscious
Hx of recent seizure
No seizure activity
  at present
]—→ Yes Urgent
    Draw blood for
      laboratory tests
    Anticonvulsant therapy

No

Known seizure disorder
Medication refill
]—→ Yes Nonurgent
    Check VS
    Walk-in clinic
      prescription

SWALLOWING DIFFICULTY

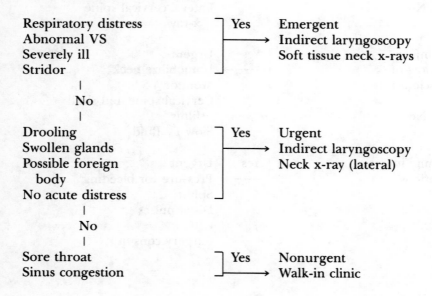

Respiratory distress
Abnormal VS
Severely ill
Stridor
]—→ Yes Emergent
    Indirect laryngoscopy
    Soft tissue neck x-rays

No

Drooling
Swollen glands
Possible foreign
  body
No acute distress
]—→ Yes Urgent
    Indirect laryngoscopy
    Neck x-ray (lateral)

No

Sore throat
Sinus congestion
]—→ Yes Nonurgent
    Walk-in clinic

URINARY RETENTION

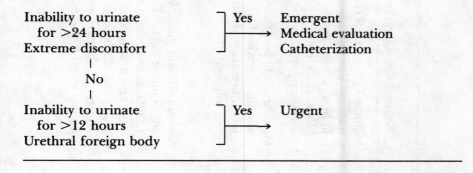

Inability to urinate
  for >24 hours   ] Yes   Emergent
Extreme discomfort   →   Medical evaluation
           | Catheterization
       No
         |
Inability to urinate
  for >12 hours   ] Yes   Urgent
Urethral foreign body   →

VAGINAL BLEEDING

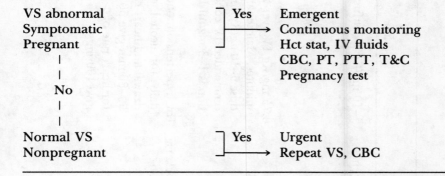

VS abnormal
Symptomatic   ] Yes   Emergent
Pregnant   →   Continuous monitoring
    | Hct stat, IV fluids
    | CBC, PT, PTT, T&C
   No   Pregnancy test
    |
    |
Normal VS   ] Yes   Urgent
Nonpregnant   →   Repeat VS, CBC

Appendix D
Emergency Medicine Drugs[a]

Generic Name (Trade Name)	Indication	Dosage	Nursing Considerations
amiodarone (Cordarone)	Ventricular and supraventricular arrhythmias	5–10 mg/Kg IV infusion	Monitor ECG and VS frequently. Use with caution in bradycardia, heart block, and CHF (IV use investigational).
amrinone (Inocor)	CHF	0.75 mg/Kg IV over 2–3 minutes. Maintenance dose 5–10 μg/Kg/min. Recommended IV concentration is 1–3 mg/ml IV fluid	Monitor for hypotension and fluid overload. If dilution necessary, use a saline solution.
atenolol (Tenormin)	Hypertension (beta blocker), alcohol withdrawal, angina, and after MI	For hypertension, one dose daily; for alcohol withdrawal and heart rate of 50–80/min give 50 mg; for heart rate of >80/min give 100 mg	Monitor BP and pulse. Use with caution for CHF, COPD, asthma, renal disease, and bradycardia. Don't discountinue abruptly. Can mask signs of shock and hypoglycemia.

Drug	Indication	Dose	Nursing Considerations
atropine	Asystole, bradycardia, heart block	0.5 mg every 5 minutes IV push (IVP) (total: 2 mg); may be given via endotracheal tube	Use with caution in patients with glaucoma and urinary retention.
bretylium (Bretylol)	Ventricular instability, ventricular fibrillation, tachycardia	5 mg/Kg via IVP (may give 10 mg/Kg to 30 mg/Kg total); for IV drip mix 2 gm in 500 ml (4 mg/ml). IV maintenance dose 1–2 mg/min	Monitor for hypotension. Nausea occurs if drug is given too fast IVP.
clonidine (Catapres)	Hypertensive state or opiate withdrawal	0.2 mg PO stat, followed by 0.1 mg PO every hour, maintenance dose 0.1–0.8 mg daily in divided doses	Monitor BP frequently. Do not stop abruptly.
diazepam (Valium)	Seizures, muscle spasms	5–10 mg slow IVP, repeat up to 30 mg in 1 hour. May be given by IV infusion to prevent seizure recurrence at a dose of 1–10 mg/hr	See nursing considerations for lorazepam. Monitor respiration; have bag/mask device available.
diazoxide (Hyperstat)	Hypertensive crisis	100 mg via slow IVP over 5 minutes × 3, or 5 mg/Kg given at 15 mg/min via IV pump	Monitor BP and I&O. May cause Na and H_2O retention and hypoglycemia.

Generic Name (Trade Name)	Indication	Dosage	Nursing Considerations
digoxin (Lanoxin)	CHF, rapid atrial fibrillation	0.25–0.50 mg IVP slowly, followed by 0.2 mg every 3–6 hours to a total of 1.0–1.5 mg	Monitor heart rate and rhythm. Hold drug and notify MD for rate < 60/min, PVC, nausea/vomiting. Check potassium and renal function.
dobutamine (Dobutrex)	Refractory CHF, pulmonary edema	1–10 µg/Kg/min via IV pump; mix 250 mg in 500 ml (500 µg/ml)	Monitor BP, I&O, and ECG. In high doses it may increase heart rate, BP, and PVCs.
dopamine (Intropin)	Shock states; low dose increases renal perfusion	1–20 µg/Kg/min via IV pump; mix 200 mg in 500 ml = 400 µg/ml	Monitor BP, heart rate, and urinary output. Do not give with $NaHCO_3$. May cause nausea or tachycardia at doses > 10 µg/Kg/min.
edrophonium (Tensilon)	Supraventricular tachycardia; test for myasthenia	1 mg slow IVP for a test dose, then up to 10 mg total	Monitor BP, heart rate, and cardiac monitor.

Drug	Indication	Dose	Notes
epinephrine (Adrenalin)	Anaphylaxis or cardiac arrest (asystole or ventricular fibrillation)	0.5–1.0 mg 1:10,000 IVP or via endotracheal tube for cardiac arrest	Monitor BP and pulse. May widen pulse pressure.
hydralazine (Apresoline)	Hypertensive crisis; reduces afterload	IM: 10–20 mg. May repeat as increased dose after 45 minutes to 1 hour; IV: 20–40 mg given slowly	Monitor BP and pulse.
isoproterenol (Isuprel)	Bradycardia, heart block	2–20 μg/min via IV pump; mix 1–2 mg in 500 ml D5W	Monitor for tachycardia. Has a chronotropic effect (increases heart rate). Will cause an increase in myocardial O$_2$ demand. Stop if chest pain, PVCs, or ventricular tachycardia occurs.
labetalol (Normodyne, Trandate)	Hypertensive emergencies	20 mg by slow IVP; 2 mg/min via IV pump until desired effect is reached; mix 200 mg in 200 ml D5W	Monitor BP frequently. Avoid use in patients with asthma. Use with caution in patients with CHF, diabetes, chronic pulmonary disease, and PVD.

Generic Name (Trade Name)	Indication	Dosage	Nursing Considerations
lidocaine (Xylocaine)	Ventricular arrhythmias, prophylaxis in acute MI	IVP: 1 mg/Kg (may repeat boluses of 50 mg IV × 3 to total of 225 mg IV), followed by 2–4 mg/min IV via infusion pump; IV drip: mix 2 gm in 500 ml D5W; may be given via endotracheal tube	Monitor BP, ECG, and CNS effects. Stop drug if dizziness, confusion, lethergy, or convulsions occur. Infusion rate over 4 mg/min is not recommended. Use with caution if patient has heart block, bradycardia, or liver disease.
lorazepam (Ativan)	Seizures	2–4 mg IM or IV	Has a longer duration of action than diazepam. Contraindicated in glaucoma, respiratory depression, hepatic or renal disease. A schedule IV controlled substance.
midazolam (Versed)	Sedation for seizures, Rx for acute cocaine abuse	0.1–0.15 mg/Kg by slow IVP	Can be given IM or IV. Monitor VS, particularly respiratory function. Have resuscitation equipment on standby in case of respiratory depression.

Drug	Indication	Dose	Notes
naloxone (Narcan)	Narcotic-induced respiratory depression	2 mg IVP; can be repeated in 2–3 minutes; may be given via endotracheal tube	May be used to rule out narcotic-related respiratory depression. Repeat doses, or continuous drip may be required until narcotic effect has passed.
nifedipine (Procardia)	Hypertensive crisis; also used to treat vasospastic and chronic angina	Break 10-mg capsule sublingually. PO: 10–30 mg tid	Monitor BP. Use with caution in patients with CHF or those taking beta blockers.
nitroglycerin (Tridil, Nitrostat IV)	Refractory angina; reduces preload and afterload	Start with 5–10 μg/min IV and increase by 5 μg/min every 5 minutes to a total of 100 μg/min	Monitor BP. Give via IV pump by using special tubing.
nitroprusside (Nipride)	Hypertensive crisis, reduces preload and afterload	0.5–10 μg/Kg/min via IV pump; mix 50 mg in 250 or 500 ml D5W	Wrap IV bag in aluminum foil. Discard solution after 24 hours. Monitor BP.
norepinephrine injection (Levophed)	Hypotension, sympathomimetic	8–12 μg/min via IV pump; maintenance dose: 2–4 μg/min; mix 8 mg in 500 ml D5W	Monitor BP and ECG frequently. Check IV site and secure catheter. Extravasation results in tissue sloughing. If it occurs, stop IV and call MD immediately.

Generic Name (Trade Name)	Indication	Dosage	Nursing Considerations
pancuronium (Pavulon)	Neuromuscular blocker, for endotracheal intubation or fighting ventilator	0.04–0.1 mg/Kg IV	See succinylcholine. Reversed by neostigmine or edrophonium.
procainamide (Pronestyl)	Ventricular arrhythmia, paroxysmal atrial fibrillation	Give 100 mg by slow IVP every 5 minutes to total 1 gm; can follow with 1–4 mg/min via IV pump	Monitor BP and ECG; may see hypotension, prolonged Q-T, and widening QRS. Avoid use in patients with heart block or known sensitivity.
propranolol (Inderal)	Ventricular arrhythmias, atrial fibrillation, supraventricular tachycardias, refractory angina	0.5–1 mg by slow IVP to total of 5 mg; PO: 10–120 mg tid or qid	Contraindicated in diabetes, asthma, bradycardia, heart block, and cardiogenic shock. Monitor BP, ECG, and heart rate. May cause acute bronchospasm. Negative inotrope—use with caution in CHF.

Drug	Use	Dose	Comments
succinylcholine (Anectine)	Neuromuscular blocker; use to facilitate intubation	25–75 mg IV	Monitor vital signs closely. Have respiratory equipment (bag/mask device, O₂, ventilator) on hand. Store in refrigerator. Patient requires close medical supervision.
thiamylal Na (Surital)	Anesthesia for short surgical procedures	1–6 ml of a 2.5% solution given by slow IV injection diluted in sterile H₂O; may be given by IV drip diluted in D5W or NS; to mix a 2.5% solution, add 5 gm Surital to 200 ml D5W	Monitor respiratory rate and BP frequently. Use with caution in patients with respiratory depression. Check IV site; extravasation into tissue may cause necrosis. Solution should be clear.
thiopental	General anesthetic, for induction to intubate	50–75 mg 2.5% solution IV; may be repeated according to response	See succinylcholine. Monitor for pain/extravasation at IV site.

Generic Name (Trade Name)	Indication	Dosage	Nursing Considerations
tissue-type plasminogen activator (t-PA, Activase)	Thrombolytic agent used to lyse coronary artery clots, indicated in acute MI of 4–6 hours old	Total dose: 100 mg IV with 60 mg given in the first hour (of which 6–10 mg are given by bolus in first 1–2 minutes), 20 mg over second hour, and 20 mg over third hour	Reconstitute with sterile H_2O only and use immediately. May be further diluted in NS or D5W. Major complications and warning—risk of internal or surface bleeding. Avoid trauma. Monitor for arrhythmias (PVC, ventricular tachycardia, bradycardia).
trimethaphan (Arfonad)	Hypertensive crisis (especially aortic dissection)	0.5–10 mg/min via IV pump; mix 500 mg in 500 ml D5W (1 mg/ml)	Monitor BP and VS frequently. May cause respiratory depression. Give O_2 while drug is in use.
vasopressin (Pitressin)	GI bleeding due to esophageal varices (also given for diabetes insipidus)	Give 20 units via slow IVP, then 0.4 units/min via IV pump	A potent vasoconstrictor. Can cause hypertension, bradycardia, arrhythmias, and pulmonary edema. May see acute water retention. Monitor BP, ECG, and urinary output.

| verapamil (Isoptin, Calan) | Atrial fibrillation, supraventricular tachycardia (also given in vasospastic angina) | Give 5–10 mg via slow IVP; may repeat in 20 minutes | Do not give in severe CHF, second- and third-degree block, in sick sinus, or with an IV beta blocker. Monitor ECG and VS. |

For drugs that can be given via endotracheal/tracheostomy tube, remember the mnemonic NAVEL:

Narcan
Atropine
Valium
Epinephrine
Lidocaine

Appendix E
Laboratory Tests and Nursing Implications[a]

1. HEMATOLOGY

Prothrombin time (PT)	12–15 seconds, <2 seconds from control	Collect 5 ml in a blue top tube; handle gently to prevent hemolysis.
Partial thromboplastin (PTT)	60–90 seconds	Collect 5 ml in a blue top tube. Used to monitor heparin therapy. Note the time and amount of last heparin dose.
Fibrinogen	200–400 mg/dl	Draw specimen atraumatically. Collect 5 ml in blue top tube and send to laboratory immediately.
Complete blood count (CBC)—hemoglobin (Hb)	M: 13–18 gm/dl F: 12–16 gm/dl	Collect 3 ml in a tube with EDTA anticoagulant (lavender top).
Hematocrit (Hct)	M: 45–52% F: 37–48%	Collect 3 ml in a lavender top tube or capillary blood in a microhematocrit tube. The patient's fluid balance state affects Hct results.
Erythrocyte count	4.2–5.9 million/mm³	
Erythrocyte sedimentation rate (ESR)	M: <13 mm/hr F: <20 mm/hr	Collect 3 ml in a lavender top tube; a number of medications and anemia can cause false test results.
Platelet count	150,000–350,000/mm³	Collect 5 ml in a lavender tube; handle gently to prevent platelet injury. Check for drugs that affect count.

Reticulocyte count	0.5–1.5% RBC	Collect 3 ml in a lavender top tube.
White blood count (WBC) differential:	5,000–10,000/ mm³	Collect 3 ml in a lavender top tube; results are affected by bacterial infection as well as a number of other factors. Increase in immature neutrophils is termed "shift to left."
Neutrophils	40–60%	
Band neutrophils	3–8%	
Lymphocytes	20–40%	
Monocytes	4–8%	
Eosinophils	2–4%	
Basophils	0–1%	

2. URINE VALUES

Acetone	0	When using a reagent strip or Chemstrip, place entire strip in freshly voided urine specimen, remove, and tap on the container to remove the excess. Compare each test in order by holding the strip in proximity to the container chart. Follow manufacturer's instructions and read in good light.
Glucose	Negative	
Hb and myoglobin	0	
pH	4.0–8.0	
Protein	Negative	
Specific gravity	1.003–1.030	Using a urinometer, spin float and read at eye level at lowest point of the meniscus. Results are influenced by excess amounts of glucose, protein, and contrast media.

3. BLOOD PLASMA OR SERUM VALUES

Acetone	0.3–2.0 mg/dl	Collect >2 ml.
Albumin	3.5–5.5 gm/dl	Collect 5-ml specimen in a red top tube.
Ammonia	5–69 μg/dl (resin) 70–200 μg/dl (colorimetric)	Collect 5-ml specimen in a gray, lavender, or green top tube; fill tube and mix well; place in ice; and send to laboratory immediately.
Amylase	4–25 U/ml 80–330 IU/liter	Collect 5-ml specimen in red top tube, and draw before medication is given.
Arterial blood gases (ABGs) pH pCO$_2$ pO$_2$ CO$_2$	7.35–7.45 35–45 mm Hg 75–100 mm Hg 22–26 mEq/liter	Seal syringe to prevent air leaks, place in container of wet ice, and send to laboratory immediately. Avoid drawing immediately after suctioning. Maintain site pressure for 3 minutes. CO$_2$ is the same as HCO$_3$.
Bicarbonate	22–26 mEq/liter	
Bilirubin	Total—0.2–1.3 mg/dl Indir—0.1–1.0 mg/dl Dir—0.1–0.3 mg/dl	Collect 5 ml in a red top tube; some medications and radiopaque dye will cause inaccurate results. Keep specimen out of strong light and handle gently to avoid red blood cell lysis.
Blood urea nitrogen (BUN)	6–25 mg/dl	Collect 5-ml specimen in a red top tube; levels are affected by a significant number of drugs and conditions.
Calcium (Ca)	9–11 mg/dl	Collect 3-ml specimen in a red top tube.

Carboxyhemo-globin	0–10%	Collect 7 ml in a green top tube. Send to the laboratory immediately.
Chloride (Cl)	95–105 mEq/liter	Collect 3-ml specimen in a red top tube.
Cholesterol	150–270 mg/dl	Collect 5 ml in a red top tube; for HDL, use tube with EDTA (lavender top). Collect in morning after NPO from evening meal.
Creatine phos-phokinase	F: 5–35 mU/ml M: 5–55 mU/ml	Collect 5 ml in a red top tube; draw as soon as possible (level rises within hours); CPK_2 (MB) is normally 0–5% of total CPK.
Creatinine	0.5–1.5 mg/dl	Collect 7 ml in a red top tube. Certain medications and dyes will interfere with results.
Glucose fasting	70–120 mg/dl	Collect 5 ml in a red top tube. A number of medications cause false results. If the patient has eaten glucose, fasting levels should return within 2 hours.
Iron, total	50–200 μg/dl	Collect 3 ml in a red top tube without hemolysis.

Lactic dehydro-genase	60–120 U/ml	Collect 5 ml in a red top tube; avoid red blood cell hemolysis, normally LDH_2 is greater than LDH_1.
Lead	<30 µg/dl	Collect 5 ml in heparin, oxalate, or EDTA anticoagulant (green, black, or lavender top tube).
Lipase	<2 U/ml	Collect 5 ml in a red top tube; food and drugs (opiates) may interfere with results; collect after NPO for 12 hours.
Magnesium	1.5–2.5 mEq/liter	Collect 3-ml specimen in a red top tube; avoid hemolysis and deliver promptly to laboratory. A number of medications will affect test results.
Osmolality	285–295 mOsm/Kg	Collect 3-ml specimen in a red top tube, and deliver promptly to laboratory.
pH pCO$_2$ pO$_2$		See "Arterial Blood Gases."
Phosphatase, acid	1–11 IU/ml	Collect 5 ml in a red top tube; avoid hemolysis and deliver promptly to laboratory.
Phosphatase, al-kaline	13–39 IU/ml	Collect 3 ml in a red top tube; patient should be NPO for 12 hours—some food will raise results. Deliver promptly to laboratory.
Phosphorus (P), inorganic	3.5–5.5 mEq/liter	Collect 3 ml in a red top tube; handle carefully to avoid hemolysis; have specimen brought promptly to laboratory.

Potassium	3.5–5.5 mEq/liter	Collect 3 ml in a red top tube; any specimen hemolysis will cause a false elevated level.

Protein, total
  Albumin
  Globulin
	6.0–8.0 gm/dl
	3.5–5.0 gm/dl
	2.3–5 gm/dl
		Collect 5 ml in a red top tube; bromsulfophthalein used in liver function tests will affect results.

Sodium (Na)	135–145 mEq/liter	Collect 3-ml specimen in a red top tube; avoid drawing on arm with IV of electrolyte solution.
Triglycerides	20–160 mg/dl	Collect 5 ml in a red top tube; test is influenced by recent diet and alcohol intake; collect in morning with patient NPO after evening meal.
Uric acid	3–7.5 mg/dl	Collect 5 ml in a red top tube.

4. CEREBROSPINAL FLUID

Pressure	60–150 mm H_2O	3–5 ml of CSF are collected in each of three or more tubes; number each in order of collection; if blood in specimen is due to trauma, the amount will decrease with each consecutive specimen. Deliver immediately to laboratory. Instruct the patient to lie flat for several hours to prevent headache; nausea and dizziness are caused by removal of CSF.
Cell count	WBC: 0–8 cells/dl RBC: none	
Chloride	100–130 mEq/liter	
Glucose	45–75 mg/dl	
Protein	15–45 mg/dl	

5. TOXICOLOGY

	Toxic Level	
Acetaminophen	>120 µg/ml	Collect 3 ml in a red top tube. Refer to Chapter 7.

Barbiturates Short-acting	>5 µg/ml	Collect 10 ml blood in a red top tube; don't shake the tube—hemolysis can cause false positive.
Intermediate-acting	>30 µg/ml	
Long-acting	>15–35 µg/ml	
Carbon monoxide (carboxyhemoglobin)	>10% saturated >60% lethal	Collect 7 ml in a green top tube. Refer to Chapter 7.
Diazepam (Valium)	>0.5 mg/dl	Collect 5 ml in a red or black top tube.
Digoxin	>3 ng/ml	Collect 3 ml in a red or green top tube.
Dilantin	20–30 µg/ml	Collect 5 ml in a red top tube without hemolysis.
Ethanol	80–100 mg% legally drunk as per state law	Collect 5 ml in a lavender or black top tube. Do not prepare skin with alcohol. Refer to Chapter 7.
Methanol (wood alcohol)	>20 mg/dl	Collect 5 ml in a black or blue top tube. Do not use alcohol for skin preparation.
Lithium	>2 mEq/liter	Collect 3 ml in a red top tube, 8–12 hours after last dose.
Salicylates	>30 mg/dl	Collect 5 ml in a green top tube with heparin for plasma or whole blood specimen. See Chapter 7.

GENERAL GUIDELINES FOR NURSING

1. Alterations in laboratory values should not be viewed in a vacuum but be considered in light of the patient's overall condition, medications, diet, etc. Laboratory results will affect the patient's nursing plan of care, as they reflect alterations in cardiac output, breathing pattern and gas exchange, fluid volume, and nutrition or potential for injury related to biochemical or drug imbalance.

2. Patient instructions should include the necessity for any food or fluid restriction when tests are prescheduled.

3. Draw specimens as atraumatically as possible, and have them delivered to the laboratory without undue delay.

4. Do not leave tourniquet in place for any longer than necessary; prolonged hemostasis may affect results.

5. Avoid drawing blood from arm with IV infusion when the IV fluid contains the factor being tested, i.e., NaCl, 5% glucose and water.

6. Consider the legal regulation or special handling required for specimens collected in conjunction with a criminal investigation. Consult the hospital procedure manual for special instructions for collection of blood alcohol, toxicology, and sexual assault specimens.

7. Refer to universal precautions ("Appendix F") for safe handling of laboratory specimens.

8. Collection tubes
   a. Red top—contains no anticoagulant or other additive
   b. Lavender—contains EDTA
   c. Blue—contains sodium citrate and citric acid
   d. Green—contains heparin
   e. Black—contains sodium oxalate (coagulation studies)
   f. Gray—contains a glycolytic inhibitor (glucose determinations)

---

[a]Data are taken from Bryne JC, Saxton DF, Pelikan PK, Nugent PM. Laboratory tests. 2nd ed. Menlo Park, California: Addison-Wesley Publishing, 1968; and from Corbet JV. Laboratory tests in nursing practice. Norwalk, Connecticut: Appleton-Century-Crofts, 1982.

Appendix F
Precautions to Prevent Transmission of Human Immunodeficiency Virus[a]

UNIVERSAL PRECAUTIONS

Since medical history and examination cannot reliably identify all patients infected with human immunodeficiency virus (HIV) or other blood-borne pathogens, blood and body-fluid precautions should be consistently used for all patients. This approach, previously recommended by CDC and referred to as "universal blood and body-fluid precautions" or "universal precautions," should be used in the care of all patients, especially those in emergency care settings in which the risk of blood exposure is increased and the infection status of the patient is usually unknown. Universal precautions are:

1. All health care workers should routinely use appropriate barrier precautions to prevent skin and mucous membrane exposure when contact with blood or other body fluids of any patient is anticipated. Gloves should be worn for touching blood and body fluids, mucous membranes, or nonintact skin of all patients, for handling items or surfaces soiled with blood or body fluids, and for performing venipuncture and other vascular access procedures. Gloves should be changed after contact with each patient. Masks and protective eyewear or face shields should be worn during procedures that are likely to generate droplets of blood or other body fluids, to prevent exposure of mucous membranes of the mouth, nose, and eyes. Gowns or aprons should be worn during procedures that are likely to generate splashes of blood or other body fluids.
2. Hands and other skin surfaces should be washed immediately and thoroughly if contaminated with blood or other body fluids. Hands should be washed immediately after gloves are removed.
3. All health care workers should take precautions to prevent injuries caused by needles, scalpels, and other sharp instruments or devices during procedures; when cleaning used instruments; during disposal of used needles; and when handling sharp instruments after procedures. To prevent needlestick injuries, needles should not be recapped, purposely bent or broken by hand, removed from disposable syringes, or otherwise manipulated by hand. After they are used, disposable syringes and needles, scalpel blades, and other sharp items should be placed in puncture-resistant containers for disposal; the puncture-resistant containers should be located as close as practical to the use area. Large-bore reusable needles should be placed in a puncture-resistant container for transport to the reprocessing area.

4. Although saliva has not been implicated in HIV transmission, to minimize the need for emergency mouth-to-mouth resuscitation, mouthpieces, resuscitation bags, or other ventilation devices should be available for use in areas in which the need for resuscitation is predictable.
5. Health care workers who have exudative lesions or weeping dermatitis should refrain from all direct patient care and from handling patient care equipment until the condition resolves.
6. Pregnant health care workers are not known to be at greater risk of contracting HIV infection than are health care workers who are not pregnant; however, if a health care worker develops HIV infection during pregnancy, the infant is at risk of infection resulting from perinatal transmission. Because of this risk, pregnant health care workers should be especially familiar with and strictly adhere to precautions to minimize the risk of HIV transmission.
7. Immunization with hepatitis B virus (HBV) vaccine is recommended as an adjunct to universal precautions for health care workers who have exposures to blood.

Implementation of universal blood and body-fluid precautions for all patients eliminates the need for use of the isolation category of "Blood and Body Fluid Precautions" previously recommended by CDC for patients known or suspected to be infected with blood-borne pathogens. Isolation precautions (e.g., enteric, "AFB") should be used as necessary if associated conditions, such as infectious diarrhea or tuberculosis, are diagnosed or suspected.

PRECAUTIONS FOR INVASIVE PROCEDURES

In this document, an invasive procedure is defined as surgical entry into tissues, cavities, or organs or repair of major traumatic injuries (1) in an operating or delivery room, emergency department, or outpatient setting, including both physicians' and dentists' offices; (2) during cardiac catheterization and angiographic procedures; (3) during a vaginal or cesarean delivery or other invasive obstetric procedure during which bleeding may occur; or (4) during the manipulation, cutting, or removal of any oral or perioral tissues, including tooth structure, during which bleeding occurs or the potential for bleeding exists. The universal blood and body fluid precautions listed above, combined with the precautions listed below, should be the minimum precautions for all such invasive procedures.

1. All health care workers who participate in invasive procedures must routinely use appropriate barrier precautions to prevent skin and mucous membrane contact with blood and other body fluids of all patients. Gloves and surgical masks must be worn for all invasive proce-

dures. Protective eyewear or face shields should be worn for procedures that commonly result in the generation of droplets, splashing of blood or other body fluids, or the generation of bone chips. Gowns or aprons made of materials that provide an effective barrier should be worn during invasive procedures that are likely to result in the splashing of blood or other body fluids. All health care workers who perform or assist in vaginal or cesarean deliveries should wear gloves and gowns when handling the placenta or the infant until blood and amniotic fluid have been removed from the infant's skin, and should wear gloves during postdelivery care of the umbilical cord.

2. If a glove is torn or a needlestick or other injury occurs, the glove should be removed and a new glove should be used as promptly as patient safety permits; the needle or instrument involved in the incident should also be removed from the sterile field.

---

[a]Data are taken from CDC. Recommendations for prevention of HIV transmission in health-care settings. MMWR 1987;36:5S–7S, and Update: universal precautions for prevention of transmission of human immonodeficiency virus, hepatitis B virus, and other blood borne pathogens in health-care settings. MMWR 1988;37:377–382.

Appendix G
Guidelines for Declaration of Brain Death[a]

I. Determination of brain death by using brain-based criteria - An individual with irreversible cessation of all functions of the entire brain, including the brainstem, is dead.

In order to declare a patient "brain dead" the following conditions must be present:

A. Coma with cerebral unresponsiveness - The patient must be in a deep unresponsive coma, with no movement or response to stimulation (excluding spinal reflexes). The pupils are fixed and dilated and do not respond to a direct source of bright light.

B. Absolute apnea - This is defined as a total lack of spontaneous respirations. The patient must not recover spontaneous respiratory function after the respirator has been turned off for 3 minutes, according to the following procedure:
   1. Patient is given room air via a respirator for 10 minutes.
   2. The respirator is then turned off and an oxygen catheter is placed either in the tracheostomy or in the endotracheal tube for delivery of oxygen at 6 liters/min.
   3. There will be enough diffusion of oxygen for an apneic patient to be adequately oxygenated during this time period of 3 minutes.

C. Lack of cephalic reflexes
   1. External ocular movement, in response to head turning and to irrigation of the ears with ice water, is absent.
   2. Blinking is absent.
   3. There is no evidence of postural activity (decerebrate or other).
   4. Swallowing or yawning and vocalization are absent.
   5. Planta responses are absent.
   6. The tendon reflexes are generally absent, but since these require only a spinal arc, a rudimentary response may be noted.

D. Electrocerebral silence - An EEG will be conducted after 6 hours of the onset of the prerequisite conditions and is adjunct to the brain function examination. The EEG should be recorded for 10–20 minutes at 25 μV/0.5 cm. No cerebral activity should be recorded during that time.

E. Irreversibility of the prerequisite conditions has been established (comatose apneic state).
   1. If possible, the etiology of the condition has been ascertained.
   2. The following reversible conditions have been ruled out:
      a. Chronic pulmonary disorder

      b. Drug intoxication

      c. Endogenous intoxication

      d. Exogenous intoxication

      e. Neuromuscular block

      f. Shock

II. Confirmatory tests

    A. Except in cases with highly evident etiology and extensive discernible brain damage, all tests are to be repeated. It is advisable for the physician to wait a minimum of 12 additional hours before the definitive brain function tests, including the EEG, the absence of cerebral unresponsiveness, lack of cephalic reflexes, and the presence of absolute apnea, are repeated.

    B. Confirmatory tests are required if the patient has small traces of sedative drugs present in the blood, the pupils remain small and nonreactive, or any question remains.

III. Procedure for the pronouncement of brain death

    A. Both a licensed physician of the primary team and a neurosurgical or neurology attending physician must certify the results of the brain death criteria.

       Note: In the event of an organ donation, these physicians can neither be involved with the actual organ donation from this patient nor be involved with any other patient who may become a potential organ recipient.

    B. The following information must be documented in the medical record by the designated licensed physician and countersigned by the attending physician:

      1. Initial observation of the onset of coma and apnea (includes date and time)

      2. The definitive brain function examination with documentation of cerebral and brainstem status and all test results establishing the diagnosis of brain death

      3. The repeat brain function examination, where appropriate, and findings

      4. The pronouncement of death

      5. Notification to the patient's next of kin, when available, of the declaration of brain death

      6. A written order by the neurology or neurosurgical attending documenting that the support system is to be disconnected as brain death criteria has been met

    C. Consent for organ retrieval, when applicable, can be made according to the hospital's organ donation policy.

IV. Applicability for children under age 3 years

    A. For children under 3 years of age, a time period of at least 72 hours must elapse from the onset of the comatose state to the pronouncement of brain death.

B. For children under age 3 years, three different brain function examinations must be performed in addition to the confirmatory test for lack of cerebral circulation.

C. Caution should be exercised in interpreting the clinical condition of children and ancillary confirmatory tests including EEGs.

---

[a]Based on Regulation 10 NYCRR 400.16 of the New York State Department of Health State Hospital Review and Planning Council.

Appendix H
Guidelines for Organ Donation

Part I. Guidelines for Obtaining Solid Organ and Tissue Donations[a]
I. Criteria for suitable candidates
  A. All tissue organ donors must meet the following minimal criteria:
    1. There should be no disease process that, based on current medical knowledge, could be transmitted to the recipient.
    2. There should be no history or presence of viral illnesses or transmittable disease: slow viruses; AIDS; hepatitis; Jakob-Creutzfeldt disease; rabies.
    3. There should be no systemic sepsis or active infection. Must have negative blood cultures.
    4. The following tissue organs may be obtained after cardiac arrest and biological death:

Organ	Time frame	Age range	Additional individual exceptions
Eyes	Up to 12 hours	12 months–70 years	None
Skin	Up to 24 hours	18–70 years	All malignancies; malnourished/obese; long-term steroid Rx; autoimmune disease; MS; diseases of skin
Bone	Up to 24 hours	15–65 years	All malignancies; insulin-dependent diabetes (>6 months); MS; known diffuse bone disease; autoimmune disease; evidence of transmissible disease

  B. All solid organ donors must meet the following minimal criteria:
    1. The patient must be unconscious, with fixed dilated pupils, and require a respirator. Brain death criteria must be met according to the hospital's policy on declaration of brain death prior to pronouncement of death and taking of organs.
    2. There must be no systemic sepsis or active infection. Must have negative blood culture.
    3. There must be no history or presence of viral illness or transmittable disease: slow viruses; AIDS; hepatitis; syphilis; Jakob-Creutzfeldt disease; rabies.
    4. There must be no malignancy, with the exception of primary brain tumor.

5. There should be no disease process that, based on current medical knowledge, could be transmitted to the recipient. (Refer to "Part II" of this appendix "Guidelines for Adult Donor Management.")

Organ	Age	Exception
Kidney	1–60 years	No history of malignant hypertension or kidney disease
		No prolonged hypotension or oliguria
		Creatinine of <2 mg% on day of nephrectomy
Heart	6 months–45 years	No history of heart disease or hypertension
		Normal cardiac examination (physical, ECG, chest x-ray)
Liver	6 months–50 years	No history of liver disease; normal liver function
		No prolonged hypotension
		No history of diabetes mellitus
Lung	12–50 years	No history of pulmonary disease or current active pulmonary disease or problem
		Normal chest x-ray, blood gas values, and tidal volumes
		No chest tubes
		Donor must be able to achieve a pO_2 of >400 on a trial of 100% F_IO_2
Heart/lung	Same criteria as heart and lung donor	
Pancreas	Same criteria as kidney donor	No history of diabetes mellitus
		No history of pancreatic disease

II. Exceptions
Organ donation should not be pursued if any of the following is known:

1. There is actual notice of contrary intentions by the decedents.
2. There is actual notice of opposition by a spouse, child, parent, sibling, or guardian.
3. There is reason to believe that an anatomical gift is contrary to the decedent's religious or moral beliefs.

III. Procedure for obtaining consent

A. The appropriate hospital administrator should be notified when a patient has been identified as a suitable candidate for organ donation. The physician, in conjunction with the transplant coordinator, will evaluate the suitability of the candidate for donation.

B. Consent is sought from the patient's next of kin. Note that the staff member obtaining the consent cannot be directly involved in the pronouncement of brain death of the donor, in the removal of the organs from the donor, or in the reimplantation of the organs to a recipient. There should be complete agreement among family members about the donation, or the donation should not be pursued.

IV. Documentation

A. As required by the Public Health Law and hospital policy, once consent for organ donation is obtained, the following medical records documentation and forms must be completed:

1. Medical record documentation of pronouncement
2. Documentation of family notification, as well as their understanding of the patient's status and the donation process
3. Consent for organ donation and record of Medical Examiner's approval, where applicable

---

Part II. Guidelines for Adult Donor Management[b]

These suggested procedures have been adapted from the United Network for Organ Sharing (UNOS) handbook. They are offered only as a guide and should be modified in accordance with practice in individual hospitals.

IDEAL PARAMETERS FOR ADULT ORGAN DONORS

Systolic blood pressure	90–180 mm Hg
CVP	8–12 cm H_2O
Urine output	1–2 cc/Kg/hr
Pulse	50–120/min
Normal or acceptable blood gases	pH = 7.40; pO_2 = 80–100; pCO_2 = 28–38

Body temperature   97–101°F

SUGGESTED ADULT DONOR MAINTENANCE PROTOCOL

Pulmonary
1. Maintain respiration with volume-dependent respirator.
2. Draw ABGs every 6 hours routinely. Adjust respirator setting to keep pO_2 80–100, pCO_2 28–38. Repeat ABG after each change in ventilator setting.
3. Chest x-ray daily.
4. Pulmonary toilet every 2 hours as necessary.

Vital Signs
1. BP every 15 minutes until stable, then every 2 hours.
2. CVP reading every 1 hour and as necessary (ideal CVP is 8–12).
3. Temperature every 4 hours.
4. Record urine output every 1–2 hours.

Fluids
1. Start 1 central line.
2. Start 2 maintenance peripheral lines.
3. Change IV fluids to D5W one-quarter NS to replace urine output cc/cc plus 1 cc/Kg/hr.
4. If serum K^+ is <3.5 mg%, add 20 mEq KCl to each liter of D5W one-quarter NS.
5. Repeat serum electrolytes every 1 hour after KCl is added to IV.
6. If additional KCl supplement is needed, 10 mEq KCl in 100 cc D5W via IV drip can be given. Repeat serum electrolytes.

Blood pressure
1. After adequate hydration, attempt to wean from all vasopressors.
2. Maintain CVP of 8–12.
3. If BP is <80–100 systolic, bolus with 500 cc NS; if no response, begin dopamine (400 mg in 250 D5W) and titrate to maintain systolic BP of 100 mm Hg.
4. Wean from dopamine, if possible, using IV fluids and volume expanders.

Urine output
1. If urine output is low (<1 cc/Kg/hr), give bolus D5W one-quarter NS 500 cc over 1 hour. Repeat as necessary.
2. If urine output does not increase sufficiently, a volume expander may also be given.
3. If urine output remains <100 cc/hr, Lasix, 20 mg IV push, may be given. If no response, bolus 500 ml Hespan over 1 hour.

DIABETES INSIPIDUS

Diabetes insipidus is often seen in patients with severe brain injury or death. It is characterized by the inability to secrete or produce sufficient amounts of antidiuretic hormone (ADH). This results in hypotonic polyuria leading to dehydration, hemoconcentration, and hypovolemia.

1. If urine output is in excess of 300 cc/hr, replace urine output cc/cc with low sodium solution.
2. Check serum electrolytes every 1–2 hours. Note that patients in diabetes insipidus will retain sodium (Na) and lose potassium (K$^+$).
3. If urine output remains >300 cc/hr, begin aqueous Pitressin, 50 units in 500 cc of D5W. (10 cc/hr delivers 1 unit of Petressin.) Titrate up to 50 cc/hr as needed to maintain urine at 200–300 cc/hr.
4. Serum glucose may be elevated () due to fluid replacement. Regular insulin IV, 10 units, may be given and repeated as necessary.

LABORATORY TESTS

Routine evaluation and maintenance of the organ donor include the following:
1. ABO.
2. Daily chest x-ray.
3. Serum electrolytes every 6 hours as baseline, including BUN, creatinine. Frequent serum electrolytes should be obtained with the administration of diuretics, Pitressin, or fluid changes.
4. Daily CBC.
5. Daily urinalysis.
6. Daily liver function tests.
7. Daily cardiac function tests.
8. Daily ECG if a potential heart donor.
9. ABG every 4 hours or after each change in the ventilator setting.
10. Blood, urine, and sputum cultures as needed and on day of donation.
11. Testing for hepatitis B, cytomegalovirus (CMV), syphilis, and human immunodeficiency virus (HIV) will be done on all donors.

---

[a]Based on Article 43A of the New York State Public Health Law (Uniform Anatomical Gift Act). This law requires hospitals to seek permission from a family member for the donating of organs from a suitable donor at the time of the potential donor death according to traditional criteria (cessation of heart beat and respiration) or brain death criteria.
[b]Reprinted with permission of New York Regional Transplant Program.

Appendix I
General Guidelines for Implementation of Do-Not-Resuscitate Orders

The following guidelines are based on the provisions of the New York State Public Health Law section 405.42 (10 NYCRR):

1. It is assumed that patients admitted to a hospital have consented to CPR unless a written and properly documented do-not-resuscitate (DNR) order is in the patient's medical record.
2. An attending physician can write a DNR order under the following circumstances:
   a. An adult patient who is deemed to have the capacity to understand the nature and consequences of the DNR order and able to participate in this decision without injury.
   b. An adult patient who lacks the capacity to understand and has a designated family member as surrogate.
   c. An adult patient who has the capacity to understand but, in the written opinion of the attending physician, would suffer severe injury from such a discussion.
   d. An adult without capacity to understand and without a surrogate when it has been determined by a concurring physician that CPR would be medically futile (the legal department should be consulted).
   e. A minor without capacity to understand, in which case consent must be obtained from parent or legal guardian. When a minor has the capacity to understand, consent must be obtained from the patient (minor) as well as from the parent or guardian before a DNR order can be issued.
3. In circumstances other than an adult with capacity to understand, the written opinion of a concurring physician is required.
4. When circumstances are not clearly applicable to the law and the hospital policy, the legal department should be contacted.
5. Special provisions exist concerning patients transferred from a psychiatric facility or a center for treatment of developmental disability.
6. Under the circumstances described in 2b, c, d and e the attending and a concurring physician must determine to a reasonable degree of medical certainty that:
   —the patient has a terminal condition; or
   —the patient is permanently unconscious; or
   —resuscitation would be medically futile; or
   —CPR would impose an extraordinary burden on the patient

in light of the patient's medical condition and the expected outcome of the CPR.

7. DNR order must be reviewed, with written documentation of the review in the patient's medical record, at least every 3 days or sooner if there is an improvement in the patient's condition.

8. Under guidelines issued previously by the Department of Health, prehospital care personnel are required to initiate cardiopulmonary resuscitation (CPR) in all instances where the patient is determined to be unresponsive, not breathing, and lacking a detectable pulse. The exceptions to this rule are:

   a. Cases of obvious death (decapitation, burned beyond recognition, and other similarly mortal injuries);

   b. Rigor mortis; and

   c. Tissue decomposition.

   The new law requires prehospital care personnel to comply with a DNR order issued by the patient's attending physician whenever the patient is being transferred from one health care institution to another. The transferring hospital must provide the ambulance service with a copy of the written DNR order.

9. In accordance with the applicable law, no civil or criminal liability shall attach for the carrying out of a DNR order in good faith and consistent with hospital policy and the law.

Appendix J
Commonly Used Antidotes

Antidote/Dosage	Uses and Indications
N-Acetylcysteine (Mucomyst): Give loading dose of 140 mg/Kg PO or via NG tube, diluted 1–3 with juice or soda. Then give 70 mg/Kg every 4 hours for 17 doses. Give same loading dose IV, followed by 70 mg/Kg IV every 4 hours for 12 doses.	Acetaminophen (Tylenol)
Activated charcoal: 60 gm PO every 2–4 hours	An adsorbent that adheres to many drugs and chemicals, used repeatedly for "gastrointestinal dialysis"
Ammonium chloride	An acidifying agent to increase renal excretion of toxic agent
Antivenin (*Crotalidae*) Polyvalent (Wyeth)	Crotalid snake bites
Antivenin (*Latrodectus mactans*) (MSD): Give 5–8 vials for minimally severe bites, 8–12 vials for bites of moderate severity, and 12–30 vials for very severe bites. Give at a rate of 1 vial every 15–20 minutes. Always call the Regional Poison Control Center.	Black widow spider bites, brady-dysrhythmias

Antidote/Dosage	Uses and Indications
Atropine: Give 1–2 mg by slow IV push until desired effect is achieved (normal heart rate, dilated pupils, dry mouth).	Cholinesterase inhibitors: Organophosphate insecticides (malathion, parathion), cholinergic agents (neostigmine, pilocarpine, methacholine), and mushrooms.
Botulinal antitoxin (ABE-Trivalent): Contact CDC at (404) 329–3753 for specific dosage instructions.	Botulism (available from local health department or CDC)
Calcium chloride: Give 10 ml of 10% solution by slow IV and repeat, if necessary, to achieve desired effect.	Oxalates, fluoride, ethylene glycol, calcium channel blockers ($CaCl_2$) should not be injected directly into soft tissues; black widow spider bites
Calcium gluconate: Infiltrate each square cm of burn with 0.5 ml of 10% calcium gluconate SC by using a 25-gauge needle.	Hydrofluoric acid burns, black widow spider bites
Cyanide kit (amyl nitrite, sodium nitrite, sodium thiosulfate): Break pearl and hold it under patient's nose; give 10 ml of 3% sodium nitrite solution IV at 2.5–5 ml/min; then give 12.5 gm of sodium thiosulfate slowly IV.	Cyanide (potassium cyanide, hydrocyanic acid, laetrile, nitroprusside sodium)

Antidote/Dosage	Uses and Indications
Deferoxamine (Desferal) DFO challenge test: Give 50 mg/Kg IM up to a maximum of 2 gm. DFO therapy: Give 90 mg/Kg IM up to a maximum of 2 gm every 6–8 hours until urine is no longer red. If hypotensive, give 15 mg/Kg/hr by slow IV infusion. Watch for drug-induced hypotension or rash.	Iron (acute and chronic)
Dextrose in water (50%): Give 25 gm by IV push. If the patient responds, or the blood glucose is under 60 mg%, give a repeat dose and begin an IV infusion of D10W.	Hypoglycemic agents, patients with altered mental status
Diazepam (Valium): Give 5–10 mg by slow IV push. Repeat as needed.	Seizures, severe agitation, stimulants
Digoxin-specific antibody (Fab, Digibind): Multiply serum digoxin concentration by 5.6 and multiply the result by the patient's weight in Kg. Divide this by 1000 and divide the results by 0.6. This gives the dose (in the number of vials) to use.	Digitalis intoxication

Antidote/Dosage	Uses and Indications
Dimercaprol (BAL, British anti-Lewisite): *Arsenic poisoning:* Give 3–5 mg/Kg by deep IM injection every 4 hours until GI symptoms resolve. *Lead poisoning:* Give 3–5 mg/Kg IM every 4 hours for 2 days; then every 4–12 hours for up to 7 additional days. *Mercury poisoning:* Give 3–5 mg/Kg IM every 4 hours for 2 days; then 3 mg/Kg every 6 hours for 2 days; then 3 mg/Kg every 12 hours for 7 additional days.	Arsenic, gold, mercury, and lead poisoning
Diphenhydramine (Benadryl): Give 25 mg by slow IV push and repeat as needed.	Extrapyramidal reactions (antipsychotics), allergic reactions
Ethanol: Give a loading dose of 0.8 gm/Kg of a 10% solution by slow IV push, followed by an infusion of 130 mg/Kg/hr. If patient is being dialyzed, give 250–300 mg/Kg/hr to maintain levels. Chronic alcoholics may require higher doses.	Methanol, ethylene glycol
Ethylenediaminetetraacetic acid (calcium EDTA): Give 50 mg/Kg/day by deep IM injection or slow IV infusion in 4 doses for 5 days. May repeat if necessary.	Heavy metals (lead, zinc)

Antidote/Dosage	Uses and Indications
Folinic acid/folic acid: Give 1 mg/Kg up to 50 mg folinic acid IV slowly, followed by 1 mg/Kg up to 50 mg of folic acid IV every 4 hours for 6 doses.	Methyl alcohol, methotrexate
Glucagon: Give 3–5 mg by slow IV push. May repeat to a total dose of 10 mg. Can be given by IV infusion at 3–10 mg/hr.	Beta blockers, calcium channel blockers, and oral hypoglycemics
Haloperidol (Haldol): Give 5–10 mg IM or by slow IV push. May repeat or increase dose to achieve desired effect.	General (as a major tranquilizer)
Ipecac (syrup of): Give 30 ml PO or via NG tube, followed by 300 ml of fluid. May be repeated in 30 minutes if emesis does not occur.	Emetic
Magnesium sulfate (Epsom Salts) or magnesium citrate: Give 30 gm PO or via NG tube. May repeat as necessary. Avoid magnesium-containing cathartics in the presence of renal failure.	General (cathartic)
Methylene blue (1% solution): Give 1–2 mg/Kg as a 1% solution by IV over 30 minutes. If cyanosis doesn't resolve, may repeat dose after 1 hour. Should not be used in a patient with a G-6-PD deficiency because it can cause hemolysis.	Methemoglobinemia

Antidote/Dosage	Uses and Indications
Naloxone HCl (Narcan): Give 2 mg IM or by IV push. Can be repeated up to a total dose of 10–20 mg. Some opiates such as propoxyphene, meperidine, and codeine may require high doses. If patient responds, give two-thirds of the total dose necessary to reverse opiate effects every 1 hour by IV infusion.	Narcotic-related respiratory depression
Nicotinamide: Give 500 mg IM or by slow IV push. Then give 100–200 mg IM or IV every 4 hours for up to 48 hours.	Vancor and rodenticide
Oxygen (oxygen, hyperbaric): Use the highest concentration possible. If the patient is breathing independently, use a non-rebreathing mask with 100% oxygen. If the patient is being mechanically ventilated, use 100% oxygen.	Carbon monoxide, cyanide, hydrogen sulfide
d-Penicillamine: Give 0.750–1.50 gm daily. Do not exceed daily dose of 2 gm. High incidence of side effects: fever, rash, bone marrow depression, and proteinuria.	Copper, lead, mercury, arsenic

Antidote/Dosage	Uses and Indications
Physostigmine (Antilirium): Give 0.5 mg slow IV push as a test dose, followed by up to 1.5 mg IV over 5 minutes to a total of 2 mg. Can cause seizures and should not be used routinely.	Anticholinergic agents and tricyclic antidepressant poisoning. Indications in anticholinergic poisoning include: SVT with hypotension, seizures and arrhythmias unresponsive to conventional agents, and extreme agitation or delirium.
Polyethylene glycol (GoLYTELY): Give 2 liter/hr PO or via NG tube. Continue administration until the watery stool is clear and free of solid matter.	Use as a general GI decontaminant to produce "whole bowel irrigation." Indicated for patients with serious ingestions who present late (after 2 hours), ingestions of sustained release medications, iron ingestions.
Pralidoxime Cl (Protopam, 2-PAM chloride): Give 1 gm by slow IV push over 5–10 minutes. If muscle weakness persists after 1–2 hours, give a repeat dose. Thereafter, a continuous infusion of 0.5 gm/hr may be used.	Given with atropine in organophosphate insecticide poisoning; contraindicated in carbamate (Sevin) poisoning; use with extreme caution in patients with myasthenia gravis, renal disease, and asthma
Protamine sulfate injection: Give by slow IV push in doses not to exceed 50 mg/10 min. Each mg of protamine sulfate neutralizes approximately 100 units of heparin. Since heparin is cleared rapidly from the circulation, the dose of protamine should be halved 30 minutes after the last administration of heparin.	Heparin

Antidote/Dosage	Uses and Indications
Pyridoxine hydrochloride: Give 100 mg IV daily for ethylene glycol poisoning. For INH toxicity, give 1 gm/gm ingested up to a maximum of 5 gm IV.	Ethylene glycol, isoniazid, mushrooms containing monomethylhydrazine
Sodium bicarbonate (5% solution): Give 2 mEq/Kg by slow IV push. Thereafter, give a constant infusion of $NaHCO_3$ in 500 ml D5W. Attempt to maintain arterial pH of 7.55 or less and a urine pH of 8–9.	Salicylates, tricyclic antidepressants, phenobarbital
Sorbitol: Give 1 gm/Kg PO or via NG tube. May be repeated, if necessary. Excessive use can lead to diarrhea.	General (cathartic, sweetener for activated charcoal)
Starch: Give PO as tolerated to bind iodine in the GI tract.	Iodine
Thiamine hydrochloride: Give 100 mg IM or by slow IV push. Indicated for all alcoholics and malnourished patients.	Thiamine deficiency, ethylene glycol
Vitamin K (Aquamephyton): Give 25–50 mg by slow IV at a rate not to exceed 1 mg/min. Can occasionally cause an anaphylactoid reaction.	Oral anticoagulants, rodenticides

Appendix K
Common Formulas, Conversions, and Other Useful Information

METRIC-APOTHECARY EQUIVALENTS

	Metric	Apothecary
Volume	1 ml (1 cc)	15 minims
	4–5 ml	1 fluid dram
	30 ml (30 cc)	1 fluid ounce
	500 ml	1 quart (approximate)
	1000 ml (1 liter)	4 quarts (1 gallon)
Weight	1 µg (0.001 mg)	—
	30 mg	gr ss (½ gr)
	60 mg (or 65 mg)	1 gr
	1 Kg	2.2 pounds
	0.45 Kg	1 pound
Distance	1 inch = 2.5 cm	
Pressure	$\dfrac{\text{cm } H_2O}{1.36} = \text{mm Hg}$	
	1 mm Hg = 1.3 cm H_2O	

TUBE SIZE (ENDOTRACHEAL TUBE)

π × Internal diameter in mm = Circumference or size in French

FORMULA FOR CALCULATING IV FLUID INFUSION RATE (DROPS/MIN)

$$\frac{\text{Drops/ml of infusion set}}{60 \text{ (min in hr)}} \times \text{Total volume per hour} = \text{Drops per minute}$$

CLARK'S RULE—FORMULA FOR CALCULATING ESTIMATED SAFE DOSAGES FOR CHILDREN BASED ON WEIGHT

$$\frac{\text{Average adult dose} \times \text{Weight of child in pounds}}{150} = \text{Estimated safe dose}$$

CONVERSION OF CENTIGRADE TO FAHRENHEIT

$$°C = (°F - 32) × 5/9$$
$$°F = (°C × 9/5) + 32$$

FORMULAS

A−a gradient — 5–10 mm Hg (up to 30 mm Hg in the elderly)

Acid-base
  a. A change in pCO_2 of 10 mm Hg = change in pH of 0.08 units. A change in pCO_2 of 10 mm Hg (increase or decrease) changes pH inversely by 0.08 pH units.
  b. A change in bicarbonate of 10 mEq/liter (increase or decrease) changes pH directly by 0.15 units.

Amylase clearance — ≤3%

Anion gap — ≤12 (if potassium not included in the calculation)
  $[Na^+] - ([HCO_3^-] + [Cl^-]) = 8–12$ mEq

A-V oxygen difference — 2–5 vol%
  a/v O_2 difference = (aO_2 saturation − vO_2 saturation) × 1.34 cc O_2/gm Hb × patient's Hb measured in gm/100 cc

Osmolarity — $2 (Na + K \text{ in mEq/liter}) + \dfrac{glucose}{180} (\text{mg/100 cc}) +$

$$\dfrac{BUN \text{ (mg/100 cc)}}{2.8} = 2(Na + K) + \dfrac{glu}{18} + \dfrac{BUN}{2.8} =$$

$$2(Na + K) + \dfrac{glu}{18}$$

Oxygen content of the blood equals oxygen carried by hemoglobin plus oxygen dissolved in the blood —
  O_2 content = 1.34 cc O_2/pts Hb in gm × measured O_2 sat + 0.003 cc O_2/100 cc blood × pO_2 in mm Hg

CARDIOVASCULAR

Blood volume: ~ 7% body weight in kilograms
Cardiac output: ~ 3 liters/min/m^2 BSA
Circulation time (arm to tongue): 10–16 seconds

Cardiac Pressures	Range (mm Hg)	Mean
Venous pressure	5–14	(6–12 cm water)
Right atrium	0–5	3 mm Hg
Right ventricle—systolic	150–30	25 mm Hg
—diastolic	0–5	3 mm Hg
Pulmonary artery—systolic	15–30	25 mm Hg
—diastolic	3–13	10 mm Hg
wedge	5–13	9 mm Hg
Left atrium	2–12	8 mm Hg
Left ventricle—systolic	100–140	120 mm Hg
—diastolic	4–12	8 mm Hg
Aorta—systolic	100–140	120 mm Hg
—diastolic	60–80	70 mm Hg

DIFFERENTIAL DIAGNOSIS OF CARDIAC CATASTROPHES BY SWAN-GANZ CATHETERIZATION[a,b]

	Pressures (mm Hg)			
	RA	RV	PA	PAW
Normal	Mean = 0–6	15–25/0–6	15–25/4–13	Mean = 4–13
LV failure	↑ or →	↑ / ↑ or ↑	↑ / ↑	[c]
RV failure (pulmonary disease)	↑ ↑	↑ ↑ / ↑ ↑	↑ ↑ / ↑ ↑	→
RV infarction	↑ ↑	↑ or →/ ↑ ↑	↑ or →/→	→
Cardiac tamponade[d]	↑ ↑	↑ or →/ ↑ ↑	↑ or →/ ↑	↑ ↑
Hypovolemia	↓	↓	↓	↓

[a]Reproduced with permission of Flomenbaum NE, Goldfrank LR. Diagnostic testing in the emergency department. Rockville, Maryland: Aspen, 1984:207.

[b]Abbreviations and symbols: RA = right atrium; RV = right ventricle; PA = pulmonary artery; PAW = pulmonary artery wedge; ↑ = elevated; ↑ ↑ = markedly elevated; ↓ = decreased; → = unchanged.

ᶜProminent "CV" wave in mitral regurgitation.
ᵈIn cardiac tamponade, all diastolic pressures are equal and elevated: (PAW = diastolic pulmonary artery = right ventrical diastolic pressure = right atrial pressure).

SUTURE GUIDEᵃ

Location	Suture Size	Days until Removal
Scalpᵇ	3–0 or 4–0	7–10
Faceᵇ	6–0	4–5
Eyelidᵇ	4–0 or 7–0	3
Earᵇ	4–0 or 5–0	7–10
Inside mouthᶜ	4–0 or 5–0	7–10
Trunkᵇ	4–0 or 5–0	10
Armᵇ	4–0 or 5–0	10
Legᵇ	3–0 or 4–0	12–14
Footᵇ—top	4–0 or 5–0	10–12
—bottom	3–0	10–12

		Days to Dissolve
Subcutaneous tissue or fascia	3–0 or 4–0	7–14 plain gut
		20–40 chromic gut
		60–90 Vicrylᵃ
		100–120 Dexonᵃ

ᵃReprinted with permission from Roberts JR, Hedges JR. Clinical procedures in emergency medicine. Philadelphia: WB Saunders, 1985:494.
ᵇA monofilament, nonabsorbable suture material (nylon or polypropylene) is preferred.
ᶜUse silk or absorbable sutures (Dexon, Vicryl, or gut).

EXAMPLES OF SUTURE MATERIALS[a]

Absorbable Sutures	Nonabsorbable Sutures	
Monofilament		
Plain gut	Dermalon[b]	Steel
Chromic gut	Ethilon[b]	Surgilene[c]
PDS[d]	Prolene[c]	Tevdek[e]
	Silk	
Multifilament		
Dexon[f]	Ethiband[g]	Surgilon[b]
Vicryl[h]	Mersilene[i]	Ti-cron[i]
Coated Vicryl[j]	Nurolon[b]	

[a]Reprinted with permission of Roberts JR, Hedges JR. Clinical procedures in emergency medicine. Philadelphia: WB Saunders, 1985:494.
[b]Nylon.
[c]Polypropylene.
[d]Polydioxanone.
[e]Teflon coated.
[f]Polyglycolic acid.
[g]Polyethylene.
[h]Polyglactin.
[i]Dacron.
[j]Polyester.

Appendix L
Useful Mnemonics

1. Acidosis
   (1) Anion gap acidosis
M	methanol ingestion
U	uremia
D	diabetic ketoacidosis
P	paraldehyde ingestion
I	iron, isoniazid
L	lactic acidosis (secondary to shock, hypoxia, sepsis, etc.)
E	ethanolic ketoacidosis, ethylene glycol
S	salicylates, solvents, starvation

   (2) Normal anion gap acidosis (hyperchloremic acidosis)
   A. Low serum K^+
P	pancreatic fistula
D	diarrhea, Diamox (acetazolamide)
R	renal tubular acidosis types 1 and 3

   B. High serum K^+
P	pyelonephritis, obstructive uropathy
A	ammonium chloride, lysine, and arginine monohydrochloride administration; hyperaldosteronism
R	renal tubular acidosis type 4

2. Anticholinergic syndrome
   Mad as a hatter
   Dry as a bone
   Red as a beet
   Blind as a bat
   Hot as a hare

3. Cholinergic syndrome
D	diarrhea
U	urinary incontinence
M	meiosis or mydriasis (with nicotinic receptor involvement)
B	increased bowel sounds, bronchorrhea
E	emesis
L	lacrimation
S	salivation

   or

S	salivation
L	lacrimation

U   urinary incontinence
D   defecation

4. Drugs that can be administered via the endotracheal tube
   N   naloxone (Narcan)
   A   atropine
   V   Valium (diazepam)
   E   epinephrine (Adrenalin)
   L   lidocaine

5. Emesis indicated with hydrocarbon ingestion
   C   camphor
   H   halogenated hydrocarbons
   A   aromatic hydrocarbons
   M   heavy metal hydrocarbons
   P   pesticide hydrocarbons

6. Radiopaque substances that may be ingested
   C   chloral hydrate, carbon tetrachloride
   H   heavy metals (arsenic, lead, iron), health foods
        (vitamins, bone meal)
   I   iodides, iron
   P   psychotropics (phenothiazines, tricyclic anti-
        depressants)
   E   enteric-coated medicine (salicylates, potassium)
   S   solvents (chloroform, carbon tetrachloride)

7. Limb ischemia - the five P's
   Pain
   Pallor
   Pulselessness
   Parathesias
   Paralysis

INDEX

Page numbers in *italics* denote tables; those followed by "f" denote figures.